COMMUNITY HEALTH SERVICES FOR THE AGED

Promotion and Maintenance

Chiyoko Furukawa
University of New Mexico at Albuquerque

Dianna Shomaker
University of New Mexico at Albuquerque

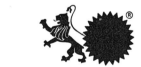

AN ASPEN PUBLICATION®
Aspen Systems Corporation
Rockville, Maryland
London
1982

Library of Congress Cataloging in Publication Data

Furukawa, Chiyoko.
Community health services for the aged.

Includes bibliographical references and index.
1. Community health services for the aged.
I. Shomaker, Dianna McDonald.
II. Title. [DNLM: 1. Community health services.
2. Health services for the aged.
3. Health promotion. WT 30 F984c]
RA564.8.F87   362.1'9897   81-19105
ISBN: 0-89443-382-2   AACR2

Library of Congress Catalog Card Number: 81-19105
ISBN: 0-89443-382-2

Printed in the United States of America

1 2 3 4 5

*To our husbands and families
for their love and support*

Table of Contents

Preface

For years the needs of the elderly were disregarded. Ironically when they were finally recognized, service providers were frustrated because many elderly refused the insensitive and regimented services. In a perplexing contradiction of values, professionals insisted that their clients' lives would be better if only they'd accept the services offered. In essence they said, "You must live better, maximize your potential—even if you don't like it." This disparity created a chasm that seemed too immense to bridge. However, analysis of current research has demonstrated that a connecting span is emerging.

This book provides a format for community health care of the aging population that is sensitive and flexible. The underlying premise of this format views aging as a stage of development and adaptation that is similar to the earlier stage of life. Society tends to perpetuate the myth that aging is a disease process, and this notion has been infused into the philosophy of health care for the elderly. The model presented here is an effort to eradicate the natural misconception that aging is a disease process without potential for quality of life. Hence, the authors' beliefs are contrary to the stereotyped misconception and focus on the elderly and their capability to maximize their full potential.

Many concerns have arisen as a result of the current increase in the number of elderly people. More people are beginning to voice dissatisfaction and frustration over the lack of attention toward, and preparation for, the care of this group. Middle-aged people are caught in a dilemma trying to provide care and guidance for both their children and their aging parents. The alternatives to care outside the nursing home are poorly defined and inadequately developed. Finally, health care delivery personnel are finding that their education pays little attention to the problems of the elderly.

Also, this complex problem is being exacerbated by the following factors inherent in present-day American life:

- Longevity is increasing.

- Inflation is consuming retirement savings and rendering meaningless many peoples' financial planning.

- Due to the mobile nature of the population, family members often do not live near each other. Thus, for the elderly, care by a family member requires moving to a new city and leaving behind known sources of support, such as friends, institutions, and familiar climate and geography.

- Many elderly are rejecting the option of nursing home care. The intensifying struggle to stay out of nursing homes is reinforcing their reluctance to relinquish their individuality, yet other options have not been developed in any depth.

The goal of this book is to outline a guide for health professionals who are concerned with improving the quality of life for the elderly residing in their communities. The authors propose a plan for the development of health promotion and maintenance services that present information and guidelines necessary to implement effective services with the elderly.

The philosophy for the health care of the elderly flows from the premise that people are basically problem-solving beings, capable of making decisions about their life styles and being responsible for such decisions. Moreover, people are unique individuals as well as complex human beings. This unique complexity is evidenced when a person considers health care. Not only is it a physiologic component of living, but it is interdependent upon environmental, cultural, societal, emotional, and cognitive processes as well. Such processes are interrelated and integrated as a holistic unit. Therefore, none of them can be dealt with individually or separately in the person.

In addition, in promoting this holistic problem-solving concept, this book is wedded to the notion that health promotion and maintenance are vital to the aged, and this philosophy should be the basis for care and education of the elderly. The authors hope to assist in minimizing the myth that aging is a disease process by deemphasizing the disease treatment approach. This process should maximize the concept that the elderly need alternatives to institutionalized care whenever inadequate adaptation to insult occurs. Moreover, it emphasizes recognition of the concept of aging as a developmental and adaptive process.

Finally, an overall goal of this volume is to encourage the development of the elderly client's potential to achieve a higher level of wellness. This may be accomplished by developing a framework for a team interaction among client, community resource persons, and the family in program planning and services. Therefore, an approach for health maintenance and promotion of the elderly is presented based primarily on the concept of high-level wellness developed by Halbert Dunn. This, together with a holistic approach and prevention of illness, implies that the client's responsibility is to maximize the quality of his or her life, and the care provider's responsibility is to maximize the process and the resources.

This book is organized into four sections, with each section contributing information toward establishment of a community health promotion and maintenance program for the elderly. In the first section a theoretical model is identified, and in the third section a pragmatic application of the same model is presented. These models are the basis for the developmental plan of health services offered to the elderly in the community. In addition, factors related to client and community involvement as well as economic and political limitations are explored. The second section focuses upon the management of the health promotion and maintenance service. This is the knowledge base upon which to deliver relevant health care to the aging population. The third section discusses the actual delivery of services. It stresses the following: (a) identifying the roles of the health professionals and volunteers; (b) disseminating information regarding available services; (c) establishing service priorities; (d) defining advocacy roles and their implications; and (e) teaching self-care. The last section offers tools, guidelines, and resources for the implementation of the health promotion and maintenance model to the aging population. Samples of health record forms, assessment outlines, and various instruments designed to provide more efficient services for the elderly are included.

We are indebted and grateful to our husbands, Paul and John, for their editorial services, typing assistance, and invaluable critique of the chapters. In addition, we would like to express our appreciation to Nellie Collins for further typing of the manuscript.

Chiyoko Furukawa
Dianna Shomaker
December 1981

Part I

Development of Health Promotion and Maintenance Service

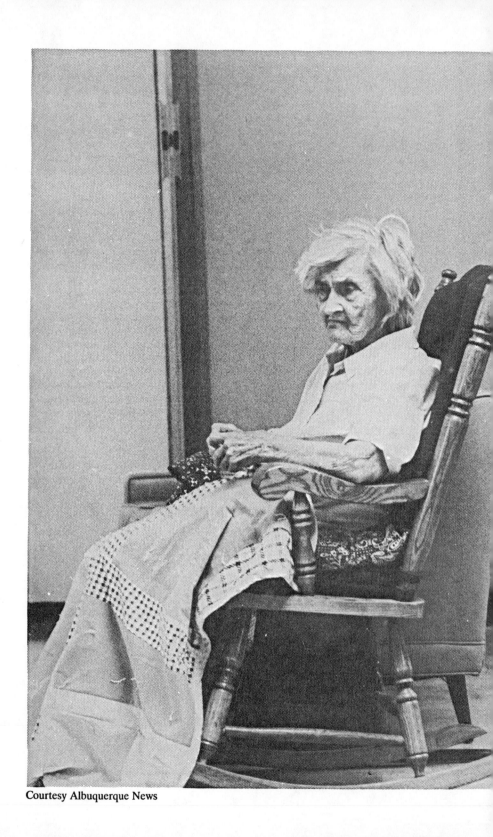

Courtesy Albuquerque News

Chapter 1

A Theoretical Model

Chiyoko Furukawa, Dianna Shomaker, and Joann Buck

PHILOSOPHICAL BASIS FOR A THEORETICAL MODEL

The theoretical model described here is an elaboration of ideas, thoughts, and experiences that best illustrate the ideal model for client relationships. To exemplify the philosophical basis, a diagram showing the factors influencing the elder's health status is presented. Furthermore, the diagram may be viewed as an underlying framework supporting the major emphasis of the philosophical foundation.

The basic diagram depicts the various relationships among individuals, families, and communities. "Community" is defined both as a geographical area and as any group sharing a common purpose, for example, mental health community, ecological community, and religious community.

Elders are central to a circle of persons with whom they are immediately and personally involved. This group can be labeled "family" with the understanding that they need not be biologically related, but rather they are by choice or obligation the first line of defense and assistance in the elder's support system.

Figure 1–1 illustrates the interdependency of seven distinct areas in which the elder's assets and liabilities are specifically and individually delineated. The categories—financial, medical, legal, environmental, mental health, activities of daily living (ADL), and self-responsibility—have been arbitrarily selected. While these areas are universally pertinent, the model can readily incorporate others. The seven areas are defined as follows:

1. Financial realities for each individual include not only the obvious income and resources, but also the eligibility for and accessibility of any free services or financial aid that might be balanced against present and potential future need.

Figure 1–1 Basic Diagram of Interrelationships of Care Components and Resources

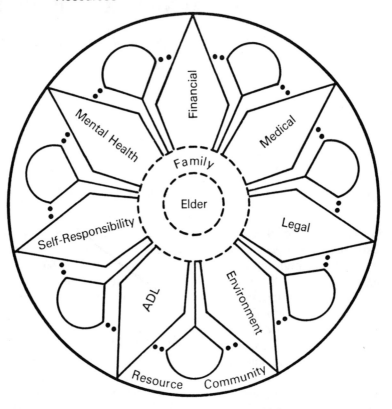

2. Medical issues encompass medical history, present state of physical health, projected probabilities for health strengths and weaknesses, and an analysis of both prescription and over-the-counter drugs.
3. Legally the elder is involved with estate arrangements: the existence of a will; the designation of a guardian should a catastrophic illness occur; and the expression of desires regarding physical care and funeral arrangements.
4. Environment is defined to include both physical and social environments. A home for the elder that is safe, comfortable, affordable, and emotionally appropriate may need to be created more than once as different levels of self-care and responsibility are experienced. The social environment includes family interaction and support, peer group contact, and a wide variety of social activities.

5. Mental health is defined in the context of high-level wellness. To be mentally healthy is to maintain the ability to cope and adapt to the realities of the aging experience, maintain a positive and loving attitude, and retain a sense of humor, self-worth, and emotional stability. Mental health also includes an individual's spiritual state. The elders that have a supportive faith have that added resource to draw upon during their aging experience. The issue of spirituality could be considered separately in the basic diagram, but because the results of spiritual and mental health can be similar, they have been combined here. In contrast, behavioral patterns that reinforce the self in misleading or negative ways are not considered mentally healthy because they lead the elder away from an ability to communicate effectively and to fulfill needs and desires successfully.

6. The ADL includes the abilities to feed, dress, and toilet oneself; to shop and cook; and to maintain or supervise the maintenance of a house.

7. Self-responsibility represents retained independence and may be defined as the continued ability to move about the community safely and effectively. Self-responsibility includes the capacity for making decisions about such movements that are effective and responsible, and the continuance of self-motivation to accomplish social activity and those errands necessary to daily living.

A shift in emphasis of one or more of the seven care components is evident in Figure 1–2. The diagram is used to show the interrelationship of the seven areas and illustrate the evolving change as the individual confronts the aging experience. At any point in time some issues will become more prominent than others. Any person's situation can be diagrammed to illustrate the areas where strengths and weaknesses exist, the aspects that need development, and the interrelationships with the various components of caring for the aged. The levels of strength can be shown by the various shadings of the segments. For instance, if the ability to care for oneself, that is, the ADL skills, declines markedly, then the living environment may become unsuitable, the financial situation may become important in the choice of a new environment, and the state of the elder's mental health may depend on an acceptable resolution.

Ideally the family initiates access to services, even if only to seek information and act in a referral capacity, gathering data about available resources and coordinating choices and implementation. The care providers and service agencies within the community constitute the next circle of support, providing specific services and supporting the inner circles of the family and individual in their continuing process of evaluation and devel-

Figure 1–2 Decline in ADL Skills, Resulting Relationships

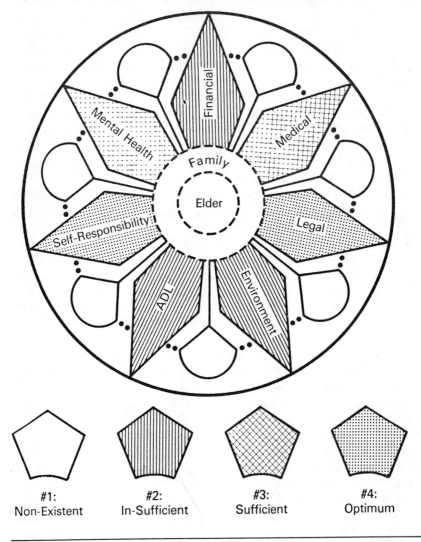

opment of the aging experience. No one course will necessarily be the central or ultimate solution, and involvement in the process is the role for each additional circle of resources. A major obligation of the resource community is the involvement holistically in the individual case. In other words, if a care provider cannot supply all the needed services, that person or agency is obligated to help direct the client and family to someone who can. That person or agency has a further obligation to follow up for results and feedback, and so attempt to close the gaps between the specific services.

Each community has a defined sphere of responsibility and support. In the issue of elder care, local definition of philosophy and responsibility will differ from area to area, thus optimizing the appropriateness and acceptability of service delivery to the local residents. The state and federal support systems seem to be largely concerned with providing and equalizing aid and the opportunities for aid within each area. The pragmatic application of the basic issues will be addressed in subsequent chapters.

In discussing the philosophical basis of the diagram, it is necessary to remember that the aging population is a group of people with special needs occasioned by their developmental stage of life. Aging is a positive and natural life process that every individual experiences in a personal way. The aging process is a complex, uninterrupted, and orderly phenomenon. The changes resulting from this process impinge on every aspect of the individual, and there is a tendency toward adaptation.

Care providers for the aged use their own philosophies about the aging group to guide their choices of service. The philosophies may not be in concert with the needs of the elderly, as is vividly illustrated by the discordant directions of the Medicare program.

Attention has been focused on the immediacy of acute care rather than on disease prevention, health maintenance, and long-term supportive care. More money is paid for in-hospital acute care than for the prevention of conditions that lead to it. However, proof is readily available to demonstrate that vulnerability to disease and chronic illness are much greater barriers to the health of the elderly than is acute episodic illness. The aged individuals, their families, and the health care professionals often expect discomfort and dysfunction as a normal course of aging. Consequently, the elderly may wait too long before seeking medical care.[1]

There is a probability that chronic disease and aging have a basic relationship. This is supported by the fact that since 1940 the death rates from heart disease and cancer have each increased by one-fourth.[2] Brotman found that 67 percent of the independent elderly living in the community have chronic conditions.[3] These individuals are the high-risk group often overlooked by the existing health care system available to the elderly. Hammerman believes the elderly are locked into the acute care system, which is ill-equipped to meet the demands of the chronic illness and long-term needs of the aged.[4]

INTEGRATION OF HIGH-LEVEL WELLNESS, HOLISM, AND PREVENTION

High-Level Wellness

The philosophical foundation of this theoretical model centers upon three major concepts: (1) high-level wellness; (2) holism; and (3) prevention. Dunn [5,6,7] developed the concept of high-level wellness to encourage the individual, family, and community to maximize their potentials in seeking to attain a quality of life suitable to their capabilities. High-level wellness goes beyond mere freedom from disease. It is more ambitious than that. It is an open-ended, progressive, upward-looking attempt to attain a higher plane of satisfaction in the use of a person's untapped capabilities. In this context the emphasis is on the individual's positive attributes rather than the negative aspects of illness. High-level wellness does not deny the existence of concurrent illness; rather, it involves the notion that a person employs remaining positive capabilities and characteristics in spite of illness.

The attainment of high-level wellness is believed to be achievable at any point in a health-illness continuum. Levels of health and illness can be thought of as tracing roughly parallel, but intermittently overlapping and diverging curves. To draw a single linear continuum is misleading because health and illness appear to be at polar extremes. This illusion is perpetuated in society's dichotomous conception of "health" as representing only the absence of sickness. In actuality both can appear simultaneously; for example, in Figures 1–3, 1–4, and 1–5, the individual has the potential for being both well and ill to some degree at the same time. In Figure 1–3, wellness is a constant almost nonfluctuating condition in opposition with an underlying low-grade illness that gradually worsens until it is more obvious than the degree of wellness. In Figure 1–4, wellness remains con-

---

Figure 1–3 Low-grade Illness Gradually Worsening

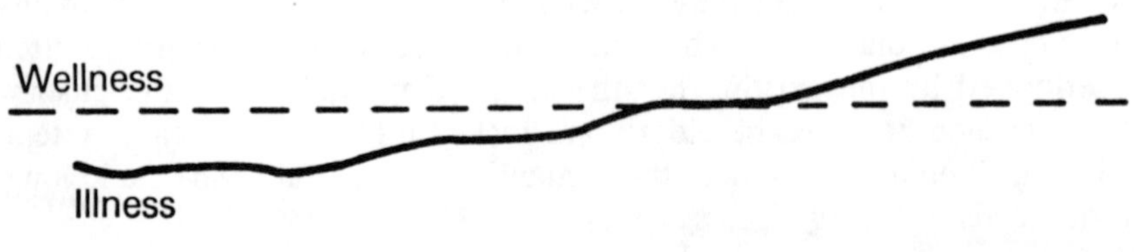

Wellness

Illness

Figure 1–4 Fluctuating Illness

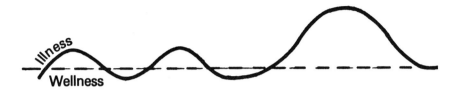

stant but at a low level, while illness fluctuates between a low-grade energy drain on the system and acute episodic incidents of varying intensity of a chronic illness. In Figure 1–5, the profile is of an acute episodic attack in which the level of wellness and level of illness buffet one another in a single, short-term dysfunction. For all three, the time frame can be expanded or contracted.

From these figures it is apparent that even when a person is very ill, there remains some degree of wellness. Terminal illness does not necessarily mean health has been terminated at some earlier stage. For example, a person with late stages of terminal illness can still be assisted to maintain a degree of positive attitude and mental composure that will allow death with peace and understanding. In such a case, the health-illness profile might appear something like that in Figure 1–6. There is a strong psychological aspect suggested here, which is what wellness is about. It's more than being "OK." After all, who's the sickest? The healthy lady who thinks she's dying of cancer, or the patient with post-myocardial infarction who's planning to carry on with happy living tomorrow?

Implementation of high-level wellness considers many factors. Health and illness are omnipresent phenomena, and interpretation of their relative positions of importance is a profound influence on other factors affecting one's life at a given moment. Many times there is no sharp demarcation between health and illness. Both require constant adaptation; they cannot

Figure 1–5 Acute Episodic Attack

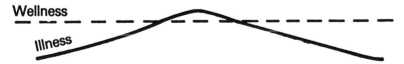

Figure 1–6 Late Stage of Terminal Illness

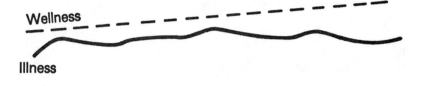

be compartmentalized. Some demands exceed a person's adaptive resources. Other demands are so slight that resources are subject to minimal drain. In addition, all degrees of wellness are unique to each individual because of the individual's uniqueness. It is necessary to understand this concept if a person is to maximize wellness; individuals not only interpret each of life's encounters based on past personal experience, but they draw the necessary energy for adaptation from a reservoir founded on genetic, environmental, psychological, and sociocultural factors.

Energy is necessary not only for recovery from illness, but for maintaining health. If coping mechanisms fail to result in adaptation, energy needs are increased even more for future success than they were in previous attempts to adapt.[8] Of course, if energy reserves are depleted during illness, the individual suffers a secondary imbalance due to this reduction. Therefore, in order to overcome this imbalance and restore wellness, energy is often diverted from other areas of functioning. This implies that a human being responds to energy demands as an integrated unit, so that stress in one component of a person's existence creates stress in another. Despite the desirability of necessary change, it will always require more energy from a system than if no change had occurred.[9] The goal in health is to restore balance in the relationship between energy use and conservation.

Holism

The concept of energy use is the basis of holism and is subsumed in the principles underlying high-level wellness. A human is viewed with a holistic context as an integrated and increasingly complex psychosocial being. Out of this integration of complex factors evolves a pattern of functioning that reflects the premise that the whole is greater than the sum of its parts, and that a person responds as a unified whole. This response of a person may lie at any point within a broad range of variation for a particular situation, and the result is an activity unique to that person. This range of variation can be identified by observing the totality of a person's reaction to a stimulus, taking into account mass, structure, function, and feelings. "The energy field underwrites the unity of man and provides the conceptual boundaries which identify his oneness."[10]

The concept of holism supports the philosophy that individuals have various roles and positions to fulfill simultaneously, and these roles involve specific rights and obligations. However, both client and health professionals may be uncertain of their roles and obligations in such an approach, and the beneficial aspects of a holistic approach to health maintenance may be unclear. Moreover, the dichotomy between the values of these two populations often obstructs development of an acceptable mechanism for achieving a smoothly integrated holistic health care pattern. The health professionals need to realize the importance of potential disparity between the perceptions, values, and beliefs of the client and those of the care provider regarding health and illness. Subscribing to the notion that a holistic approach minimizes the amount of energy necessary for health maintenance will aid in alleviating some of the differences in these perceptions.

Prevention

The third concept of concern here is prevention. It is believed to play a vital part in achieving high-level wellness; the concepts are consistent and mutually supportive. For example, both require a conscious choice on the part of the individual, both are energy efficient, and both are coterminous in maximizing wellness. Prevention has two major components: primary prevention and early detection of asymptomatic health-threatening conditions. Primary prevention aims to decrease or eliminate the chances of illness. The use of immunizations, provision of adequate nutritional intake, and avoidance of hazardous materials such as cigarettes are some examples of primary prevention. Early detection, on the other hand, facilitates timely treatment to stop, curtail, or delay the development of chronic conditions. Pender views preventive behavior as action taken by individuals to minimize the potential threat of illness and is neither curative nor remedial in nature.[11] Furthermore Pender outlines three factors—personal, interpersonal, and situational—that influence the decision making to seek preventive care. Personal factors are the individual's perceived vulnerability and estimation of the seriousness of his or her condition and of the effectiveness of action taken. The value placed on health and the psychological makeup of internal versus external control also significantly influence preventive behavior. Interpersonal factors are often the influences that facilitate or deter primary prevention and/or early detection.

The concerns shown by a significant other, the established family pattern for seeking preventive health care, expectations conveyed by friends, and information provided by health professionals are examples of interpersonal factors vital to the notion of prevention. Situational factors also weigh heavily in the acceptance or rejection of preventive health. Health norms are established by the individual's referent group and by information about health received via the media as commercials or public health care advice.

In Pender's model of preventive health behavior, cues are required during the action phase to encourage the individual to participate in preventive health care. Cues may come from a number of sources including the internal perception of fatigue, external influence of advertisement on billboards, and knowledge of health care facilities that provide screening services. It is known that for preventive health care, behavioral cues must be more intense than for those seeking illness care. In order to be effective, cues must be positive and acceptable rather than negative and overwhelming, because the tendency for discouragement may prevent a person from taking any action.

Preventive health behavior is individualized and determined on a voluntary basis. This is closely aligned with the individual's right to seek a level of wellness. This also implies that the responsibility for decision making is the individual's domain and requires identification of needs and priorities and one's level of readiness. Health care providers assume an advocacy role in assisting individuals in understanding and accepting both rights and obligations toward their own level of health. Effectiveness of decisions correlates highly with a person's degree of understanding. A role of the health professional is to make clear that every act has more than one consequence; the choice of the action with its subsequent consequences is the client's; and the choice may change as new information is introduced.

OPTIMUM INDIVIDUALITY OF CLIENT

The integration of these three concepts—holism, high-level wellness, and prevention—into a workable model optimizes client individuality in several ways. Individual strengths are built upon to develop solutions to elder-care problems. Individual weaknesses are identified as areas needing attention or compensation in the development of a solution. Indeed, individuality becomes an asset in this model and is encouraged and supported. This is in contrast with prevailing systems, which must minimize individual differences in order to provide the same services to all recipients and do so in an economically efficient way.

Solutions based on individuality are likely to be more successful in that the elder is recognized as a viable and worthy person, which increases an elder's sense of self-worth and self-confidence. Moreover, solutions based on individuality are likely to be more successful because they reflect the specific needs of each client.

The integration of high-level wellness, holism, and prevention underscores the individuality of the elderly client. Each concept supports the uniqueness of the person and emphasizes the expectation and acceptance of the differences among these aged persons. The person working toward the achievement of high-level wellness is allowed to seek the optimum level of function unique to that individual. For example, an elder with a mobility problem would not be expected to walk the same number of blocks for exercise as an elder with normal ambulatory function.

In giving support to attain the goal of maximum function, all dimensions (biophysical, psychological, sociocultural, and environmental) that make up the total person are considered in the holistic approach. Holism provides a more complex base upon which to guide the client as decisions are made. For example, those with impaired mobility have the right to determine the degree of mobility they will tolerate. When considered in a holistic manner, appraisal must include factors from all dimensions. This will provide a total profile of a client's limitations and resources. The approach directs health professionals to give credence to all aspects of the individual as these attributes contribute to the optimum individuality of the client.

The concept of prevention as applied to the individual differs in the level of health achieved, since a person makes choices based on numerous and complex variables, such as cultural biases and beliefs. Indeed the choices made in subscribing to preventive measures are as divergent in the aged as they are in younger population groups. Nevertheless, the notion of prevention allows for optimum individuality for the client to select whatever health services are of particular value.

OPTIMUM COMMUNITY RESOURCES

In response to criticism regarding deficiencies in existing programs, the White House Conference on Aging gave impetus to communities in raising the consciousness of their constituents to optimize community resources for the elderly. Many communities sought federal funds, which were available through various grants, to establish community agencies for the aging. However, this well-intended activity lost its direction, and these agencies tended to "do their own thing" without coordination within the community. Often the result was fragmented services and duplicated care to the community's aged. In some instances the gap in the services to the aging grew. Thus, the outcomes from these services are viewed as less than adequate support to the elderly as a group, even though significant amounts of tax dollars were exhausted. In this day of limited resources, communities must analyze critically the mix of services available to the elderly. It is essential to develop coordinated community services so that direct financial benefits and the service agencies will contribute significantly to the aging group's quality of life.

The establishment of optimum community resources depends upon the strengthening of the conceptual approach, which helps identify specific comprehensive needs of the aging. Moreover, the high-level wellness, holism, and prevention concepts help in the development of positive attitudes toward the aging. These concepts also assist in the delineation of relevant services and provide encouragement to the elderly to remain in the community and thus be allowed their chosen life styles. The community that accepts high-level wellness will offer various levels of services in order to match the specific needs of the elderly.

Without the use of holistic approach to service, the impact and ramifications of the problems of the aging could be easily overlooked. This situation is vividly demonstrated by a community's choice for separate recreation and nutrition programs. If these services were joined, the elderly could enjoy both nutrition and organized recreation in one location, thus meeting several related needs in a single program.

Another glaring omission is in the area of preventive health services to maintain and sustain the aged. As mentioned earlier, the elderly as a group require an ongoing service, rather than an episodic one, to monitor conditions that may vacillate between an acute phase and a chronic one. Services based on the concept of prevention contribute to reassurance of the aged, and more importantly, convey a care component that the elderly desperately need.

RELATED PRINCIPLES: RESPONSIBILITY, DECISION MAKING, AND ADAPTATION-COPING

Responsibility

The theoretical model for the development of the health promotion and maintenance service integrates the concepts of responsibility, decision making, and adaptation-coping. These principles not only occupy a pivotal position for the philosophical basis of the model, but are also significant in the clarification and justification of the theoretical model.

The principle of responsibility is central to the delivery and acceptance of health care. Hence, responsibility implies active participation by the consumer and the health professional. Webster defines responsibility as a state or quality of being responsible, accountable, and reliable. Implicit in this definition is that the individual who accepts responsibility is answerable and amenable to obligations. Responsibility involves a continued relationship rather than a one-time contact. Ethically, responsibility implies the character of a free moral agent. Frequently, one is responsible, answerable, or accountable for something, often to some person or authority. Claus and Bailey have similiar thoughts and note that responsibility is specific and task-oriented.[12] A task is delegated by an authority, and the person has a duty to perform the task adequately. Responsibility in Claus and Bailey's view is an expression of one's obligations of performance. Using the definitions by Webster and Claus and Bailey, it may be concluded that responsibility is reciprocal in nature and involves a degree of understanding as to the necessary task and upon whom the obligation to perform the task is to fall. Further, it strongly implies a commitment between the concerned parties.

Feelings of conflict and guilt also influence the distribution of responsibility. The clarity of responsibility is imperative if the health professional and the client are to understand their respective roles in achieving the health care goal. The professional's responsibility is to structure health care practices and data-gathering, whereas that of the client is to make decisions as to the degree of involvement. This is particularly difficult for the professional, who in the past assumed full responsibility for decisions involving the client. Moreover, it is equally difficult for the client, who has often preferred to delegate decision making to the care provider. The responsibility of the professional is to assist with the pros and cons of health care and to provide adequate information in order that the client may make an intelligent decision.[13] The opportunity for the elderly to participate in decisions about health care leads to acceptance of responsibility and to follow up on the prescribed interventions.

Decision Making

The aging process itself often causes the elderly to be stereotyped as incapable of making decisions about the significant aspects of their daily lives. Health professionals, family members, and friends unknowingly force the elderly to become inactive, nonparticipating, and dependent. The recurring issue of whether to continue living independently or in a supervised environment is often settled without input from the elderly.

Each person's decision-making capability must be evaluated on an individual basis rather than on the myth that intellectual loss is universal with aging. A literature review supports the contention that cognitive abilities do not cease with the aging process. Seymour reports many older people are able to perform tasks at rates comparable with those of younger people, and older people continue to have the ability to think and make decisions.[14] The elderly tend to solve problems on the basis of past experience and knowledge, rather than through experimentation with new solutions.[15] This is understandable because the elderly have reservoirs of many life experiences, including successful decisions made during their lifetimes. In selected circumstances where new and complex decisions are necessary, people may be less likely to analyze the problems they face. Instead, they approach solutions in previously tried ways. For some, this is compounded by the aging process. Some evidence proposes that the older persons' thought processes lean more toward simple association rather than toward analysis.[16]

Aging itself doesn't necessarily change one's ability to make decisions. Those who were adequate decision makers when they were younger will continue to use such talents. Conversely, those who deferred decisions to others in youth will prefer passive roles as elders. There are many factors involved in decision making, not the least of which are education, experience, communication, genetic composition, and physical disposition.

Archer and Fleshman view decision making as an essential and ubiquitous part of living.[17] It is an inescapable process for individuals, and there are adverse consequences if decision making is delayed. If the delay is long enough, the result often is that others usurp one's right to decide, and alternatives become fewer. Eventually only one course may be left from which to "choose." Crisis situations may result from prolonged delay in the decision making that is necessary for planning for the future. Implicit in the decision-making process is consideration for eventuality and anticipatory planning to cope with the problems or to prevent them from occurring.

The concept of decision making and the freedom to participate in the process is extremely important to the elderly. Independent status and having an intact self-concept and self-esteem are generated and nurtured by the ability to make decisions. This was vividly demonstrated by Beaver in her study of the decision-making process and its relationship to relocation adjustments by the elderly.[18] Beaver's findings suggest that the elderly are able to participate in the relocation decision making despite the fact that this event is stressful. The findings emphasized the resourcefulness and the self-reliance of the relocating elderly to seek and select a support system to rely upon before and after the move. The most successful adjusters to the relocation were people who received support from relatives or who had more than one choice of living arrangement. More important, the fact that the elderly were allowed to choose places to live from the beginning apparently influenced the successful or unsuccessful outcome of the relocation. The study results clearly showed that the freedom to participate in the decision-making process had an impact upon the elderly's wellness state.

Adaptation-Coping

When discussing the process of adaptation, the term "coping" is frequently used. This is misleading. These terms are not synonymous, but are sequential. Coping leads to adaptation. The two terms appear to be constructs that, to date, have no universal definition, yet everyone recognizes the use of such postulates in attempting to understand the unchanging law of human behavior in a seeming paradox that says change will occur. Adaptation is most often defined as a constant change, internally and externally, that allows survival of the organism. It is also positive, continuous, and constructive. It allows the individual to function successfully as an integrated unit.[19] These behavior patterns have a common goal and vary with individuals, family, and community, and are influenced by age, sex, culture, education, religion, and experience.[20]

The most common areas of adaptation are psychosocial and biological. In both there is a definite change in the organism that allows it to survive in a particular environment. This is a more complex, long-term, permanent response than mere accommodation or adjustment to a stimulus. Several assumptions are implied. Adaptation is constantly necessary for survival. Adaptation patterns are established, but can change.[21] An individual has the capacity to change because the mind controls much of the body's behavior. People cope with many stresses at once, often adjusting or accommodating to the environment on a short-term basis, even though adaptation is a long-term process.[22] Perception of a stimulus is influenced by a person's values and past experiences. Moreover, the same stimulus does not always elicit the same response in an individual, nor can it be predicted that two individuals will have the same perceptions and adaptation to a single, common stimulus. The adaptive process employs coping mechanisms that result in adaptation,[23] but there are times stimuli surpass a person's capability to adapt.[24]

Coping is not synonymous with adaptation per se. Coping is a series of mechanisms and behaviors employed by an individual when attempting to confront or avoid a stimulus in order that adaptation can occur. That is, coping is the mechanism that allows the individual to move toward change.

Adaptation is seen as a feedback system by Goosen and Bush.[25] In this system one perceives the problem and appraises it on the cognitive level. If it is resolved there, social adaptation occurs. This cognition becomes one of an individual's coping mechanisms. If adaptation does not occur, then one attempts to cope in other ways, many of which may be unconscious, successful patterns of the past. Initially, coping is through previously established patterns. However, when old patterns are not useful, finding new methods of coping can be a great venture in creativity.[26] If the response to the problem is mature, the problem is resolved and adaptation occurs. However, if the problem is not resolved at this point, secondary problems are often created due to the inadequate coping mechanisms. This activity taxes the system, compounding the energy drain and depleting the system through increased arousal of physiologic responses. If adaptation fails to occur, the energy drain continues to increase in proportion to intensification of arousal until, if unchecked, maladaptation creates changes in body systems and destruction to tissue. This ultimately results in secondary damage or death. Each stage of increased stress from a stimulus requires greater effort to resolve the problem.[27.28]

The elderly do not approach problems with the naiveté of naked youth. The repertoire of coping mechanisms that accompanied them into old age has allowed them to survive all these years.[29] To continue to survive they often employ patterns of coping that leave many younger people scratching their heads. Silverstone and Hyman see stubbornness and avoidance of change used by many to fight forces that disrupt their lives. This is a coping mechanism that is secularly successful and designed to improve one's feeling of security. Stubbornness is often demonstrated in refusal to try new things, new ideas, make new friends, and go new places. It becomes a protective armor to ward off change and minimize insecurity. Even though it seems contradictory, such behavior is repeated in a stubborn pattern to retain independence. Stubbornness is also seen in such responses as the overcautiousness of double-checking before leaving the house. The security of the structure increases one's own sense of security.[30]

Some behaviors only allow constructive adjustment for a period of time and then, if not changed, become maladaptive. This leads to actual physical or biological change within the body. In other words, people with chronic illness can often become crippled by their coping devices, not by the disease with which they are coping. The end result is maladaptive, although it was possibly adjustment or accommodation at an earlier stage of illness. This is often seen postoperatively, and is seen in diseases such as arthritis, stroke, and heart attack.[31]

NOTES

1. Cary S. Kart, Eileen S. Metress, and James F. Metress, *Aging and Health*, Social Perspectives (Menlo Park, Ca.: Addison-Wesley Publishing Co., 1978), p. 29.
2. U.S. Department of Health, Education and Welfare, *Working With Older People, A*

Guide to Practice, Volume II (Rockville, Md.: Bureau of Health Services Research, 1974), Perspective.

3. Herman B. Brotman, "Fastest Growing Minority: The Aged," *American Journal of Public Health* 3, no. 3 (March 1974): 251.

4. Jerome Hammerman, "Health Services: Their Success and Failure in Reaching Older Adults," *American Journal of Public Health* 3, no. 3 (March 1974): 225.

5. Halbert L. Dunn, *High Level Wellness* (Arlington, Va.: R.E. Beatty, Ltd., Fourth Printing, 1969), pp. 1-7.

6. Halbert L. Dunn, "What High-Level Wellness Means," *Canadian Journal of Public Health* 50, no. 11 (November 1959), pp. 447-57.

7. Halbert L. Dunn, "Points of Attack for Raising the Levels of Wellness," *Journal of National Medical Association* 494, 4 (July 1957), pp. 225-35.

8. Gerald M. Goosen and Helen A. Bush, "Adaptation: A Feedback Process," *Advances in Nursing Science* # 1, no. 4 (July 1979), pp. 58-59.

9. Marjorie L. Bryne and Lida F. Thompson, *Key Concepts for the Study and Practice of Nursing* (St. Louis, Mo.: The C. V. Mosby Co., Second Edition, 1978), p. 27.

10. Martha Rogers, *Introduction to the Theoretical Basis of Nursing* (Philadelphia, Pa.: F. A. Davis Co., 1970), p. 46.

11. Nola J. Pender, "A Conceptual Model for Preventive Health Behavior," *Nursing Outlook* 23, no. 6 (June 1975): 385-390.

12. Karen Claus and June Bailey, *Power and Influence in Health Care* (St. Louis, Mo.: The C. V. Mosby Co., 1977), p. 68.

13. Carolyn C. Clark, *Mental Health Aspects of Community Health Nursing* (New York, N.Y.: McGraw-Hill Book Co., 1978), p. 42.

14. Eugene Seymour, *Psychosocial Needs of the Aged: A Health Care Perspective* (Los Angeles, Ca.: The University of Southern California Press, 1978), p. 17.

15. U.S. Department of Health, Education and Welfare, *Working With Older People,* p. 29.

16. Ibid., 30.

17. Sarah Archer and Ruth Fleshman, *Community Health Nursing Pattern and Practice* (North Scituate, Mass.: Duxbury Press, 1979), p. 286.

18. Marion L. Beaver, "The Decision-making Process and its Relationship to Relocation Adjustment in Old People," *The Gerontologist* 19, no. 6 (June 1979): 567-74.

19. Bryne and Thompson, *Key Concepts,* p. 22.

20. Ibid., p. 57.

21. Ibid., p. 22.

22. Ibid., p. 26.

23. Paula Sigman, "Student Viewpoint: A Challenge to the Concept of Adaptation as 'Health.' " *Advances in Nursing Science* # 1, no. 4 (July 1979), pp. 85-94.

24. Goosen and Bush, "Adaptation," pp. 53-59.

25. Ibid.

26. Wendell Johnson and Dorothy Moeller, *Living With Change: The Semantics of Coping* (New York, N.Y.: Harper and Row, 1972), p. 9.

27. Barbara Silverstone and Helen Kandel Hyman, *You and Your Aging Parent* (New York, N.Y.: Pantheon Books, 1976), pp. 90-91.

28. Bryne and Thompson, *Key Concepts*, p. 28.
29. Goosen and Bush, "Adaptation," pp. 56-58.
30. Silverstone and Hyman, *You and Your Aging Parent*, pp. 90-91.
31. Bryne and Thompson, *Key Concepts*, p. 28.

Chapter 2

Community Health Promotion and Maintenance Model

Chiyoko Furukawa

One common misconception about the aged is that they are all ill, infirmed, or failing mentally.[1] This is not the case in reality as most older people are living and functioning independently in the community. However, there are varying amounts of disability among the elderly due to chronic illness or the aging process, and experience has indicated that most older individuals could benefit from services designed to promote and maintain their health.[2]

The aged's health care needs evolve from deviations and losses primarily in the psychological, social, environmental, and physical factors. The interdependency of these factors, which are more or less taken for granted in youth, becomes a major challenge to life adjustments as aging progresses. The adaptive capabilities lessen with longevity while occasions requiring optimal accommodation increase. Thus, an older person becomes especially vulnerable to changes of or deviations from normal functions. The timely assistance by the family and/or community to supplement the elderly's reduced coping behaviors becomes essential for health promotion and maintenance. Unfortunately, this assistance is not available to all aged individuals because of differences in family structure and relationship, or the nonexistence of community services in some parts of the country.

Morgan indicates that the relative newness of gerontology combined with the need for communication between the researcher and the program providers has contributed to the slow development of community services for older adults.[3] Consequently, most elderly persons and their families struggle to find health maintenance care in any possible way, and they are likely to pay monetarily, physically, and emotionally for the cost of such care. Those able to afford services benefit and are generally aided to function at optimal levels. Others, without resources, suffer the consequences of declining health and struggle to maintain their life styles.

Current state and federal systems are unresponsive to the health needs of older people, and the changes for inclusion of health promotion and maintenance benefits in the Medicare and Medicaid regulations appear to be progressing slowly. Since there is no simple and quick solution to altering this status, one alternative is the community approach to health programs. These locally supported programs are advantageous because they allow for greater flexibility and fewer restrictions than state- or federally-based services. Another positive aspect of the community-supported approach is the opportunity for face-to-face communication with the people who make decisions about funding for social and health programs. Thus, the astute fundseeker can exploit local political viewpoints in a favorable way to ensure funding. These activities also permit each community to examine the feasibility of developing health services and to tailor individual programs to fulfill the specific needs of the older population. Until government agencies can provide full care of the aged, health professionals must identify substitute ways to alleviate the lack of needed health services.

The comprehensive health care needs of the elderly require a systematic approach to program planning and implementation. Moreover, it is essential that a theoretical basis that applies to the developmental needs of the older population be used to guide the evolvement of the health program. A practical model for health promotion and maintenance care, which includes concepts for elderly care and a step-by-step procedure, is proposed to assist in the initiation of a comprehensive health service.

A PRACTICAL MODEL

A health promotion and maintenance model is a useful tool to initiate, plan, and implement services in community settings. A schematic diagram of a proposed model is shown in Figure 2–1.

As indicated in the figure, the philosophy of care is central to all activities leading to the establishment of the health program. The activities essential for conducting health services for the elderly begin with assessment and are followed in sequence by program goals, planning, implementation, and evaluation. One complete cycle terminates with the evaluation process; however, this does not preclude the evaluation findings from providing feedback to modify or improve the care component in the assessment function. The degree of this feedback (suggested by the broken line in Figure 2-1) can vary depending upon such factors as the success of initial implementation, complexity of elders' needs, size of population served, ethnic makeup, effectiveness of professional staff, and cooperation from community resources. More detailed discussions of each component activity from the practical model is presented in the following sections.

Figure 2–1 Community Health Promotion and Maintenance Model

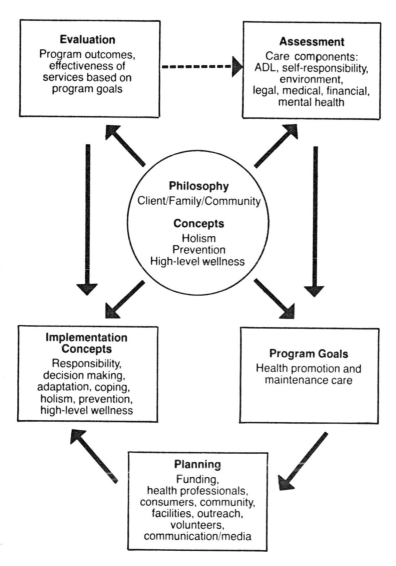

PHILOSOPHY

An initial and pivotal item for a health promotion and maintenance service is a clearly written philosophical statement. It should provide the basis for the program and be the guiding force for all essential tasks and functions from the inception to the final evaluation of the services.

The model presented here proposes that the philosophical statement embody the concepts of holism, prevention, and high-level wellness to serve as a rubric for the elders' health needs and to convey the provider's understanding and commitment to the services essential for comprehensive care. The priority and decision making for important care components are guided by the belief that preventive services are necessary to achieve high-level wellness. Early detection of problems and surveillance of health status are equally required to attain optimal health. All these care activities must be offered within the context of the holistic needs of the older person.

The application of the concepts of holism, prevention, and high-level wellness for elderly care requires the interaction of the client, family, and community because this approach to multidimensional care depends on shared responsibility. Each party has a role in meeting the elder's health needs, and the philosophical statement should support this to achieve optimum individuality for the aged and maximum use of community resources.

ASSESSMENT

The initiation of holistic care for the elder begins with an assessment of the client's assets and liabilities. The assessment is determined on the basis of the care components shown in Figure 2-1, namely, activities of daily living (ADL); ability for self-responsibility; adequacy of environment; and need for legal assistance, medical care, financial aid, and mental health. The care components are used to identify the individual's problem areas so that appropriate services may be instituted. The suggested care components are by no means all-inclusive, and other care needs may be added or substituted for those proposed. Whatever vital care components are selected, they serve as a foundation for program goals and are important for an older person's health promotion and maintenance needs. The definition of each care component for implementation of services is outlined in Chapter 1.

PROGRAM GOALS

Program goals give direction to accomplish the necessary tasks and are useful as mechanisms to communicate the intentions of health services. In addition, the goals help to legitimize the existence of an organization, develop program structure and processes, and provide measurements for evaluating the success of a health program.[4]

In the proposed health promotion and maintenance model, the program goals identify relevant services for elderly consumers. The statement of goals conveys the philosophy of care and logically follows the assessment functions that delineate specific care components that apply to the health of the community's aged group.

The program goals should have measures of specific outcomes that can be used as evidence of effective health care. These measures may require both objective and subjective inputs from the consumer and the provider of the health services. Another statement of the goals should address the consumer-provider partnership to establish clear lines of responsibility and to avoid misunderstanding of individual roles in the partnership approach to health care. This is especially important for evaluating the degree of partnership involved in health promotion and maintenance care.

Other possible goals might include the utilization of the community's legal resources for problems requiring judicial information, monitoring ADL to evaluate abilities necessary for continued independent living, and assisting to obtain appropriate medical care as required for a person's well-being.

PLANNING

The planning process is guided by the goals established from the assessment of comprehensive requirements for the care of older people. The planning activities are primarily a cognitive process to decide on the essential elements for program implementation. Planning should be done on a long-range basis to include accommodations for the changing needs of the population.[5] This procedure may begin prior to, or be a part of, the proposal to seek funds. In either case, it involves decisions on different aspects of the program for the delivery of services, for example, the selection of the professional staff, identification of an accessible and environmentally safe facility, utilization of volunteers and outreach services, determination of methods to disseminate information about health services, and participation in planning by the community and client representatives.

The planning group should ideally include an appropriate mix of consumers, professionals, and community representatives. Selection of members should be based on the kinds of input needed, and the size of the group must be most conducive to accomplish the tasks at hand. If a large group is necessary, subgroups may be formed to expedite discussions and completion of tasks. Each subgroup would then report its findings and recommendations to the entire group for final decisions.

The importance of including members of the target population in the planning group cannot be overemphasized since significantly different opinions about service needs can exist between the provider and consumers.[6,7] In this instance, it is imperative that orientation to the planning process and support during deliberations be provided to encourage and solicit maximum contributions from elderly participants. Older people tend to lack experience in working with planning groups; thus, they may be reluctant to express their opinions to professionals because of the feeling that they are powerless and their ideas are not significant.[8] Lauver also emphasizes the social class and cultural differences that exist between the client and clinician. She suggests conscious effort be made to explore the differences in values so that client's needs can be accurately assessed to plan appropriate approaches to health care. Along similar lines, Rundall and Wheeler[9] reported that senior citizens perceived susceptibility to disease and the amount of danger associated with receiving swine flu immunization as the most important determinants for using health services in a selected community. Thus, input from the elderly group about their beliefs regarding health care are important in the selection of services for the older person.

A definitive list of services and specific care to be offered by an agency must be determined and based on the human, financial, and other resources available to support one or more health programs. A successful program in one community does not assure a workable system in another, because necessary support in terms of professional staff, facilities, and so on may not be available, and client needs and wants may differ. For example, requirements for social services may be minimal in smaller communities where members have longstanding associations with one another, while health-related services might be in demand. An extensive discussion of the basic health and social programs necessary for comprehensive care of the community's elderly population is presented in Chapter 4.

Selection of Health Professionals

The selection of staff members for health promotion and maintenance programs is generally determined by the agency receiving funds. Moreover, the current trend in elderly health care is the team[10] or multidisciplinary approach with one professional taking the leadership and/or coordinating role. The physician or nurse practitioner is most frequently in this role; however, this does not exclude professionals such as a nutritionist, physical therapist, clinical psychologist, social worker, recreational director, and others from participating as leaders and coordinating the services of physicians and nurses. For example, a nutritionist at meal sites for the elderly can readily institute a multidisciplinary health care program in conjunction with the nutrition service. Whatever the situation, proper staff assignments in health programs depend on a firm understanding of the roles of the professionals and their potential contributions to the total needs of the program.

There are a number of approaches to planning health services for the community's elderly, and each locale must decide upon the array of professional services to use in its health program. One important consideration is to be aware of overlapping roles of professionals. A preservice agreement about each professional's responsibilities should be clearly identified whenever the team approach is used. Furthermore, an explicit communication and interaction system must be established to facilitate collaboration and consultation among the professionals. The use of a record system, client care conferences, and regularly scheduled staff meetings are additional ways to enhance the team approach.

The Role of Physicians

A geriatric care system should be based on clinical, preventive, curative, and psychosocial aspects of illness in the elderly.[11] This denotes that in practical settings, medical and social units should function as a team that includes physicians and other health professionals. The physician who assumes the leadership for elderly care must be an expert not only in medical sciences, normal aging, and the pathology related to aging, but also in the treatment of illnesses specific to the aged. A physician should also possess the ability to manage multiple health problems and recognize unusual symptoms as well as changes in responses to treatment that are characteristically seen in the aged. Frequently, a clinical diagnosis may be merely one of many health problems facing the elderly, and further exploration might be required to institute appropriate therapy and to prevent complications.

Specific preventive health maintenance for the elderly should include periodic and systematic assessment of the physical, mental, and social status.[12] Health screening by the medical staff should focus on the status of immunization; the early detection of cancer, hypertension, and obesity; and hazards related to smoking, alcohol, and drug consumption. Other essential preventive services that could be performed by the physician are providing nutrition counseling to assure adequate dietary intake, determining motor activity to ascertain capabilities for daily living activities, checking on the status of hemoglobin to detect anemias, assessing cardiovascular functions to identify early signs of heart problems, appraising bowel functions to prevent constipation, and identifying common sensory problems of hearing and vision loss. In addition, the exploration of psychosocial status is necessary to prevent or minimize the effects of social isolation and depression. Physicians can also offer early assistance with problems associated with retirement, finances, sex, meaning of life, and/ or impending death.

In order to implement health maintenance care and provide for an effective and efficient geriatric service in primary care settings, physicians may find the following suggestions by Morrison[13] helpful:

- Use allied health professionals such as nurse practitioners and physician assistants for data collection and to review areas of importance before, after, or separate from physician's visits.

- The episodically initiated health maintenance care should be included whenever chronic illness visits are made.

- Use a health maintenance flowsheet or checklist to remind physicians and other allied health professionals to supervise health maintenance care systematically.

The Role of Nurses

The current trend of nursing in elderly health care is the emergence of gerontological nurse specialists who have completed additional education beyond the basic nursing program and, in most cases, possess a master's degree. There are also other nurse practitioners who have attended a nondegree certificate program to increase their knowledge about the care of the aged.

The gerontological nurse specialist is knowledgeable about the elderly's health promotion, prevention and treatment of illnesses, and rehabilitation care. The aim of gerontological nursing is to assist older persons to achieve and maintain the level of physical and social functioning appropriate to their life style and environmental needs.[14] The focus of nursing care is on wellness, mobility, independence, and interdependence for the client.[15]

The nursing functions for the care of healthy older adults, as outlined by the American Nurses' Association,[16] provide for the following:

- Work and social activity—Assist older people to remain active socially, avoid isolation, and maintain ties with family members and friends.

- Exercise—Encourage regular physical activity for older adults such as daily walks that result in physical and psychological benefits, and help maintain flexibility and balance important for the prevention of falls.

- Nutrition—Recognize that older people have special dietary needs and that particular care should be taken to include the proper nutrients for health maintenance.

- Preventive services—Promote periodic health checkups (at least one physical examination every two years until age 75 and annually thereafter) to detect early health problems. Screening activities should include blood pressure checks, hearing and vision tests, hematocrits, pap smears, stool examinations, dental care, and foot care. When possible, preventive services should be provided at a single location.

- Medications—Older people take numerous medications; a periodic review of prescribed drugs with their physicians should be encouraged.

- Immunization—Urge older people to consult their physicians about immunizations, especially for influenza and pneumonia.

- Home safety—Institute home safety evaluations to suggest measures to prevent injuries from lack of ample lighting, unsturdy railings and steps, slippery floor surfaces, and inadequate fire protection and detection.

- Services to maintain independence—Assist in the use of community services to maintain an older person's independence.

The gerontological nurse may be characterized as a professional who works collaboratively with health professionals and others to assist in meeting the elderly's health needs. The nurse is capable of obtaining a health history, performing physical examinations, prescribing selected medications according to established standard orders, making decisions prospectively and cooperatively with the physician, providing traditional nursing care, and teaching or counseling patients and families about the aging process in health and illness.[17]

The Role of the Nutritionists

The nutritionist's major contributions in the health care of older people are directed to solving problems related to obesity, diets low in essential nutrients, and modified diets.[18] The need for interventions for these dietary problems is well recognized. Kelly et al. found the intake of calcium, vitamin A, and ascorbic acid was 40 percent below the recommended daily allowance among the older people.[19] Low intake of vitamin A and calcium was also identified in another study of the rural elders.[20] With regard to weight problems, a preliminary finding revealed that more than 25 percent of black and white women between the ages of 45 and 74 were obese, and for both groups, obesity was associated with low income.[21] However, the occurrence of obesity was found to be higher among black women than white women regardless of income. Finally, a study on the cause of eating difficulties showed that 41 percent of those surveyed blamed special diets as a primary problem.[22] These findings also substantiated the belief that the need for the services of nutritionists in health promotion and maintenance care centered on counseling, teaching, and nutritional assessment.

Rae and Burke suggest that successful dietary counseling must consider the total personal and social situations.[23] Factors to keep in mind during dietary counseling are that inadequate income is affected by inflation, transportation, or mobility problems; the variety of foods available in the stores may create difficulty in choosing the best buys; and the inability to carry groceries may be associated with limited facility to store, prepare, and eat nutritional meals. Also, eating by older people is influenced by other factors such as failing physical and mental health, decreased functioning of taste buds and saliva flow, long-established likes and dislikes of foods, and loneliness.[24] Although multiple nutritional problems are found in the elderly group, researchers have found that with appropriate interventions, appetite and food selection can be improved.[25]

Another indication confirming the need for a nutritionist's services is that Templeton found that older people seek advice on balanced diets, best food dollar buys, food preparation, food storage, new products, and food stamps.[26] This suggests that older people do desire assistance in maintaining their health despite adversities that affect their eating patterns contrary to popular beliefs that elders as a group show little interest in seeking new information. Furthermore, there is concern among many elders about the efficient use of limited finances and ways to supplement income. For example, 70 percent of the people who requested food stamp information had one or more nutrient deficiency in their diet, and 48 percent of these respondents listed their income as less than $3,000 per year.[27]

Since nutrition provides the energy and building materials essential for life, the inclusion of a nutritionist is a priority in any elderly health promotion and maintenance service. Nutritional needs are also supported by the legislation for the National Nutrition Program for Older Americans under the auspices of the Administration on Aging. This legislation provides for community nutrition sites where daily meals are served to older people. It might be noted that these sites offer the nutritionists potential settings for teaching and counseling about proper dietary intake, coordinating comprehensive care, and seeking assistance in health services from other professionals.

The Role of the Physical Therapists

Physical therapy has been and is still primarily aimed toward rehabilitative measures for fractures, cerebral vascular accidents, and severe immobility caused by arthritic conditions. This approach to practice is the result of a prescriptive relationship with physicians established when therapists began as a technical occupation; however, it overlooks the health promotion and maintenance aspects of care so desperately needed by the elders. More recently, physical therapists have moved toward a more independent practice with specific areas of expertise and competence. The American Physical Therapy Association legitimized this status in 1969 by voting a referral relationship with the physician for direct patient care.[28] This decision gave impetus to participation by physical therapists in community health programs where the functional abilities of older people could be assessed and adaptation programs implemented.

The physical therapist may undertake safe and effective applications of exercise techniques with adaptation to meet individual needs. Instituting regular programs of physical activity and exercise has been recommended to assist in the prevention or reversal of problems related to inactivity.[29] Physical activities like walking, selected calisthenics, and rhythmic exercises have been found to improve mobility and to strengthen the cardiovascular and respiratory functions. The result is an increased sense of well-being for the elders.

The optimal time for initiating a preventive physical therapy program is while the aged person is living independently in the community. Once older individuals are instructed and alerted to potential problems, they are self-directed and follow the recommended exercises and postural practices with minimal supervision.[30] This approach to activity maintenance encourages independence, retards regression of functions for daily living, and deters health problems associated with immobility.

The physical therapist in health promotion and maintenance services may focus on the evaluation of an older person's health history, life habits, complaints, and personal requirements.[31] This evaluation requires critical observations of exercise performances and movements as there are many ways in which these activities can be accomplished. The rationale as well as the expected results for specific exercise programs may be offered at this time. These planned exercises are especially appropriate when conducted at recreational sites, particularly when additional physical therapy consultation could be provided to the recreational directors about the functional abilities and safe limits of elders participating in physical activities.

Another health professional closely aligned to the physical therapist is the occupational therapist, who may also be considered as part of the staff of health promotion and maintenance programs. The occupational therapist's role is similar to that of the physical therapist's but with greater emphasis on improving physical capabilities for performing daily living activities, for example, compensating for loss of functions from illness or injury by capitalizing on the remaining capabilities. The occupational therapist is also an expert in identifying devices that assist in achieving optimal level of functioning for impaired extremities.

The Role of the Social Workers

Whenever inadequate income or other social needs are identified, the social worker is contacted for consultation and resolution of these client problems. Although a number of health professionals' educational background may include some content relative to social work, it is generally not sufficient to meet all aspects of human service needs. Thus, most health professionals rely heavily on the social worker for interventions in the psychosocial and environmental dimensions of client care.

The roles and functions of the social worker center on an understanding of human behavior and relationship, and knowledge of social problems, welfare programs, and needs of older people.[32] Some attributes required of a social worker are expertise in conducting interviews, ability to communicate clearly, skill in working cooperatively with others, competence in supervisory activities, and ability to provide consultation services to clients and other health professionals.

Social workers are the prime source of assistance in obtaining appropriate benefits for clients from government sources. Their aid in filing applications, providing interpretations, and facilitating the benefit process is extremely important to the welfare of older people. Clearly the need for these activities will continue as health and social service benefits to older people are expanded.

In addition to providing for the social welfare of the elders, the process of applying for benefits is useful in identifying persons who may also need health promotion and maintenance services. Furthermore, the experience introduces the elders to new resources of assistance when alternative plans for independent living become a requirement. For example, assistance with decision making about a health facility and preparation for admission to an institutional setting may be available to an older person and family from the social worker. The support during the pre-admission waiting period is a valuable service to assure a smooth transition and to minimize the shock of relocation. The guidance provided effectively by social workers is essential to elders' health promotion.

The educational requirement for the professional social worker, who serves as a consultant for policy decisions and initiation of services, is generally a graduate degree. On the other hand, professional workers with only baccalaureate degrees provide services to individuals who need assistance for improvement of health and social problems. These second-level social workers often provide the client and family with services necessary for health maintenance, prevention of illness, or rehabilitation.

Both levels of social workers can provide inputs to planning, policy making, and the delivery of services to elders in health maintenance programs. Currently, most professional social workers are in leadership positions in long-term institutional settings. The expertise and experience gained from these positions and settings may be useful for other community-based programs that are designed to assist the more independent older population. The continued survival and maintenance of the aged persons' life style in the community will depend on the availability of social services. The social workers provide the essential human needs to supplement the work of the health professionals.

The Role of the Clinical Psychologists

It is only in recent years that the clinical psychologist has become involved with the psychological counseling of older people. Historically, the development of mental health care for the aged has evolved slowly. Perhaps one reason for the lag in psychological care for the older population was influenced by Freud's belief that people over the age of 50 were not amenable to treatments because of long-established mental processes.[33] As gerontological knowledge increased, it has become apparent that elders could benefit from psychological care. The interrelationship between mental and physical health care is so closely bound that it is difficult to determine which of these two areas of care is more important. For example, the frustration and anxiety associated with demands for adaptation to new situations result in tension that leads to serious mental problems such as a depression. It is necessary to be cognizant of the lessened defenses the elders experience against physical and psychological illnesses and the influence of these factors upon the effectiveness of therapeutic plans.[34]

The role of the clinical psychologist may be viewed primarily as a consultant and collaborator with other health professionals in providing effective holistic care. Referrals to clinical psychologists are indicated when complex mental or emotional problems, which require more specialized service than most health professionals are able to give, are identified. The expertise of the clinical psychologist is necessary to conduct clients' interviews to elicit factors that affect the levels of activities and interests, reactions to past and present life circumstances, attitudes about self, and feelings toward the environment. An additional key function of the mental health professional is to conduct extensive psychological tests and interpret the results of the examinations.

The psychological examination for gathering data to plan counseling strategies should consider the following areas:[35]

- mental capabilities and responses to intellectual stimulation;
- special skills and/or aptitudes that suit vocational pursuits or hobbies;
- general personality characteristics and self-concepts;
- social interests and activities;
- viewpoint about family members and their attitudes and behavior toward the elderly person;
- outlook and hope for the future;
- motivation for and ability to work on new interests, activities, and social adaptations;
- possible need for psychotherapeutic or other forms of psychosocial services.

The lack of specifically designed standardized tests for the elderly group is acknowledged, but some selected tests are currently used to determine the psychological makeup of older people. The more frequently used tests may include the Wechsler Adult Intelligence Scale, the Catell Personality Test, the Sentence Completion Test, and the Kuder Preference Record and Activity Check List.[36]

After completion of psychological testing and before proceeding with the therapy sessions, the clinical psychologist makes a determination about the person's ability and willingness to cooperate with the therapy, to participate in self-evaluation, and to identify realistic goals that are congruent with the individual's personality. Frequently, interviews with family members are also used to verify an elder's interaction pattern and capability to participate in family relationships. These preliminary activities are used to assess whether therapy sessions will be acceptable and to provide some indication of the potential benefit to the client.

The clinical psychologist is academically prepared at the doctoral level and in most states is required to complete board examinations successfully before being certified and licensed to practice. Clinical psychologists differ from psychiatrists in that they do not attend medical school. Thus, prescribing medications is not a function of the clinical psychologist, and clients requiring drug therapy are referred to psychiatrists. In many instances, these two mental health professionals work as a team for the treatment of emotional, intellectual, social, and personality problems.

A particular specialty area of the clinical psychologist is conducting group or individual counseling sessions for ego support or encouragement, and assistance with specific personal problems of the older person. A major emphasis of this care is to gain information about self-interest areas, exploring and interpreting life stresses and feelings about life experiences. This type of group therapy for the elders is reported to decrease depression and somatic complaints, and increase social activities.[37]

The Role of Dentists

Dental care as a part of elderly health care is minimally emphasized by the responsible agencies. The current health care plans for the aged, that is, Medicare and Medicaid, fail to include the dental needs of older people. Although teeth are necessary for mastication of food, the process of digestion, articulation, and aiding one's appearance, they are considered to be unessential for survival.[38] This notion is reinforced by the low priority that dental care receives in an elder's health care budget allocation, particularly when finances are limited.

The inclusion of dental care in health promotion and maintenance care is imperative because the inability to chew adequately affects nutritional intake and may lead to serious health problems. Dental care may be provided on a consultation basis or by a referral system that offers services for a reduced fee. A thorough examination of the oral cavity and the condition of the teeth, and proper fitting of dentures is necessary for maintaining the overall health status of older individuals. Periodic dental examinations for early detection of dental caries, periodontal diseases, stomatitis, glossitis, bone lesions, miscellaneous benign and malignant neoplasms, moniliasis, and other pathology are particularly significant for health promotion and maintenance care. Furthermore, the examination of the mouth allows the dentist to evaluate the mobility of the mandible and the status of facial muscles, and to identify creptitus of the temporomandibular joints associated with generalized arthritis. All of these dental assessments are vital not only to determine the health status, but also to institute treatment in a timely way.

The Role of Podiatrists

The team approach to elderly health care includes a podiatrist who specializes in maintenance of ambulation. This relative newcomer to the team serves to achieve three important goals in gerontology, namely, to limit disability, to preserve maximum normal function, and to restore the highest possible level of independent activity for the individual.[39]

Podiatrists working in concert with other health professionals can make significant contributions to health maintenance care. For example, they can provide expertise on foot problems such as thickened toenails, callouses, corns, and common mechanical malfunctions resulting from anatomical deformities (for example, Morton's toe and calcaneal spurs). Recommendations of appropriate footwear for support or various devices to redistribute pressure for protection can also be provided by the podiatrist to maintain the elders' ambulatory capabilities.

In most states, podiatrists are licensed practitioners who may or may not be required to treat clients in consultation with the physician. State boards of health professionals are ultimately responsible for regulations and licensing of podiatrists. Some recognition of the podiatrist as a health care provider has been shown by the recent approval of third party payment for podiatric services as a benefit of Medicare.

Selection of Facility

Following the selection of the health care team, the planning group must decide upon the setting for the health services. The size and location of the facility are determined by the number of health care team members who will be giving care and by the accessibility of the site for the clients.

One of the first considerations in choosing a health care facility is to survey the existing sites where services for the elders are offered. Frequently, community organizations responsible for senior citizens' activities welcome the addition of health services for their participants. The senior citizens' centers and nutritional sites are especially ideal locations to consider. Advantages associated with these sites are twofold: first, the potential users of the services are accustomed to the environment; and second, the transportation problems to the location are resolved or minimal in nature.

The team approach to health promotion and maintenance care is enhanced by the use of existing senior activity sites because comprehensive services can be offered within a single setting. Moreover, it is a cost-effective approach in terms of rent, utilities, custodial services, building maintenance and repairs, and so on, because these expenses could be shared or budgetarily considered as a contribution to the health program. Another favorable reason to use existing settings is that, in most instances, environmental barriers and hazards such as those created by excessive stairs that impede the mobility of the elders have been eliminated or minimized.

Other environmental assessments should address the adequacy of space for conducting interviews, personal discussions, and physical examinations. Privacy and confidentiality of information given by the clients must be protected by using portable screens and allowing ample distances between the interviews taking place and other waiting clients. Another important element is the availability and accessibility of bathroom facilities so that sanitary practices could be exercised for the health protection of all clients. Such facilities are also necessary for procedures such as screening for urine and blood tests.

A specially designed new facility is the most desirable for community health promotion and maintenance care programs although other buildings, such as those built only for health services, can be used. However, it should be noted that in the latter case, health services for the ambulatory healthy older people are generally viewed as part of informal, quasi-recreational activities rather than a formal setting representing the traditional more serious health care environment. From the perspective of the elders, these formal settings are mostly associated with and used for illness rather than for health promotion activities.

Vacated neighborhood stores, residential or mobile homes, and recreational vehicles may be potential facilities for health maintenance services. These settings would be notably less costly than the rental of a health care facility; however, there are advantages and disadvantages. To illustrate, a store setting may not have adequate bathroom facilities to provide safe services and to accommodate all of the clients. Some expense for constructing partitions to make separate rooms or offices may be necessary. Heating and cooling systems may be antiquated and cause difficulty in maintaining the proper temperature. On the other hand, the store may be located where a large portion of the target population lives; thus, the clients would be more familiar with the setting, and transportation problems would be minimal or nonexistent. Since there are a number of factors involved in selecting sites and facilities, each community should include professional and client inputs to decide on the arrangement most advantageous for its purposes.

Publicity for the Health Services

Dissemination of information about health services to the greatest number of people requires the full use of the communications media. This approach should save staff time and help direct efforts to other essential program activities that cannot be delegated. Publicity through the media also reaches more potential users of the health services who otherwise might be missed.

The benefits of a well-written news story, feature article, or a television spot cannot be underestimated. Frequently, the publicity may result in responses from listeners and readers who are willing to become volunteers for the programs or contribute valuable ideas, money, time, and so on. The most important outcome from the publicity may be the attainment of community support. This support is most welcomed and may be needed at a later time when the initial funding terminates and new monetary sources for continued services must be found.

Important considerations for the development of an effective publicity campaign is succinctly described in the *Public Information Manual for Human Services*, published by the New England Gerontological Center of the University of New Hampshire.[40] This publication outlines in detail the essential processes and components for the effective use of the media to advertise newly developed health services.

Television as a means to publicize health programs should be given priority because studies have shown greater television viewing by the aged as compared to the middle-aged or young adult groups.[41] In addition, the preference for television programs among older people has consistently centered around news and public affairs programming.[42] This suggests that the elders have greater desires to know about the environment in which they live. The aged seem to prefer more practical information rather than entertainment; their information seeking is focused on issues concerning health, housing, income, and other matters that become important to living and life styles as aging advances.[43] However, the extent to which the elders are gratified by the communications media for getting information or compensating for the loss of social contact is unclear. Further study and analysis of the individual's perceived assistance or lack of fulfillment need to be pursued.[44]

A novel approach to meet the health information needs of the elders and to improve communication between the health care providers and consumers has been reported.[45] A variety of programs on health topics of interest to the elders has been produced by using television personalities and older people as performers. The benefits of improved self-image and self-esteem were noted by the elderly participants in these productions. Moreover, there was evidence to suggest that the opportunity to participate in the programs may have contributed to the reduction of isolation.

After television, newspapers and radio are the media most frequently used by the elders to seek information. The newspaper is preferable for obtaining local news and probably offers a better means to reach the target population to publicize new health programs.

Another method to promote publicity is to design and distribute brochures that outline and describe the important aspects of the available health services. The content should clearly convey the benefits of the services, but be brief. The size of print must be large enough to meet the needs of the visually handicapped, and the brochures should be colorful and attractively presented. If possible, pictures of clients receiving some service such as a blood pressure check may be appropriate to show peer participation in the health services. In communities where minority populations are found, brochures in each native language should be printed to ensure proper communication and participation by the individual groups.

The distribution of brochures may be done in cooperation with the senior citizens' activities and through professionals who work with older people. Other settings useful for the placement of brochures are the neighborhood grocery stores, post offices, churches, subsidized housing projects, and other locations where older people live or visit on a regular basis. An excellent opportunity to disseminate information on the available health services is provided whenever any professional staff member accepts a community speaking engagement. The occasion can also be used to distribute the brochures not only to the aged, but to others who have elderly parents, relatives, neighbors, or friends.

Regardless of the methods chosen to publicize community health programs, it is important to be aware that peoples' perceptions of an event or information depend on psychological processes. Thus, certain communication techniques can be exploited to encourage or reinforce acceptance of information. Three methods that can be employed to enhance acceptance of a new health program are: (1) selective exposure to raise the consciousness and to bombard the community with the message; (2) selective attention to increase interest level through the use of mass media and by personal contacts; and (3) selective retention facilitated by reemphasizing the positive aspects of the service and by demonstrating peer groups' participation.[46] These methods are well worth remembering when health programs are initiated and there is a requirement to conduct the publicity phase in an expeditious manner to promote acceptance of health care by potential consumers.

Volunteer and Outreach Services

The recruitment and retention of volunteers in local service programs benefit not only the volunteers, but also the agency. The agency's allocated funds are used judiciously when volunteers assist with assignments not requiring the staff's expertise. The procedure is seen as a long-range support for the programs because it demonstrates that local tax monies are used only for essential staff services. Often a knowledgeable volunteer's report about a program's effectiveness is more desirable at budget request sessions than an agency staff's justification on client needs.[47] Somehow the volunteer's report seems to convey more credibility than the statistics submitted by the agency personnel. Volunteers also have an advantage over the staff in that they are freer to contact legislators and other elected officials to solicit continued funding.

The most successful volunteer programs are usually supported by a key community person who can motivate others to continue with their commitment. In some communities, this key person manages the volunteer organizations and locates individuals with interest and preference to become involved with specific service agencies. When individuals are recruited, the agency staff must train, assign, and supervise with consideration for the volunteer's needs. Since the volunteers do not receive pay, job satisfaction is an important element that motivates them to continue their involvement. It is also important to keep them informed about agency events, particularly in the areas that affect their work. Finally, input should be solicited from the volunteers on topics for which they can provide some answers.

Administrative and operational are the two basic types of volunteers used in services designed for the aging population.[48] The administrative volunteers serve as board or committee members who assist in planning, resolving organizational problems, or suggesting policies. The operational volunteer assists by supplementing the staff's work, including some possible fund-raising activities. Most organizations need both types of assistance; the volunteers' gratification from serving in these positions must evolve without feelings of being overburdened, particularly when the assignments have the potential to extend talents and/or time. The volunteer coordinator or the responsible agency person must continuously evaluate the effectiveness of volunteer usage both from the perspective of the agency and with regards to the volunteers' satisfaction.

The use of older volunteers for elderly services is becoming more known and accepted. The contributions and benefits to individuals and organizations are well documented in a publication by the Ethel Percy Andrus Gerontological Center in Los Angeles.[49]

Outreach services, as with volunteer programs, require careful planning and implementation. The basic purpose of outreach is to locate and provide information to older people about specific services available in a community. Specific outreach functions are determined by health agencies and may range from simply giving the names of service agencies to actual delivery of care, the extent of which depends on the outreach worker's qualification and experience. In some instances, outreach may include follow-up actions to ensure that services were indeed delivered to the needy client.

Other outreach activities might involve conducting a door-to-door neighborhood canvas where large numbers of older people live, or locating and contacting isolated persons. The outreach methods are often determined by the availability of financial and human resources as well as the overall purposes of the program. Locating the truly isolated elder requires the efforts of many service agencies and the use of various outreach methodologies.

IMPLEMENTATION

The implementation of a health promotion and maintenance program is the actual delivery of services to the consumers. Our model uses the concepts of responsibility, decision making, adaptation, and coping to guide the implementation process. These concepts were selected to augment those of holism, prevention, and high-level wellness, which serve as the philosophical basis for the health services.

Since most health promotion activities require full participation of the clients, responsibility and decision making about the acceptance or rejection of care must be shared. If this notion is accepted, the health worker must be ready to offer any information essential for making health care decisions with the elder. Generally, health promotion activities allow clients to make choices, as there is no immediacy for interventions as seen in life-threatening conditions. In this instance, the professionals are primarily in a position of partnership to encourage and guide clients to participate in health promoting activities. The benefits clients receive are future-oriented rather than resulting in an immediate change in their health status. Since each person has unique adaptation and coping capabilities, individual assessment and exploration of ways to match client abilities with health promotion activities must be pursued. For instance, anticipatory guidance for controlling dietary intake to maintain a given health status may be appropriate to prevent complications from chronic illness. Individuals with heart problems or other long-term health conditions may benefit from this type of care. Teaching and counseling about self-care may also become a priority and contribute to an eventual optimal level of functioning. The day-to-day health maintenance activities are assumed by the elderly clients, and the professionals provide continuing support and consultation to ensure self-care is implemented correctly.

The implementation of health services must deliberately attend to the early detection of health problems. This can be accomplished by activities such as taking a health history, performing examinations, and using screening procedures. In addition, this approach to periodic health assessment must incorporate the holistic view of the aged with investigations of problems associated with the psychological, sociological, and environmental aspects of the person.

Documentation of this health information requires that a definitive record system be designed before beginning the implementation phase. The records may be used not only to communicate information among the professionals, but also for continuity of care and to record a person's health status. The records also become a means for gathering data about a health program and can be used as evidence to support the evaluation procedures. Thus, the items in the records should be chosen to reflect the care components and program goals. These activities are illustrated in Figure 2–1 where arrows indicate that the components of care do have a relationship to the implementation phase.

It is critical that some method for tabulating service information and a data retrieval system be clearly established before implementation of services. The protection of clients' rights to privacy and confidentiality of information must be adhered to within the retrieval system by the use of appropriate techniques, for example, employing identifying numbers rather than names. Names of individuals should only appear on the original health record and not be used for gathering information about the health services.

The referral services and follow-up care by other agencies are additional activities that must be addressed in the implementation phase. To establish an effective system and minimize inappropriate referrals, the professionals should be knowledgeable about community resources and the eligibility requirements for obtaining services. A well-planned system not only ensures delivery of services, but is a prerequisite for providing comprehensive care for elderly clients.

Another function of the implementation phase, which contributes to an effective and efficient health service, is to devise ways to minimize client waiting periods. The employment of an appointment system or service on a first-come basis are two options, and the method in use, or to be used, by each service agency must be clearly communicated to the clients. If the latter method is used, some system such as assignment of numbers should be devised so clients are served in an orderly fashion. When the health service is offered in conjunction with recreational or other activities, clients might be encouraged to participate in their interest group while they are waiting.

Another important aspect of the implementation phase is the development of relationships with the client, family, and community by the professional staff to encourage the use of the health services. Effective communication skills are needed for this and other activities conducted to assist the older people and to promote a partnership approach to health care. This is a new experience for many of the elders; thus, it will require the professional to show patience, support, and understanding to foster the partnership and to share responsibilities, decision making, care information, and so on.

Finally, implementation of a team approach may necessitate the establishing of guidelines for the professionals to follow in providing health care. For example, protocols might be enacted for the care of individuals with abnormal health screening results or any other deviations from normal profiles. These protocols should be defined by the professionals involved with the specific health care and should be regarded not as inhibiting professional decision making, but rather as a way to standardize health services.

EVALUATION

The plans for evaluation activities should be written, addressing the components of the health promotion and maintenance model, and be in place before the implementation of the health services. The evaluation process must be accomplished in a systematic way, which means that program goals should be explicitly stated with standards of measurements identified or defined before the evaluation process begins.

Since evaluation is a complex task and remains problematic, the concepts used as the theoretical basis for the health promotion and maintenance model are recommended as guidelines for the evaluation process. For example, the concept of prevention could be a guide to determine the number of services given in this special area and to identify some measurement that would indicate improvement of a client's health status. In this way, some outcomes of preventive care may be elicited. This process involves a retrospective study of actions, primarily of behavior changes, to determine the effectiveness of client care. Inherent in this procedure is the understanding that subjectivity about behavior changes on the part of the professional and the client is a shortcoming of this type of human assessment. Although every effort is made to minimize biases, no method has yet been found that gives a completely objective evaluation.

Other evaluation issues to consider are health services utilization based on various categories, number of health services rendered, and clients' perceptions about the appropriateness of and satisfaction or dissatisfaction with the available care. These results are often useful to generate information and data that may justify future funding requests or proposals for health care research.

Funding sources are interested in obtaining both subjective and objective data that show that past funds were properly used. Most often, data related to total numbers of clients served, types of care given, and the results of care are presented as justifications for expenditures. It is necessary for all professionals who have participated in the health promotion and maintenance care programs to contribute to the evaluation process in order to provide an accurate accounting of the available health services and the care delivered to the elderly population.

NOTES

1. Ollie A. Randall, "The Aging and the Aged in Yesterday's, Today's and Tomorrow's World," in Minna Field, ed., *Depth and Extent of the Geriatric Problem* (Springfield, Ill.: Charles C. Thomas Publisher, 1970), p. 22.

2. Chiyoko Furukawa, "Adult Health Conference: Community-Oriented Health Maintenance Care for the Elderly," *Family & Community Health* 3, no. 4 (February 1981): 105–121.

3. John C. Morgan, *Becoming Old* (New York, N.Y.: Springer Publishing Co., 1979), p. XII.

4. Eleanor M. White, "Conceptual Basis for Nursing Intervention with Human Systems: Group and Complex Organizations," in Barbara R. Weaver and Joanne E. Hall, eds., *Distributive Nursing Practice* (Philadelphia, Pa.: J. B. Lippincott Co., 1977), p. 148.

5. F. Anthony Bushman and Philip D. Cooper, "A Process for Developing New Health Services," *Health Care Management Review* 5, no. 1 (Winter 1980): 41.

6 Pat Keith, "A Preliminary Investigation of the Roles of the Public Health Nurse in Evaluation of Services for the Aged," *American Journal of Public Health* 66, no. 4 (April 1976): 379–81.

7. Raymond Leinbach, "The Aging Participants in an Area Planning Effort," *The Gerontologist* 17, no. 5 (October 1977): 453–58.

8. Diane Lauver, "Recognizing Alternatives: A Process for Client Centered Health Care," *Health Values: Achieving High-Level Wellness* 4, no. 3 (May/June 1980): 134–38.

9. T. G. Rundall and J. R. Wheeler, "Factors Associated with Utilization of the Swine Flu Vaccination Program Among Senior Citizens in Tompkins County (New York)," *Medical Care* 17, no. 2 (February 1979): 191–200.

10. Emmanuel Margolis, "Changing Disease Patterns, Changing Values," *Medical Care* 17, no. 11 (November 1979): 1121.

11. Ibid., p.1121.

12. John D. Morrison, "Geriatric Preventive Health Maintenance," *Journal of the American Geriatric Society* 28, no. 3 (March 1980): 133.

13. Ibid., p.135.

14. Thelma J. Wells, "Nursing Committed to the Elderly," in Adina M. Reinhardt and Mildred D. Quinn, eds., *Current Practice in Gerontological Nursing* (St. Louis, Mo.: C. V. Mosby Co., 1979), p. 189.

15. Ibid., p. 190.

16. American Nurses' Association Congress for Nursing Practice, "Healthy Older Adults," *Quality Assurance Update* 4, no. 1 (May 1980): 1.

17. J. D. Brocklehurst, *Geriatric Care in Advanced Societies* (Baltimore, Md.: University Park Press, 1975), p. 108.

18. C. L. Templeton, "Nutrition Counseling Need in Geriatric Population," *Geriatrics* 33, no. 4 (April 1978): 59.

19. L. Kelly, M. A. Ohlson, and L. J. Harper, "Foods Selection & Wellbeing of Aging Women," *Journal of the American Dietetic Association* 33, no. 5 (May 1957): 466–70.

20. H. A. Guthrie, K. Black, and J. P. Madden, "Nutritional Practices of Elderly Citizens in Rural Pennsylvania," *The Gerontologist* 12, no. 4 (August 1972): 330–35.

21. C. L. Templeton, "Nutrition Counseling Need in Geriatric Population," p. 59.

22. Ibid., p. 60.

23. J. Rae and A. L. Burke, "Counseling the Elderly in Community Health Care System," *Journal of the American Geriatrics Society* 26, no. 3 (March 1978): 130.

24. Ibid., p. 130.

25. Ibid., p. 130.

26. C. L. Templeton, "Nutrition Counseling Need in Geriatric Population," p. 65.

27. Ibid., p. 65.

28. Jessica A. Hopkins, "The Role of Physical Therapy in the Care of the Geriatric Patient," in Austin B. Chinn, ed., *Working with Older People, Volume IV* (Rockville, Md.: U.S. Government Printing Office, 1974), p. 375.

29. Helen D. Skeist, "Role of Physical Therapy in Physical Activity Program in Nursing Homes: A Survey," *Journal of the American Geriatrics Society* 28, no. 3 (March 1980): 125.

30. Jessica A. Hopkins, "The Role of Physical Therapy in the Care of the Geriatric Patient," p. 373.

31. Ibid., p. 374.

32. Elaine M. Brody, *Long-Term Care of Older People* (New York, N.Y.: Human Sciences Press, 1977), p. 246.

33. Ralph J. Kahana, "Strategies of Dynamic Psychotherapy with the Wide Range of Older Individuals," *Journal of Geriatric Psychiatry* 12, no. 1 (1979): 72.

34. Samuel Granick, "Psychological Study in the Management of the Geriatric Patient," in Austin B. Chinn, ed., *Working with Older People, Volume IV* (Rockville, Md.: U.S. Government Printing Office, 1974), p. 322.

35. Ibid., p. 330.

36. Ibid., p. 332.

37. Joseph Richman, "A Couples Therapy Group on a Geriatric Service," *Journal of Geriatric Psychiatry* 12, no. 2 (1979): 203–13.
38. Cary S. Kart, Eileen S. Metress, and James F. Metress, *Aging and Health: Biological and Social Perspectives* (Menlo Park, Ca.: Addison-Wesley Publishing Co., 1978), p. 77.
39. A. E. Helfand, "Podiatry and the Elderly Patient," in Austin B. Chinn, ed., *Working with Older People, Volume IV* (Rockville, Md.: U.S. Government Printing Office, 1974), p. 377.
40. David C. Riese, *Public Information Manual for Human Services* (Durham, N.H.: The University of New Hampshire, 1977), p. 3.
41. Robert W. Kubey, "Television and Aging: Past, Present, and Future," *The Gerontologist* 20, no. 1 (February 1980): 16–35.
42. Thomas J. Young, "Use of Media by Older Adults," *American Behavioral Scientist* 23, no. 1 (September/October 1979): 119–36.
43. Constance Swank, "Media Uses and Gratifications: Need Salience & Source Dependence in a Sample of the Elderly," *American Behavioral Scientist* 23, no. 1 (September/October 1979): 95–117.
44. Edward Wallenstein and Carter L. Marshall, "Telecommunications: An Approach to De-isolation of the Elderly," *Perspective of Aging* 3, no. 6 (June 1974): 3–6.
45. Ibid., p. 5.
46. Gustavo M. Quesada, "Campaigning for Health Program," *American Journal of Nursing* 80, no. 5 (May 1980): 952–53.
47. Jerry E. Griffin, "Local Volunteerism," in Lorin A. Baumhover and Joan D. Jones, eds., *Handbook of American Aging Programs* (Westport, Conn.: Greenwood Press, 1977), p. 91.
48. Ibid., p. 93.
49. Mary M. Seguin and Beatrice O'Brien, eds., *Releasing the Potential of the Older Volunteer* (Los Angeles, Ca.: University of Southern California, 1976).

Chapter 3

The Changing Relationship of the Elderly as a Group to Society as a Whole

Dianna Shomaker

There are always a few people older than the vast majority of the society. The significant size of the older aggregate is increasing in most industrialized societies, where modern technology has minimized mortality rates and increased the number who are surviving well into their seventh decade of life.

Technological advances have complicated the roles of persons in these societies. It takes less time to produce the same output. Technology has increased the need for new skills and has often required mobility from those seeking employment. The elderly, who were educated a long time ago, have been retired in deference to the younger workers, creating a "surplus" of unemployed older people.[1]

In evolutionary terms, the elderly can be said to have specialized in a work niche that became outmoded. Time was too short for many to learn new skills. The young, who were not yet highly specialized, learned to adapt to new niches of technology, leaving the elderly behind. Longevity also increased, and, as a result, family patterns and roles changed for those who were living longer.

The three areas that most markedly reflect the evolution of the role of the aged are population change, urbanization, and advancing technology. Within this structure there are shifts in kinship; in dependency and labor patterns, which represent evolutionary processes of adaptation for more efficient use of environment; and in refinement of role for survival.

DEMOGRAPHICS OF THE INDUSTRIAL REVOLUTION

The Industrial Revolution began in England in the early 1800s, where preindustrial patterns were evolving into what is now considered the industrial pattern. There were population shifts from rural to urban; an

47

economy and society that were regional became national; and scientific knowledge about control of disease was increased. Cities that were once small and depended on rural agricultural production for livelihood became larger as populations became more densely situated in urban areas.

The industrialization of the United States began later in the 1800s and was further influenced by waves of immigration. Agriculture was the prevalent means of livelihood, but the young country had a new government, a sense of forward progress, a pioneering pattern already established, and an intense entrepreneurial spirit. There were vast resources to be tapped and immigrants seeking work.

As young people emigrated from Europe to the United States, they often left their elderly behind. As a consequence, the mean age of the population of the United States lowered; that of the European nations increased. The majority of all populations on both continents lived in rural agrarian economies. At least three-fourths of the preindustrial population was involved fulltime in agricultural activity. Where there was mining, it was a small-scale, simple operation run by the landowner.[2] Families worked together as a production unit in a basically patriarchal structure where specific rules of inheritance, power, rights, and responsibilities of family members were well established. Not only were children advantageous as producers, but they offered family continuity and security as the adults grew older and relinquished manual chores to them. These multigenerational households were most often bound by blood-ties of loyalty and respect. The elderly were usually maintained on the farm, working as their capacity would allow and needs dictated.

The Agricultural Revolution had allowed people to gather in more dense aggregates, but it was not until the Industrial Revolution that populations multiplied at any significant rate. Until then, population growth was very slow. Few lived to be old. The decreased mortality rate and increased longevity that the Industrial Revolution brought about was probably due to improved reliability of food supply, change in food production, improved housing conditions, and progressive medical and sanitation facilities.

The United Nations has analyzed the age structures of populations of nations and arbitrarily classified them according to age structure as "young," "mature," and "aged." [3] Today, a young nation has less than four percent of its total population over 65 years of age. A mature nation, on the other hand, has four to seven percent of its population over 65 and is still in the stage of rapid industrial development. In these mature countries the birth rates are relatively high, and life expectancy at birth is about 64 years of age. Compare this with aged countries, which are economically more developed, such as those of Europe and North America, where more than seven percent of the population is 65 and over. These countries share the commonality of lower birth rates and a life expectancy at birth that is about 71 years of age.[4]

Throughout the industrialization process, the marriage and death rates have gradually declined. In contrast, the birth rate has fluctuated in response to economic and environmental factors. Generally, however, statistics suggest that a lower death rate will precede a lower birth rate during industrial growth. In the United States decreasing birth rates were recorded from 1870 to the 1930s, but rates rose again in the 1940s in what is commonly referred to as the postwar baby boom. This pattern again reversed in the 1950s.[5]

In the past, the birth rate was high because of a need for children as producers and to offset death rates, which were high due to poor nutrition, epidemic diseases, and general lack of medical technology, especially in the context of public health and sanitation. In the cities the death rates were even higher due to atmospheric pollution from factories and increased population density.

With the advent of chemotherapy and immunization, mortality rates declined, especially for infants and the elderly.[6] However, life expectancy for those over 75 increased only by a few years. The bulk of increase in longevity was really added to the life of the young and the middle-aged, even though to some degree it has increased the proportion of those receiving pensions.[7] Mortality rates for those under a year and those over 45 years of age did not see a noticeable improvement until the early 1900s.

The long-term effect of decline in mortality rates was to increase longevity and create a shift in the age distribution.[8] Not only did the population increase, but the number of elderly was significantly greater in proportion to the bulk of the population. This age proportion was seen in all industrial nations following the two World Wars along with significant increases in the imbalance of the male-female ratio.

These disproportions upset family structure, and in turn affected the status of the aged. Mobility of young adults increased as they pursued new industrial occupations. Households shrank from a multigenerational to a nuclear structure. The old patriarchy was undermined as an economic unit. The patriarch was no longer a supreme authority, employer and manager of sons and hired men. Economic independence guaranteed by ownership of a farm was greatly diminished. The elderly who sought outside employment found their skills could not compete with new machines. Moreover, employers could dismiss workers without an obligation of support as had been previously guaranteed by the arrangements in multigenerational households.[9]

"The general effect of industrialization [was] to break up the extended family into independent nuclear units with the extended family no longer a closely knit unit but rather a network as demonstrated by Bott." [10] Fertility rates were closely connected to industrialization. In Western Europe and the United States, population growth leveled off, but death rates declined before birth rates. As a result there were more old persons than in the past, but it became more difficult for their children to offer them security. This was partly due to decreased opportunities for children as laborers since the need for family farm labor was declining. Furthermore, children were now urban consumers instead of rural producers, and as such, large numbers of them were a disadvantage. Not only were they a financial burden, but they limited the mobility of young adults, who were seeking increased education and employment. [11]

The implications of these demographic changes are twofold. First, a larger number of people now live significantly beyond 50 years of age and are subject to death in later years due to chronic illness and degeneration, rather than to epidemics of communicable diseases as in the past. The second implication arises from the marriage and dependency patterns.

When children marry younger, they are often not economically secure before bearing children. In addition, their parents and grandparents are living longer into retirement, which increases the dependency ratio. Young adults find themselves in the impossible dilemma of needing to support dependent children as well as dependent elderly.

CURRENT POLITICAL AND ECONOMIC DILEMMA

In Western cultures, where industrialization and urbanization have accelerated rapidly, the political and social action to meet the needs of the changing conditions of the elderly has begun to be intensified. This is particularly true in Great Britain, where medical and psychosocial services for the elderly are highly developed. [12] The U.S. is just beginning to develop services that cover more than financial support.

In countries where industrialization and urbanization have been late in developing, governmental and social action in recognizing the needs of the elderly has also been slow. [13] In the Soviet Union, virtually no interest has been developed in the psychological aspects of aging. If any needs of the elderly have been recognized, they have no doubt been financial. For example, continuation of employment beyond retirement age has been allowed, but it has been due to the labor shortages of the country, not to the humanitarian considerations of economic needs of the aged. Anderson sees the Soviet Union as a young country, still evolving in the early stages of industrialization. [14] The country's major focus is on children, adolescents, and young adults. Aging has not yet strained the adaptability of the Soviet system enough to become a significant social problem. When it does, more attention may be turned toward it.

Burgess maintains that societies develop stages in which they attempt to meet the basic needs of the elderly.[15] These stages can be viewed as types of adaptation within a niche. The U.S. has established a retirement age and subsequent pension plan. That is part of the first stage, that is, to accommodate economic needs through social insurance or pension plans. The second stage is to supply health care and special housing. And, as the society evolves, it also provides leisure-time activities.

Ultimately a new pattern of social relations emerges in which independence and autonomy in both younger and older generations replaces the old patriarchal, dependent, extended family of the past. This new family and kinship relationship is an adaptation to the actualities of urban life, and culture changes into an extensive collaboration of social ties that complement one another in a network system.[16] These networks, often seen in rural areas of industrialized society, extend beyond kin into groups of people with shared interests, needs, and resources.[17] "Consequently, the network stands between the family and the total social environment." [18] This serves as both a buffer and a support system in the interrelationship of family and society.

As the families change structure and function, they must constantly adapt if they are to survive. "Culture is man's means of adaptation."[19] It is a system shared among a plurality of individuals, and its main purpose is survival of the species.[20] A process analogous to general evolution of a species takes place as a culture moves to a higher, more complex, level of technology and capture of energy. Cultures were basically agrarian in the sixteenth and seventeenth centuries. However, after people were able to capture energy more efficiently through use of machines, evolution was again moved forward and into the industrial era, and considered to be a higher level of energy capture than the agrarian pattern that preceded it.

Within each of those major levels of development, people adapted specifically to an environmental niche. However, when the niche had no more potential for adaptation and a person stabilized, there was little chance for movement to a higher level of evolution by those stabilized species.

If the niche is tested beyond its capability though, it must either evolve, adapt, or expire. Those whose adaptive qualities are superior achieve a general dominance over lesser species. They will retain this dominance, pushing lesser species aside until their positions are usurped by a newer innovative adaptation. When the maximum potential of the niches of a level of evolution has been exhausted, the species will then evolve to a higher level of evolution.[21]

Often those who surge ahead, passing up old forms of adaptation, are what Service refers to as those with "privileged backwardness." Service applies his Law of Evolutionary Potential and the notion of privileged backwardness to growth of nations that forge ahead in inventiveness and new use of their remaining potential of a level of evolution. Also these nations are the ones that push a culture to move to new levels of general evolution. This is especially so in rapidly changing societies. "Youth is served, and the experienced elders, adapted to the outmoded cultural forms, become merely old fogeys."[22]

In the long run, the adaptive capacity of a given species allows higher levels of general adaptability and greater degrees of specific adaptation.[23] Therefore, as the U.S. moved from an agriculturally-based society to an industrially-based society, there were increases in technology, complexity, and integration. That is, in the higher level of evolution, there was an accompanying higher order of segmentation—more parts—and the whole was more effectively integrated, making the culture less dependent on its environment.[24]

The family members were no longer isolated patriarchal units locally controlled, but a series of individuals segmented but nationally controlled. They were interdependent on one another for survival because of increased specialization. The elderly, no longer the heads of local patriarchal autonomous units, were no longer provided for solely by their families, but by institutions within the central government, for example, pensions, housing, health care, and leisure organizations. The blood ties of reciprocal obligation became contractual ties.

This does not mean that the extended families became extinct, but merely changed their ways of adapting. Communal households were less common, but emotional ties still existed, and were perhaps stronger, as they extended across vast miles. The patriarchal family government was replaced by a more egalitarian process. The reciprocal obligations of services were perhaps less apparent but not obliterated. Nonkinship networks outside the household took on the intensity of reciprocal family obligations eulogized in the past.

CURRENT DEMOGRAPHY

The United States has had a noticeable increase in the age of its population, paralleling its industrialization. This, in part, is due to a decline in the birth rate between 1885 and 1975, an influx of a large number of immigrants below the mean age of Americans, and a major advance in life expectancy.

The population of the U.S. increased from 23,191,876 in 1850 to 203,211,926 in 1970. Of these, there were 958,792 people 65 years and older in 1850, and by 1970 there were 20,065,502.[25] It has been projected that by the year 2000 the population over 65 years of age could be as great as 32 million, or in a ratio of one elderly person to five total. The median age would be in the mid-30s.[26] Eisdorfer, in a lecture on aging, maintained that by the year 2020 this ratio could be as great as 1:3.

As of 1974, the population pyramid for the United States was as shown in Figure 3-1. The significant information in this pyramid is the pattern of the elderly, with their disproportionate number of women to men. This is a relatively new trend. In 1935, the elderly population of 7.8 million people was evenly divided between men and women. This was when the Social Security Act was passed. Of those over 65, "42 percent (were) 65 to 69 years old; 28 percent 70 to 74; and 30 percent 75 and over."[27] By 1955, there were 115 aged women for every 100 aged men. By 1985, this will have increased to 138 women to 100 men.[28] It is clear that women outlive

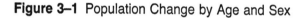

Figure 3-1 Population Change by Age and Sex

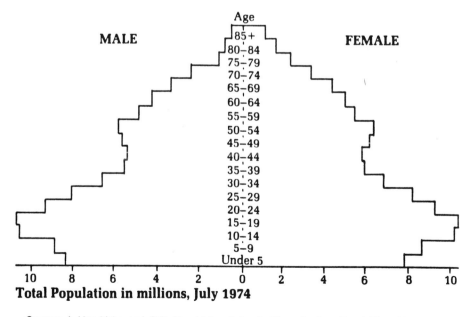

Source: J. Hendricks and C.D. Hendricks, *Aging in Mass Society* (Cambridge, Mass.: Winthrop Publishers, Inc., 1977)

men. In 1900 the average length of life for white males was 48.2 years, but for white females it was 51.1 years.[29]

Today that dichotomy is even greater. Life expectancy is about 72 years at birth, having increased 19.5 years since 1901. The highest percentage of all persons over 65 lived in the western and the southern regions of the country.[30] The largest increase was in the Pacific states. There, general population increased 50 percent, but the population over 65 in the same area increased 56 percent due to large migrations earlier in the century. (See Figure 3–2.)

Not only was the trend of migration away from the northeastern and central states, but it was from the rural to the urban areas. This was a trend common to industrialization everywhere. For many of the elderly the migration has been because the South and West were less expensive and warmer, because members of their families had moved in search of work, and because the urban setting put many resources together in a

---

Figure 3–2 The Impact of Migration on the Aged: 1940–1950

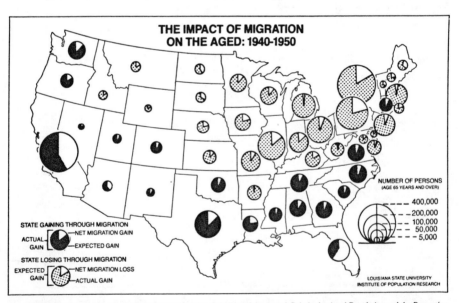

The Proportion That the Estimated Net Migration Gain Was of the Actual Gain in the Aged Population and the Proportion That the Estimated Net Migration Loss Was of the Expected Gain in the Aged Population, by States, 1940-1950.

Source: *Studies of Aged and Aging: Population*, Volume XIII (Washington, D.C., U. S. Government Printing Office, 1956)

smaller area. The bulk of the migration was during the early part of the twentieth century, when industrialization was just beginning. The timing is probably not accidental. This migration pattern is shown in Figure 3–2 and Table 3–1.

In 1977, 41.7 percent of those 65 years and older lived alone. Table 3–2 shows a slight decline of those who were household heads and an increase in the percentage of widows and widowers in families of which they were not the household heads. Of these elderly, 57.8 percent were living in families, 40.8 percent were the primary individuals, 8 percent were employed, and only 5–7 percent were at any point institutionalized.[31] The dependency ratio has also increased from 11 per 100 over 65 years of age in 1940 to 18 persons per 100 in 1980.[32]

Table 3–1 Urban-Rural Distribution of the Total Population and of the Population 65 Years and Over, 1900-1950

		Urban		Rural	
Year and age	Total	Number	Percent of total	Number	Percent of total
All ages:	Thousands	Thousands		Thousands	
1900	73,095	30,160	30.7	43,835	60.3
1910	91,972	41,999	45.7	49,973	34.3
1920	105,711	54,158	51.2	51,553	48.8
1930	122,775	68,955	56.2	53,820	43.8
1940	131,669	74,424	56.5	57,246	43.5
1950[1]	150,697	90,468	54.0	54,230	36.0
63 and over:					
1900	3,080	([2])	([2])	([2])	([2])
1910	3,950	1,693	42.0	2,257	57.1
1920	4,933	2,339	47.4	2,594	52.6
1930	6,634	3,524	53.1	3,110	46.9
1940	9,019	5,073	56.2	3,946	43.8
1950	12,270	7,826	63.8	4,443	36.2

[1] The urban and rural population data for 1950 are not comparable with data for earlier periods because of changes in the definition of urban residence which added densely settled urban fringe areas and unincorporated places of 2,500 inhabitants or more. As a result of the changed definition, the figure for the total urban population in 1950 is about 8 million larger than it would have been under the 1940 definition.

[2] Not available.

Source: U.S. Department of Commerce, Bureau of the Census: 1900-1940, all ages, Historical Statistics of the United States. 1739-1945; 65 years and over, Sixteenth Census of the United States. 1940 Population. vol. II, Characteristics of the Population. 1950, 1950 Census of Population, vol. II, pt. 1, United States Summary, table 38

Table 3–2 Living Arrangements of Elderly Widowed Persons: 1968 to 1977

Widowed Persons	Household Head				Not a Household Head		
	Total (1,000)	Percent primary family head	Percent primary individual		Total (1,000)	Percent in families	Percent secondary individuals
			Living alone	Living with non-relatives			
1968: Total	4,902	24.5	71.8	3.7	2,047	91.2	8.8
Widow..............	3,948	24.5	72.2	3.3	1,013	92.2	7.8
Widower	954	24.3	69.8	6.0	434	87.6	12.4
1970: Total	5,296	22.3	74.8	3.1	1,984	89.4	10.5
Widow..............	4,344	22.2	75.0	2.9	1,519	92.2	7.7
Widower	952	22.9	73.0	4.1	465	80.0	19.8
1975: Total	6,117	18.6	78.9	2.5	1,583	92.3	7.7
Widow..............	5,110	18.8	78.7	2.4	1,407	93.5	6.5
Widower	1,007	17.3	79.4	3.2	181	82.9	17.1
1977: Total	6,440	17.4	80.4	2.2	1,607	92.3	7.7
Widow..............	5,425	17.4	80.3	2.2	1,325	94.6	5.4
Widower	1,015	16.9	81.1	2.1	282	81.6	18.4

Source: U.S. Bureau of the Census. *Current Population Reports*, series P-20, No. 323, and earlier issues

ROLE OF AGING IN PRESENT DAY SOCIETY

Traditionally, families have supported their elderly. Now, however, increasing numbers of people over 65 are being supported by persons who also have to support their own children, and this is a toll too heavy for the general middle-aged populace to bear.

In evolutionary terms, adaptation has become very specialized. A person supported elderly parents for very few years when longevity was minimal. Many had no parents to support because of the short life span. However, as the numbers of elderly who reached 65 have increased and the number of years they lived beyond retirement age has also increased, it has become more and more difficult to attend to the financial needs of the aging parents without compromising the care given the children. Also many persons must travel to other locales in the country in pursuit of career opportunities. These new locations are often great distances from their elderly, making three-generational households physically impossible. The present pattern is that one-fifth of all Americans over 65 are impoverished and in need of help[33] in contrast to one-fourth who retire because they can afford to.[34]

During the 1930s the American family seemed to be in transition. The extended kinships in multigenerational households were dissolving. Some propose they were only temporary at best even earlier; others say they were never very prevalent. But now industrialization and urbanization and its resultant mobility were operating to divide families and complicate financial support. Attempts to legislate family responsibility gave way to private and federal pensions beginning with the 1935 Social Security Act. The elderly were not destroyed by this series of events, but adaptation tactics changed. Blood ties and their responsibilities were challenged, and many such relationships were replaced by contracts between the elderly and various pension programs. The Index of Pensions for the U.S. is reflected in Table 3–3. It has risen by a factor of 2 in 9 years in the U.S., but 2-1/2 times in 9 years in the United Kingdom. The wage index was slower in rising in both countries from 1965 to 1974. In the U.S. private pensions are not widespread, and ensuring oneself of economic security after 65 is difficult.

If you remain in good health and stay with the same company until you are 65 years old, and if the company is still in business, and if your department has not been abolished, and if you haven't been laid off for too long a period, and if there is enough money in the fund, and that money has been prudently managed, you will get a pension.[35]

Table 3–3 Indexes of Pensions, Average Weekly Earnings, and Consumer Prices, Selected Countries: 1965 to 1974

Country and Index	1965	1970	1972	1973	1974
United States:					
Pensions..........	107	130	184	184	205
Wages............	120	149	172	185	197
Prices...........	107	131	141	150	167
Austria:					
Pensions..........	109	141	162	178	203
Wages[1]...........	143	213	270	304	390
Prices...........	121	142	158	170	187
France:					
Pensions..........	173	254	310	344	379
Wages............	143	219	268	322	347
Prices...........	120	149	166	170	203
Germany, Fed. Rep.:					
Pensions..........	148	203	237	264	293
Wages............	153	219	260	297	311
Prices...........	115	131	145	155	162

Country and Index	1965	1970	1972	1973	1974
Netherlands:					
Pensions..........	232	381	473	547	645
Wages............	148	229	287	325	370
Prices...........	118	140	173	187	204
Sweden:					
Pensions..........	154	209	245	259	205
Wages[1]...........	148	212	249	264	321
Prices...........	120	149	169	181	198
Switzerland:					
Pensions..........	173	260	285	519	649
Wages............	140	196	246	276	310
Prices...........	117	130	158	172	189
United Kingdom:					
Pensions..........	160	208	270	310	400
Wages............	127	182	228	261	309
Prices...........	119	149	174	191	221

[1] Average monthly wage.
Source: U.S. Social Security Administration, *Social Security Bulletin*, November 1976

Home care of the ill elderly has also undergone a similar change. Instead of the elderly being cared for at home, they are temporarily hospitalized or placed in nursing homes. In addition, federal and state governments pay for many of the services. Family members have assumed that role in earlier decades. The actual assumption of medical assistance for the elderly from 1970–1977 has more than tripled for only double the number of recipients over 65. (See Table 3–4.) Not only has the government assumed increasing responsibility for the elderly, the general citizenry finds this appropriate. One study shows that 81 percent of the people agree with the notion of aiding older people from general tax funds; 85 percent agree that Social Security benefits should parallel increases in the cost of living and that the government should provide income for nonworking older people.[36]

Another area where evolutionary processes among the elderly can be identified is in their power and social activity, two factors that mesh throughout history. In the patriarchal family structure of the past, the eldest male was head of the household with total authority. His wife was subject to his decisions, but she also held a secondary position of power. The family unit and its accompanying entourage made up the structure that supported most social activities. Later this entire group also socialized within the confines of the church. Today units are smaller, the eldest male is often without power over multigenerations, only over self and conjugal family at most.

For the elderly, who seem to have lost the most expansive power, a new pattern is emerging in clubs and politics. During the transitional time around the 1920s and the 1940s, there was no power either place, that is, home or community. Now the American elderly are such a large bloc of people with voting rights and multiple needs that they have created a visible political force that is wooed by politicians and acknowledged by government. Further, instead of allowing others who were often younger and did not always have the needs and best interests of the elderly at heart to form and run organizations for the elderly, they have begun their own organizations, which have gained national recognition and lobby to serve the needs of their peers. These groups include the Senior Citizens, Retired Teachers of America, and so on. This evolving adaptation has allowed the elderly greater control of their time and resources, and greater effectiveness in their communities and government. Again, they have increased their adaptation to their niche and control more of their environment.

SUGGESTIONS FOR CHANGE

There appears to be a good deal of confusion still about the role of the family in an industrial society. Even though there is an agreement as to

Table 3–4 Medical Assistance (Medicaid) under Social Security—Average Monthly Recipients and Payments: 1970 to 1977

Basis of Eligibility	Recipients (1,000)					Payments (mil. dol.)				
	1970	1974	1975	1976	1977	1970	1974	1975	1976	1977
Total	5,376	3,070	8,884	0,180	9,018	422	913	1,124	1,253	1,085
Age 65 and over	1,534	1,969	2,040	2,087	2,046	159	344	420	451	505
Blindness	42	52	46	45	45	3	7	7	8	8
Permanently and totally disabled	608	1,076	1,217	1,348	1,392	87	210	271	326	378
AFDC[1] program, total	2,824	4,369	4,972	5,078	4,996	140	298	357	388	416
Children	(NA)	2,099	3,020	3,105	3,037	(NA)	146	176	194	207
Adults	(NA)	1,670	1,952	1,973	1,959	(NA)	152	181	194	208
Other	347	604	608	621	569	32	34	69	79	79

NA Not available.

[1] Aid to families with dependent children.

Source: U.S. Health Care Financing Administration, *Medical Assistance (Medicaid) Financed Under Title XIX of the Social Security Act.* Report B-1, annual

the importance of the family as a unit, there is considerable consternation over the function and place of the elderly in relationship to that unit. However, not only have health care programs of the past neglected the philosophy of holism and primary prevention for the major consumers in a family, it has neglected its integration for the elderly as well. The limitations imposed by previous rigid standards and patterns have stifled the flexibility necessary to meet the needs of persons as their bodies age and as they move from a preponderance of acute illness impositions to chronicity.

Health care in the past meant care at home by family members. But that was often brief in parallel to shorter longevity. Then longevity increased, and with it came the norm of hospitalization for illness. For some it was accompanied by the increased use of nursing home facilities to relieve families of taking care of their elderly. Today the mounting costs of medical care that compounds chronicity and longevity must be faced, and alternatives to institutional care must be realized.

Health education for the public will stave off some expenses through primary prevention and will give persons better knowledge of how they can assume responsibility for care in the home. Health educators to date have only scratched the surface of such a program, the importance of which has only been partially acknowledged by a select few of the citizenry in any age bracket. The need to decrease dependence on medical advice and prescriptions, and increase individuals' abilities to more readily care for themselves is crucial to the thrust of the argument and the process. A physician in the Midwest gave his patients a set of guidelines of what to do before calling him. The list told the patient basic things to do; that is, first do this for x condition, then, if the results are such and such, do a, b, c. If the condition persists, call the physician. This approach was applauded by his patients for increasing their self-confidence and sense of responsibility by sharing the curing process with them. It decreased the number of unnecessary visits to his office and increased his rapport with his patients when they came for serious problems. He was still their physician in time of need. His sharing of his process of evaluating their problems minimized the gap between his cognitive ability and theirs and his responsibility and theirs, and increased their sense of sharing the health problem.

It is not only the dependence for medical advice that fills the physician's waiting room. For some people the physician is one of a select few who can give care and can be a quasi-social contact in an empty day. For these people, shopping and visiting physicians' offices are a major socializing pattern. It gives a sense of purpose and worth to the day, and reassures the person that he/she is in fact still alive, and someone has recognized this. These socializing processes need to be rechanneled into a more whole-some pattern.

The public is capable of much more self-care than has been assumed. Dependency on the physician for all decisions has minimized the degree to which people think and act on their own cognizance. In turn, it has often clogged the physician's office with trivia. In the original issue—that of care of the elderly—the same is true.

Many elderly, who are a paradox to their family, are hospitalized or placed in nursing homes. Perhaps they could be cared for at home if family members knew how to approach the organization of such care.

One of the major problems of aging is confusion. There appear to be many causes, both organic and environmental, for this condition, but there is little profound evidence to allow diagnosis of specific cause. So many have erroneously equated confusion with aging, as though it should be accepted as normal because of hereditary factors or personality predis-position. The manifest symptoms of this condition are prevalent in nursing homes and home care. If these elders are going to assume any quality of life, vast amounts of research need to focus on the depths of the issue.

In the future, community health nurses will need to be augmented by outreach staff from nursing homes and hospitals to organize effective home care of the elderly. By teaching elders how to make sensible decisions regarding care, the awesome mystique of that part of daily living presently given over to the medical profession can be removed. In a sense this is a return to the approach that the elderly received before the consequences of industrialization.

Another factor for the future is to change the image and function of the nursing homes. Presently, nursing homes carry the image of a holding-place that harbors the totally incapacitated until death. Many who enter seem to give up living once they pass the doorway. Others resign themselves to waiting for death in a limbo-type of existence.

Nursing homes are capable of a much greater creative potential. Without the negative stigma, they could be used as temporary shelters in a sequential process of care for the elderly; that is, someone who enters the hospital for an acute episodic illness might be transferred to a nursing home during the recuperative period at a cost much less than that of the hospital. This places the nursing home in line with hospital and home, not as a dead-end aside. It also would alleviate some of the depressive air of nursing homes if patients were discharged to a fuller life process, rather than resigned to a waiting process. People need not assume that nursing homes have no exit in this newer connotation.

On the other hand, those who stay because they have no place to go could be taught to assume greater responsibility for their own health promotion and maintenance, ultimately allowing for greater flexibility of life patterns among residents. For those who are discharged, nursing homes can also send workers into the homes to teach and organize extended care, offering support and guidance to the family and client.

The implication of such changes would allow nursing homes in the community to become more creative and dynamic. Such institutions have the potential to become the motivational force for improving the quality of life for persons in the community as well as for those who need temporary care. Their potential has scarcely begun to be explored. To date persons are admitted to nursing homes for 24-hour care. Why is this necessary? The positive results of day care centers for the frail elderly have been proven, but more of them are needed. Finding facilities and staff to increase the availability of these daytime centers has been a barrier to expansion of this vital concept. Why can't nursing homes with a new perspective be a partial solution? Clients could come to nursing homes on an 8-hour basis while still living at home with their families. Nursing home personnel could monitor the client's activities, while giving the family a welcome respite. In total, this individualized care would cost less than fulltime institutionalization and would provide untold psychological relief. The aim would be to serve the individuality of the elderly, not the average.

NOTES

1. Jon Hendricks and C. Davis Hendricks, *Aging in Mass Society* (Cambridge, Mass.: Winthrop Publishers, Inc., 1977), p. 4.
2. J. Patten, ed., *Pre-Industrial England* (Kent, England: Wm. Dawnson & Sons, Ltd., 1979), pp. 11–22.
3. Hendricks and Hendricks, *Aging in Mass Society*, p. 29.
4. P. Hauser and L. Schiore, eds., *The Study of Urbanization* (New York, N.Y.: John Wiley and Sons, 1966), pp. 31–32.
5. R. Mitchison, *British Population Change Since 1860* (London: Macmillian Press, Ltd., 1977), pp. 19–20; J. Habakkuk, *Population Growth and Economic Development* (Leicester, England: Leicester University Press, 1971), pp. 37–40.
6. Ibid., pp. 46–49.
7. Ibid., pp. 76–77.
8. Ibid., pp. 39–40.
9. E. Burgess, "Western European Experience in Aging as Viewed by an American," in Jerome Kaplan and Gordon Aldridge, eds., *Social Welfare of the Aging* (New York: Columbia Univ. Press, 1962), pp. 349–52.
10. Ibid., p. 351.
11. Hendricks and Hendricks, *Aging in Mass Society*, pp. 6–7.
12. Burgess, "Western European Experience," p. 277.
13. Ibid., p. 352.

14. J. Anderson, "Research on Aging," in E. Burgess, ed., *Aging in Western Societies* (Chicago: University of Chicago Press, 1960), p. 371.

15. Burgess, "Western European Experience," p. 352.

16. Ibid., p. 353; also Gluckman in E. Bott, *Family & Social Network*, 2nd ed., (London: Tavistock, 1971), pp. xxv–xxvii.

17. E. Bott, *Family & Social Network*, 2nd ed. (London: Tavistock, 1971), p. 288.

18. Ibid., p. 98.

19. M. Sahlins and E. Service, eds., *Evolution & Culture* (Ann Arbor, Mich.: University of Michigan Press, 1973), p. 24.

20. T. Parsons, "Evolutionary Universals in Society," *American Sociological Review* 29, no.3 (1964): 339–57.

21. J. Kaplan and G. Aldridge, eds., *Social Welfare of the Aging* (New York: Columbia Univ. Press, 1962), pp. 69–77.

22. Sahlins and Service, *Evolution and Culture*, p. 105.

23. Ibid., p. 22; Parsons, "Evolutionary Universals," pp. 339–41.

24. Sahlins and Service, *Evolution and Culture*, p. 22.

25. *Historical Statistics of the U.S.* (Washington, D.C.: U.S. Government Printing Office, 1975), p. 15.

26. Ibid.

27. *Studies of Aged and Aging, Fact Book on Aging*, Volume XI (Washington, D.C.: U.S. Government Printing Office, 1957), p. 77.

28. Ibid., pp. 75–77.

29. Ibid.

30. *Studies of Aged and Aging, Population: Current Data and Trends*, Volume VIII, (Washington, D.C.: U.S. Government Printing Office, 1956), pp. 41–44.

31. Ibid., pp. 59–76.

32. Ibid.

33. Hendricks and Hendricks, *Aging in Mass Society*, p. 245.

34. L. Harris, *The Myth & Reality of Aging in America*. (Washington, D.C.: National Council on Aging, 1975), pp. 82–88.; Hendricks and Hendricks, *Aging in Mass Society*, p. 71.

35. Hendricks and Hendricks, *Aging in Mass Society*, p. 245.

36. Harris, *The Myth & Reality of Aging in America*, pp. 222–24.

Chapter 4

Maximizing Community Resources

Chiyoko Furukawa

Health promotion and maintenance programs are in the rudimentary stages of development compared to programs for the treatment of disease conditions. Many factors can be blamed for the deficiency of programs designed for the prevention of illness. Torrens contends that the "lack of money, lack of detailed experience in multiple-disease prevention, lack of adequate means of measuring results, and lack of psychological and professional rewards to individual practitioners have all combined to give prevention a relatively low priority for the public, for health professionals, and for the American health care system."[1] This status of the health care delivery system perpetuates the scarcity of health promotion services and affects the elderly population more than any other group.

The maximization theory from a political perspective stresses attaining power;[2] when combined with the findings for elderly care, this aspect of the theory suggests that health care power and resources are directed to inpatient care. This fact is substantiated by the public fund payment report for elderly health care, which shows that areas of risks are unevenly distributed. The fund met 86.1 percent of the elderly's hospital bill, 71.3 percent of the physician's bill, 60 percent of the nursing home costs, and only 23 percent of the combined expenses for dentists, drugs, eyeglasses, home health, and other services.[3] Clearly, the thrust of elderly health care is on acute illness care with minimal attention to health promotion and preventive and rehabilitative needs. However, if old age is believed to be physiological instead of pathological, it can be theorized that diseases of old age may be avoidable, minimized, or arrested by timely diagnosis and treatment.[4] The social science theory of maximization supports the notion that human behavior is somehow oriented toward maximization of some desired end.[5] The outcome sought here is to provide health services that match the needs of the elderly.

With respect to maximal use of community resources, studies on the utilization of community services by the elderly showed varying degrees of participation in the available services.[6,7] Hanssen and her group found that for increased use of the senior center, information and a full explanation about the services of the center should be communicated to the target population by their peers.[8] In addition, the center was not fully used because it lacked health promotion and maintenance care to assist the elderly with health problems. These findings clearly indicate the need for community organizations to put forth a concerted effort to inform as well as provide comprehensive services for the multiple needs of the elderly.

With regards to the types of community services needed for the elderly, a different perception of priorities was found to occur between the provider and the consumer.[9] The provider viewed social activities to decrease loneliness as important, while the elders' highest priority was those services that assisted them to maintain their independence. Maximizing community resources to meet the needs of the aged requires that essential services be considered from the perspective of the elderly. In addition, it is important that the services fulfill the needs of the client because, as indicated by the economic theory of maximization, human wants are unlimited, and people constantly strive to maximize their satisfaction.[10]

Another concern for maximizing community resources deals with agencies whose services are limited to a small segment of the elderly population. In order to optimize allocation of scarce community resources, these agencies must implement strategies to reach more consumers. They also need to determine whether their services are meeting consumer needs. For example, are services offered only during traditional working hours rather than in the evenings or weekends when consumers are more likely and able to participate? Another inquiry might question whether people know where and how to receive services. This is frequently a problem with the elder who is uninformed or unfamiliar with the structure of a bureaucratic system.

When health professionals continually meet their own needs rather than the consumer's, it can lead to less than optimal use of community resources. These situations occur when consumers' inputs concerning their needs are disregarded, and irrelevant services are delivered. Such incidents are not only demoralizing to the elderly, but, even more tragically, they may cause elders to refuse services even though the need exists. Thus, to ensure effective use of community resources, agency professionals purporting to provide services to the aging must continually evaluate the quality and relevancy of their services, cost effectiveness, and appropriateness of the agency goals and purposes. Any purposeful or goal-oriented professional behavior with priorities of choice implies a maximization theory.[11]

Maximizing community resources requires: (1) identifying the target population for whom services are planned; (2) determining available community resources for assistance in locating clients and offering comprehensive services; (3) interfacing community resources to coordinate services; and (4) achieving commitment from community resources for continuing needed services to consumers.

IDENTIFYING THE TARGET POPULATION

Demographic information is necessary to identify and locate the target population to whom services are to be provided. A broad overview of the population may be obtained from references such as the U. S. Bureau of Census publication, *Census Population, General Population Characteristics*. This document, which is a separate publication for each state, presents population characteristics by county, city, town, village, and so on. The information provided is separately identified as population distribution by age, income, minority ratio, major transportation system, and educational level. Because this publication depends on the census collected every ten years (shortly to become every five years), the information needs to be updated when it is obsolete or when the most recent information is required. Updated information may be obtained from the *Current Population Report*, which is also published by the Bureau of Census for states and communities. This document is published more frequently and is appropriate for validating the distribution of population for a given community. Both documents are useful for planning health care services in that they grossly define where a large portion of the elderly reside within a community.

Once a general location of the target population is determined, then more specific and detailed population characteristics may be sought through community-based sources, for example, local housing authorities, social and health agencies, Social Security offices, area aging councils, city and county planning offices, regional councils of government, health systems agencies, and longtime residents. The schools of business in some universities are also excellent resources for population statistics.

Often descriptive data about a community contribute to the statistic about a target population by amplifying the personal characteristics of a group. For identifying target populations, Klein suggests using an assessment of the physical characteristics of the community, that is, the geographical location of cities, towns, or barrios that influences transportation to health care settings and availability of resources to the residents.[12] He sees the size of the community, its physical dimensions, and population density as influences on service accessibility and therefore suggests that all must be a part of the health service planning.

Another aspect of the target population that affects the use of services and requires consideration is the religious and cultural influences of the community that affect the health-seeking behavior of individuals. The planned strategies for promoting health services and identifying acceptable services must be done with these basic factors as guidelines. Holmes and associates confirm the need to assign minority staff to neighborhoods to overcome any cultural, language, and transportation barriers that hinder minority persons from using needed services.[13]

A somewhat unconventional way to search for the target population is through the exploitation of social relationships developed by the elderly. Barnes and Bott refer to such relationships as networks and view them as a multidimensional system of relationships of the elderly with relatives, friends, and neighbors.[14,15] Since interpersonal relationships are important to the elderly and they tend to accept information from people known to them, the network approach to locate the aged seems useful. Specifically, this approach uses the categories of uniplex and multiplex relationships within the social network.

The uniplex network is asymmetrical and a one-way activity that predominantly occurs in service-oriented events. In theory, the recipient of service neither reciprocates in the interaction nor is expected to do so. The representatives or providers of essential services are considered primary resources for demographic information on the elderly because they are in a position to assist in identifying unknown potential users of health services. These service personnel are represented by the postal worker, police, firefighter, meter reader, city service worker (for example, trash collector, bus driver, and maintenance worker), druggist, grocery store worker, health and social workers, and voluntary agency worker.

The multiplex network differs from the uniplex network in that the social relationship is more reciprocal in nature with attitudes, roles, and transactions becoming more complex, having several purposes for the interaction, and requiring symmetrical exchanges. In other words, it is not a one-way relationship such as the uniplex where the clients are only recipients of specific services. The elder's neighbors, friends, and relatives are the primary resources in the multiplex network; thus, the network can be used to locate the target population and to disseminate information about specific services and/or outreach purposes.

After all possible demographic information is compiled, the actual locating of the target population requires the selection of a person to recruit assistance from individuals and groups; to plan and direct tasks, functions, and survey methods (for example, door-to-door or telephone canvass); and to assign survey areas (for example, census tract, block, precinct) of the community to assistants. These activities are designed to organize and conduct the work to identify the target population.

In some communities a variety of health and social service organizations exist that can provide assistance in terms of human resources to conduct surveys. However, the volunteers from these community organizations often need orientation about survey methods and information about the characteristics of the population they are to contact. Harbert and Ginsberg offer some helpful suggestions about communicating with older persons for the first time about community resources.[16] Their hints are summarized as follows:

- Try to give some prior notice of the visit before appearing at the home of an older person.

- Avoid rushing the visit, try to spend more than 15 minutes, be conversational, and show interest in the person.

- Do not apply pressure communication; if the person is not ready to communicate, reschedule the visit.

- Be ready to offer assistance rather than just talk; if an opportunity arises, doing a small favor will break down suspicion and reluctance.

These hints are especially meaningful for planning an approach to meet the aged, to develop rapport, and to communicate pertinent information. An additional suggestion to the volunteers is to make them realize that rejection of communication by some aged is a possibility and must be dealt with realistically. For example, when people are unreceptive to verbal communication, leaving a brochure or only a telephone number of service agencies is an alternative. Moreover, the volunteers will need support and reassurance that the elderly's rejection is not necessarily a reflection on them, but rather due to the suspicious, cautious, and reluctant response to strangers on the part of the clients.

IDENTIFYING COMMUNITY RESOURCES

In the present context, community resources are considered as new or existing support services that fulfill the health and social needs of the community residents. The resources in different communities may be similar or divergent depending on the community's age distribution, philosophy, and priorities of community services. For instance, a community with a large population of young families is more likely to focus on the development of resources such as baseball parks, soccer leagues, swimming pools, and tennis courts, which are more suited to their life styles. In such a community, activities like the senior center, shopping assistance, or a friendly visitor program may be of low priority or nonexistent. Thus, it might be said that community resources evolve from the needs of the residents, and their continuity and survival depend on the rate of use and the benefits received by the users.

Comprehensive community resources assist some elderly groups in maintaining independence. The identification of available resources is often the key to their survival, but many elders do not know about the existence or availability of community services. This lack of information may lead to frustration for the elderly because without it, they may not see any way to resolve their needs. An up-to-date information and referral source to alleviate these shortcomings is a necessity in communities where the elderly live. Furthermore, the involvement and leadership of professionals working with and delivering services to the elderly are needed to organize and implement a system to provide comprehensive service information. The senior citizen center, volunteer coordinating agency, central office of United Way agencies, social service agencies, and area office of aging are possible sources to assist community professionals in developing information and referral services. Generally, these agencies have interest in the aging and frequently possess the capabilities and associations to implement activities such as the gathering of all essential information on community resources.

In compiling information and referral data of community resources, it would be advantageous to list both the formal and informal health services so as to offer a variety of choices including material assistance, for example, clothing, ambulatory devices, and beds. Initiation of an information and referral resource system should include:

- Name, address, and telephone number of the agency, business, or individual providing the service or resource;

- Eligibility requirements to obtain assistance;

- Nature, amount, and duration of the service or resource offered;

- Name of the contact person with the agency or business, and the hours designated for inquiry and arrangement for services.[17]

The information and referral services may also serve as a clearinghouse where information can be obtained to prevent duplication of services or to ascertain whether demands exceed the availability of a specific resource.

Another important aspect of an information and referral service is the continual updating of a community's available resources. This can be accomplished by service organizations and individuals communicating any changes in eligibility requirements, the scope of services, personnel, telephone numbers, and so on that affect service implementation.

Dissemination of Information

It is essential to disseminate information on community resources to the elderly, and, in this regard, the primary concern is those individuals who might be unaware of the availability of community assistance or reluctant to use such services. Thus, concerted efforts must be directed to ensure that not only information about the services but also about their availability are properly communicated to the isolated elderly. A variety of media including newspapers, television, radio, and newsletters of organizations can be employed to transmit such information directly to the elderly or through other groups who have contact with the aged. In addition, a publication listing the resources of information and referral services may be printed and placed in locales where the information has a high probability of reaching the elderly such as the grocery store, library, Chamber of Commerce office, Social Security office, post office, nutrition site, health care facility, and senior citizens center.

Community Resource Needs of the Elderly

The availability and appropriate use of community resources are often the deciding factors in whether an elder continues to maintain independence or needs to be institutionalized. The resources must support the physical, psychological, and social conditions of the elder to alleviate the inadequacies created in these areas by the aging process. Generally, the kind of resources communities must consider are personal care, supportive health services, personal maintenance, counseling, and linkages.[18] Personal care resources are those services for body cleanliness, namely, bathing, dressing, and grooming. Supportive health services involve the physician and other professionals who monitor health status. Personal maintenance services are the functions necessary to maintain independence, for example, providing a healthy environment with housekeeping assistance, shopping for and preparation of food, and so on. Counseling activities include attentive listening, providing care and assistance, and offering guidance in the effective use of available resources. Linkages are a combination of services that facilitate the efficient use of community resources by the elderly and consist of transportation, outreach, information, and referral services.[19] Thus, the short- and long-term community resource planning requires that a variety of options be available so the elderly may choose the appropriate service or services to sustain them within the community.

Untapped Community Resources

Maximizing community resources demands an evaluation of the community for untapped resources that might be potential contributors of additional services. There may be many people who would be willing to assist the less fortunate but are unaware of the need for their services. A potentially promising group of untapped resources is the military personnel in a number of communities, particularly in sparsely populated areas. As an example, the military personnel at Minot Air Force Base in North Dakota were not attuned to the needs of the elderly until they were introduced to the Minot Commission on Aging. Since then, the volunteers have assisted the commission in keeping the senior citizens in the city of Minot and the surrounding communities independent. Their program, known as the Military and Senior Citizens Operating Together (MASCOT), included delivering hot meals to the homebound, helping with minor home repairs, and adopt-a-lawn and check-and-chat services. For most of the volunteers, this was their first experience in working with the elderly; however, the providers and the recipients of the services both acclaimed benefits from their relationship. The elderly not only enjoyed the specific services, but also the interaction and relationship with the younger volunteers and their families. For many elderly this relationship provided a substitute for their own family who no longer lived near them. In return, the military family, who also lived away from their parents and grandparents, benefited because their children were given the opportunity to relate to older people and learn to love and respect them. The commission director commented that "MASCOT helps keep the elderly independent for as long as possible and has significantly increased the number who are able to continue a life style they are accustomed to. We could never have offered the number of programs we now have without them."[20]

Another untapped resource that could contribute significantly to service programs is the healthy older people who could assist the less healthy peers. The employment of these "young-old" persons is a way to enrich their life styles by adding meaningful years of continued productive work different from their previous employment. Many believe that older people require and should fulfill roles different from those they experienced in the earlier periods of their lives; failure to structure these new roles may be related to physical and mental problems that require social interventions.[21] Thus the involvement of the "young-old" in service to the community benefits them as well as others through contributions of their talents.

To enlist the "young-old" resource, Payne suggests community centers ought to plan, coordinate, and provide support services for these older volunteers.[22] The assistance may include supporting and helping restructure their new social role, providing continuity for and maintaining the different roles, and developing new skills for those who are willing to accept challenges.

Aside from the organized volunteers of all ages, a sometimes overlooked community resource is families, friends, and neighbors. However, the elderly may not readily share these potential resources with professionals because of the elder's independence and reluctance to burden others. Combined with this, these valuable resources may not be fully utilized because of overzealous efforts on the part of the professionals to use traditional resources to provide the needed services. Skillful exploration with the aged about these potential resources of assistance is necessary to maximize community resources.

Whenever a family member, friend, or a neighbor assists an elderly in health or maintenance care, it is important that some mechanism of relief (that is, release from any task obligations) be decided before assistance is instituted. This is particularly essential for long-term assistance because changes in life circumstances may not allow continuation or completion of care. Therefore, it is imperative to identify tasks to be performed and the duration of the service commitment so that other community resources may be arranged for continued services.

In the case of family members, all concerned must be clear on their respective responsibilities in caring for an elder. In particular, efforts should be made to prevent the buildup of antagonism by family members who assume the primary caretaker role toward other family members who are nonparticipants for whatever reasons. Health professionals, as outsiders to the family structure, are frequently in a better position to facilitate discussions between an elderly person and family members concerning needed services.

Maximizing community resources to assist the community's elderly may also require seeking volunteers from another segment of the population whose interest is generally directed toward meeting their own immediate age-specific needs. This group consists of students from junior and senior high schools and universities. These younger individuals could assist in filling existing gaps in community resources with services to support the elderly's independence, for example, carrying out trash, visiting, running errands, performing yard maintenance, providing transportation, and other similar tasks. In some communities, young volunteers serve institutionalized elderly by assisting with recreational functions, making favors for meal trays, writing letters, or entertaining on holidays and special occasions.

Community organizations, notably the Junior Chamber of Commerce, Kiwanis, churches, and Lions, whose memberships may include community leaders, contribute services and funds to assist the less fortunate. These organizations provide supplemental services and aids that the health and social agencies cannot offer, and they may be capable of more contributions. Thus, communities should continue to inquire about additional assistance from these organizations to maximize resources.

Individual professionals are another untapped community resource. This group comprises persons who are aware of the aging's plight and have interest in contributing their professional expertise on a voluntary basis. Many community professionals who are willing to assist in meeting the needs of the community are psychologists, nurses, dentists, doctors, nutritionists, and other health professionals. Their assistance may be obtained through their respective associations or by individual contact.

INTERFACE WITH COMMUNITY SERVICES

Interface is a process whereby care providers aim to mesh or dovetail their services with other programs to meet the comprehensive needs of the consumers. Thus, in terms of maximizing community resources, the goal is to interface as many agencies as possible to supplement existing services, to provide comprehensive care, and to minimize duplication of health programs for the elderly. Another benefit of interfacing services is cost containment of health services by making efficient and effective use of available community resources. In interfacing with other existing services, each agency remains separate and keeps its own identity while contributing to the total service needs of the older people.

The cooperation required to achieve interface may be referred to as linkages or networks.[23,24,25] Linkages were discussed earlier in relation to the assistance the elderly needed for support and maintenance. Along this line, linkages of services prevent fragmentation of care and ensure the holistic needs of the individual. Linkages also facilitate the maintenance of a chosen life style for the elderly receiving services from a variety of community resources.

For instance, consider a person living in a rural community and lacking the transportation to obtain needed medical care. When an agency provides transportation for the client to attend a medical facility, the medical and transportation services are linked because the latter is essential to receiving medical care. Also, transportation may be linked with life essentials such as dental care, shopping, and other like needs. In this way, the physical, social, psychological, and environmental needs are met through linkages of services.

Moe identifies 23 types of activities or tasks that can serve as components of the interface process to implement networks or linkages.[26] These activities include functions such as service purchasing, technical assistance, loaner staff, referral, *ad hoc* coordination, joint program development, and multiservice centers. In addition, the concept of networks as proposed by Moe is similar to linkages and consists of three essential services for the elderly, namely, basic, supplementary, and facilitating.[27] When these three services are combined, they become the network to prevent fragmentation of services. Moe's explanation of the service categories within the network is comparable to the description of the linkages of service offered in the earlier section on the community resource needs of the elderly. The basic services comprise those essentials that contribute to the quality of life and include minimal income, health and medical care, safe housing, and legal assistance. Supplemental services complement and extend the basic services and are represented by such activities as consumer education to ensure prudent use of finances; early hospital discharge made possible by supportive services; easy access to recreational centers and meal sites; and arrangements for friendly visitors and telephone assurance services. Facilitating services assist in the use of basic and supplemental services and include counseling, transportation, information, and referral. Moe comments that "the relationship between the services and the interrelationship between agencies providing services is basic to an understanding of the emerging networks in aging."[28]

In support of Moe's network concept, a vivid example of interfacing with community services was reported by Brickner and his group.[29,30] They initiated a health care delivery system designed for the community elderly in cooperation with the Department of Community Medicine at St. Vincent's Hospital of New York, Visiting Nurse Service of New York, community groups, and individuals. The system used referrals from local churches, settlement houses, block associations, tenants' councils, police precincts, and nurse volunteers to locate the isolated elderly. Clinics were conducted in residences of severely restricted but not homebound individuals, that is, persons who functioned with some limitations but only required health care at their home. Home maintenance and preventive health care were provided by the nurses who assumed an independent role stressing primary care and shared collegial responsibility with the physician for planning, decision making, and evaluation. The nurses also evaluated referrals, made screening visits to determine needs for other service programs, and made arrangements for supplemental or facilitating services.

The delivery of comprehensive care requires interfacing services to develop interrelationship and cooperation for exchanging information about clients and agency services. The nature and extent of services available from an agency is particularly important when a new agency joins a network or linkage to initiate the interface process. This information on the new member organization should not only outline its services, but also preclude duplication of existing services. This opportunity should additionally be used to establish the extent of collaboration that the network could expect from the new agency and vice versa.

Since health promotion and maintenance programs are relatively new in communities, concerted effort is needed to educate the public and consumers about the exact nature of the services and to solicit support from other community resources. In this regard, Dewore and Kreuter state: "Health promotion must acknowledge and take advantage of relationship with related programs in the health and social services field. Health promotion will be most effective when integrated with traditional public health and private medical care endeavor."[31] This process encourages the formation of linkages or networks to achieve interface of community resources.

Another related thought is offered by Giorgi, who encourages the use of team approach to health care.[32] This involves interfacing the different skills and backgrounds of the professional, nonprofessional, and paraprofessional members of the team. If collaboration and cooperation are achieved, each group of the health care team becomes a contributing member to the consumer's care.

MEANS OF ACHIEVING COMMITMENT FROM COMMUNITY RESOURCES

A commitment is an open expression or agreement to work together, which, in some instances, can lead to a published statement of purpose with the participants pledging themselves to the defined purpose.[33] Commitment, however, goes beyond the written statement or spoken words in that participants must exhibit a determination to continue involvement despite success or failure. Biddle and Biddle stress that a vital factor in developing commitment is the determination that must come from within and be a fundamental motivation of each group member.[34]

Motivating others to gain determination is a difficult task with no sure methods. With respect to community groups, motivation involves a group process requiring an entrusted leader with the ability to instill genuine interest and to create a need in others to participate in the proposed activity. The choice to participate evolves from an individual's belief in the undertaking and the advantages gained by the involvement.

Sharing information about agency services, program goals, and assistance needs is an approach to gain involvement from the people resources of a community. Mutual concerns and goals emerge through the group process, the sharing of such information, and most importantly, the agency's contributions to the community services. The recognition of each contributor offers motivation for an agency to join others in their commitment to support one another.

The motivation of individuals results in some participants' developing a stronger and more genuine commitment to a program than others. This is due to differences in individual characteristics and in the degree of willingness to work together as community resource representatives. This latter outcome, which might take months or years of adjusting, balancing, or discouraging events to achieve, forms the core of interested individuals who are essential for the group commitment to continue and to achieve set goals.[35]

In most communities, the senior citizens service organizations appear to be a logical choice to take the initiative for acquiring commitment from other community resources. The process may begin with a meeting of one or more health and social agencies who provide services to the aging. Since the participants of such a meeting are generally perceived to be important members of the community, they could serve as a nucleus to attract other service groups. This strategy uses agency representatives with common interests and enthusiasm in beginning interagency relationships and teamwork to benefit the aging consumer of community services.

Community health agencies might also assume the leadership role in soliciting commitments from community resources, since they employ health professionals concerned with the health and social welfare of older people. In many instances, an informal agreement with some community resource is established by the health professionals through referral activities on behalf of their clients. Thus, the seeking of an official commitment may only require efforts to encourage the remaining service agencies to join with the health agency to benefit the aged cooperatively.

Another possible strategy to seek commitment from resources is by the community development process, which relies upon the people concerned with the need of social improvement for the local residents. A side benefit to the process of seeking this improvement is that the participants frequently develop self-confidence and accept the responsibility for the changes required to meet community needs.[36] With personal development and growth, incentives are provided that encourage individuals to continue with various programs although the initial leadership is terminated.

A summary of the steps to achieve commitment from community resources is outlined in Exhibit 4–1. The process has four phases, each with a specific goal, and possible activities that might be employed to achieve each goal are suggested for individual phases. The outline is offered only

Exhibit 4–1 Steps to Achieve Commitment from Community Resources

Phases	Activities
1. Initiation	Invite administrators and/or personnel of community agencies.
Goal: Introduce the notion of commitment.	Share information about agency services and status.
	Explore:
	• gaps, overlaps, and positive aspects of services;
	• possible group structure and organization;
	• rationale for commitment;
	• extent of commitment from agency participants.
2. Dialogue	
Goal: Solicit commitment.	Solicit expressions and/or demonstrations of commitment.
	Discuss:
	• goals for the group;
	• solutions for service gaps and overlaps;
	• strategies to involve nonparticipants;
	• group structure and organization.
3. Structure Identification	Reiterate commitment.
Goal: Solidify commitment.	Select leadership.
	Formulate goals or purposes for group.
	Formalize group by making decisions on:
	• by-laws, guidelines, functions, or agreements;
	• agency roles and functions;
	• roles of agency personnel, consumers, and so on.
4. Implementation	Obtain agreement (verbal or written) on commitment and coordination of services.
Goal: Implement commitment activities.	Obtain agreement on shared resources (consultation, facilities, personnel, and so on).
	Establish communications system.
	Select mechanism for evaluating commitment by community resources.
	Demonstrate continued commitment.
	Decide on future direction for the group.

as a guide; thus, some of the suggested activities might be deleted and others added depending on the group participants and the needs of the community.

The steps to achieve commitment should have a flexible time schedule because community groups will progress at different rates depending on the characteristics of the individual groups involved and the ability of the participants to function as a unit. In any case, the ultimate purpose of achieving commitment from community resources is to maximize and ensure comprehensive services to the elderly consumer.

SUMMARY

Maximizing community resources requires that the target population be identified, located, and informed about the services that are specifically designed for its benefit. This process enables the elderly group to choose those services that are most meaningful to them. There are several ways to disseminate information about the available or new programs including information and referral services; newspaper and other communication media; community agencies; business establishments; and neighbors, friends, and relatives of the older people.

Untapped or little-used community resources should be employed to increase or optimize services or to eliminate gaps in assistance to the aged. The comprehensive needs of the older people are personal care, supportive health services, personal maintenance, counseling, and linkages. Maximizing community resources ensures that these needs are fulfilled by the interfacing of appropriate agencies or organizations. The interface activities, which mesh community programs, promote the coordination of services and the optimal use of community resources to serve the elderly.

Finally, achieving commitment from community agencies is important to facilitate communication, cooperation, and collaboration among those programs involved in health promotion and maintenance care of the older population. However, the commitment must be made with sincere motivation and determination on the part of the participants in order for community resources to be used efficiently and effectively.

NOTES

1. Paul R. Torrens, *The American Health Care System* (St Louis, Mo.: The C. V. Mosby Co., 1978), p. 65.
2. Robbins Burling, "Maximizing Theories and the Study of Economic Anthropology," in Edward E. Le Clair and Harold K. Scheider, eds., *Economic Anthropology* (New York: Holt, Rinehart, & Winston, Inc., 1968), p. 181.

3. Jerome Hammerman, "Health Services: Their Success and Failure in Reaching Older Adults," *American Journal of Public Health* 64, no. 3 (March 1974): 255.

4. Ibid.

5. R. Burling, "Maximizing Theories and the Study of Economic Anthropology," p. 179.

6. John O'Brein and Donna Wagner, "Help Seeking by the Frail Elderly: Problems in Network Analysis," *The Gerontologist* 20, no. 1 (February 1980): 78–83.

7. Michael A. Smyer, "The Differential Usage of Services by Impaired Elderly," *Journal of Gerontology* 35, no. 2 (March 1980): 249–55.

8. Anne M. Hanssen et al., "Correlates of Senior Citizens Participation," *The Gerontologist* 18, no. 2 (April 1978): 193–99.

9. Pat Keith, "A Preliminary Investigation of the Roles of the Public Health Nurse in Evaluation of Services for the Aged," *American Journal of Public Health* 66, no. 4 (April 1976): 379–81.

10. R. Burling, "Maximizing Theories and the Study of Economic Anthropology," p. 183.

11. Ibid., p. 183.

12. Donald Klein, "Assessing Community Characteristics," in Barbara W. Spradley, ed., *Contemporary Community Health Nursing* (Boston, Mass.: Little, Brown, 1975), pp. 415–24.

13. Douglas Holmes et al., "The Use of Community-Based Services in Long-term Care by Older Minority Persons," *The Gerontologist* 19, no. 4 (August 1979), pp. 389–97.

14. J. A. Barnes, *Social Networks: Module in Anthropology* (Menlo Park, Cal.: Addison-Wesley, 1972), pp. 2–5.

15. E. Bott, *Family and Social Networks*, 2nd ed. (London: Tavistock Publications, 1971), pp. 248–330.

16. Anita S. Harbert and Leon H. Ginsberg, *Human Services for Older Adults: Concepts and Skills* (Belmont, Cal.: Wadsworth Publishing Co., 1979), pp. 88–89.

17. Ibid., p. 218.

18. Stanley J. Brody, "Evolving Health Delivery Systems and Older People," *American Journal of Public Health* 64, no. 3 (March 1974), pp. 245–46.

19. Ibid., p. 246.

20. J. McKee, "The Luckiest People," *Airman* 24, no. 5 (May 1980), p. 15.

21. Barbara P. Payne, "The Older Volunteer: Social Role Continuity and Development," *The Gerontologist* 17, no. 4 (July 1977), p. 356.

22. Ibid., p. 360.

23. S. J. Brody, "Evolving Health Delivery Systems and Older People," p. 245.

24. Marcella B. Weiner, Albert J. Brok, and Alvin M. Snadowsky, *Working With the Aged* (Englewood Cliffs, N.J.: Prentice-Hall, Inc., 1978), p. 203.

25. Edward O. Moe, "Agency Collaboration in Planning and Service: The Emerging Network on Aging," in Adina M. Reinhardt and Mildred D. Quinn, eds., *Current Practices in Gerontological Nursing* (St. Louis, Mo.: C. V. Mosby Co., 1979), p. 183.

26. Ibid., p. 183.

27. Ibid., p. 181.

28. Ibid., p. 183.

29. P. W. Brickner et al., "Outreach to Welfare Hotels, the Homebound, the Frail," *American Journal of Nursing* 76, no. 5 (May 1976), pp. 762–64.

30. P. W. Brickner et al., "The Homebound Aged: Medically Unreached Group," *Annals of Internal Medicine* 82, no. 1 (January 1975), pp. 1–6.

31. Richard B. Dewore and Marshall W. Kreuter, "Update: Reenforcing the Case for Health Promotion," *Family and Community Health* 2, no. 4 (February 1980), pp. 103–18.

32. Elsie A. Giorgi, "Utilizing the Health Team in the Care of the Aged," in Eugene Seymour, ed., *Psychosocial Needs of the Aged* (Los Angeles, Cal.: The University of Southern California Press, 1978), p. 73.

33. William Biddle and Loureide Biddle, *The Community Development Process* (New York: Holt, Rinehart & Winston, Inc., 1965), p. 95.

34. Ibid., p. 96.

35. Ibid., p. 116.

36. Ibid., pp. 101–02.

Chapter 5

Financial Dilemmas

Dianna Shomaker

Old age and the end of the working career often bring financial changes and uncertainty. Retired persons find themselves in the dilemma created by technology, bureaucracy, and longevity. At retirement almost everyone encounters economic decline, and many who never before experienced true financial hardship suffer economic deprivation and actual poverty. The plans to provide for financial security often offer more insecurity: pension funds become defunct; health costs more than illness; poverty becomes more than loss of money; and arguments to resolve the issues are confusing.

A discussion of financial dilemmas of aging in the United States must consider the impact of retirement on income, as well as the mixed blessings of Social Security and Medicare. All three are designed to allow planning for the future. All three are relatively new concepts to which the entire population is still adjusting. None are as idyllic as envisioned when initiated; they cannot be, given the fact that they involve a continually increasing population.

RETIREMENT AND INCOME

Kreps asserts that retirement is possible because of increased technology.[1] Not only has technology brought about better medical knowledge, nutrition, and shelter, which perpetuate life by ten or more years beyond retirement age, but it has provided a means of increased productivity with less personnel. "In a less productive economy, retirement is not possible . . . output per man hour is so low that all persons are required to work practically all their lives."[2] Hence, this increased productivity increases leisure time and the standard of living, while decreasing the need for such belabored working hours. However, Kreps points out that this is a dubious blessing for those who retire, because increased leisure time is coupled with a decreased income. Moreover, living expenses do not always decline in parallel with income. Given the fact that length of life is indeterminate and needs uncertain, how does an individual plan for financial security?[3]

For some, retirement will be the first time they have ever experienced deprivation. Others will merely live with it in greater severity. Less than 70 percent will have incomes above the poverty level, and few of these will be comfortably well off. Older, single women are the hardest hit because they live longer, have often been dependents and not wage earners, and have not handled the financial affairs of the family.[4] According to the 1980 census information, 14.0 percent of all persons 65 and over are below the official poverty level;[5] and the per capita income of those over 65, regardless of race and sex, is $5,312 a year.[6] The remainder of the approximately 30 percent whose incomes are below the poverty level are those who are totally supported by others, usually family members, and are not directly reflected in the census statistics.

Economically, elders' incomes are less than half that of younger people, with less possibility of increasing those incomes.[7] There is little opportunity to engage in leisure-time activities that require a lot of money since 80 percent of their income goes for food, housing, transportation, and medical care.[8] Many who owned their own homes find increased taxes and maintenance are too costly, and they seek alternative housing in smaller houses, apartments, or mobile homes.[9]

Saving for retirement is difficult during any stage of a career because of inflation. Regardless of the amount saved, it will not yield a comparable value at retirement unless it is invested for growth and the investment is unusually successful. To invest in order to make money grow requires a lot of knowledge and experience, which many people, regardless of age, do not possess. Unfortunately these persons' few resources and anxieties to expand them make them prime candidates for fraud such as land swindles and home improvement and business scams. If these people are in poor health, the money may go for "wonder drugs." If they are lonely, marriage schemes and lonely hearts clubs may become the subtle means of swindle.[10]

Kreps has observed that systematic savings beyond life insurance and purchase of a home begins at about 50 years of age.[11] Early investment is impeded by the needs of a growing family. This means that the average individual saves for retirement for 15 years for a potential 10 to 15 years of retirement. In order to retain the preretirement standard of living, a person would have to set aside an amount greater than presently used for daily living needs. This is partly due to inflation and increased medical needs. There may be some buffer to income loss for the small percentage of persons between 65 and 69 years of age who continue to earn up to a third of their income in the labor market. The major reason to keep working is to avoid a decreased income. At the same time it is most often those with better occupations and education who have the choice to continue working.[12] However, after the age of 70, the vast majority of persons retire and live on assets and Social Security benefits.

The income of all groups has been rising steadily. In 1950, the mean income was $2,961 for men and $1,296 for women. By 1977, it had risen to $12,063 for men and $5,291 for women. Persons 55 years of age and over begin to show a decline compared to other age groups of the same year and they continue to decline in earnings as they move into retirement age groups. (See Table 5–1.) The average income of persons increased from entrance into the employment market until about age 55, when that average began gradual decline. This is a standard pattern across the nation and across all races. However, along with the overall rise in income has come a similar increase in baseline income of working persons, regardless of age. It is reasonable to expect that our highest income will accrue at the end of worklife. Those who are younger but earning more, do so not because of actual decline in the financial status of the older worker "but because they entered the labor force in a later, more productive era . . . and thus will have higher incomes at any age, than we did at that age."[13] This clouds the issue of adequacy of retirement income and masks the true extent of poverty among those who retire on a fixed income relative to self-progress and to others when compared to that of the same persons at an earlier age. On the one hand the progressive increase in income over a lifetime suggests success and gain, but in comparison to other slightly younger workers it suggests financial decline. However, regardless of the means of measuring financial success the reality is that retirement is most commonly accompanied by lowered economic access. The income of retirees declines with retirement relative to younger families, and to their own employment history. "While the money incomes of all age groups have been rising since 1960, those of older families have not increased as much as the incomes of the under-65 age group. . . . Since 1962, the median income of elderly individuals has risen 16 percent, which is about half the percentage increase for younger persons."[14]

The question economists are asking now is "to what extent and through what mechanism are retired persons to share in the growth of the national product?"[15] Some have suggested tying Social Security benefits to the cost of living, which will help during inflation.[16] Others propose a one percent rise in retirement benefits every year.[17]

Table 5–1 Income Distribution 1950–1978, Age and Sex

MONEY INCOME OF PERSONS—PERCENT DISTRIBUTION BY INCOME LEVEL, MEDIAN AND
MEAN INCOME, BY SEX, 1950 TO 1978, AND BY RACE AND AGE, 1970 AND 1978

[Persons 14 years old and over as of **March** of following year. Based on Current Population Survey; see headnote, table 744. For definition of median and mean, see Guide to Tabular Presentation. See *Historical Statistics, Colonial Times to 1970*, series G 257–268, for percent distribution by income level, and median income]

SEX, YEAR, AGE AND RACE	All persons (mil.)	Total (mil.)	Under 2,000 [1]	2,000–2,999	3,000–4,999	5,000–6,999	7,000–9,999	10,000–14,999	15,000–24,999	25,000 and over	Median income (dol.)	Mean income (dol.)
MALE												
1950	52.6	47.6	37.1	21.7	30.6	6.6	2.0	2.0			2,570	2,961
1960	60.4	55.2	27.6	10.4	23.0	21.6	11.2	4.1	1.4	.6	4,080	4,617
1970	70.6	65.0	18.7	6.9	13.0	13.7	20.9	17.7	6.8	2.3	6,670	7,537
1975 [2]	77.6	71.2	12.9	6.1	11.3	10.4	14.6	21.8	17.5	5.4	8,853	10,429
1978 [2]	81.0	75.6	10.6	5.2	9.5	8.7	12.0	18.4	24.7	11.0	10,935	13,113
14–19 yr	12.3	7.8	61.4	12.5	13.0	5.8	4.4	2.4	.4	.1	1,315	2,264
20–24 yr	9.7	9.4	12.9	8.0	14.1	14.6	19.6	19.7	10.3	.8	7,059	7,732
25–34 yr	16.7	16.5	3.3	1.9	5.0	7.1	13.1	26.9	34.3	8.4	13,410	14,305
35–44 yr	11.9	11.9	2.5	1.6	3.5	4.7	8.7	19.4	39.2	20.3	16,572	18,571
45–54 yr	11.0	10.9	3.2	2.5	4.5	5.1	8.3	18.8	35.5	22.1	16,574	18,874
55–64 yr	9.7	9.7	3.6	3.7	8.4	7.6	11.6	19.7	29.1	16.3	13,624	16,334
65–69 yr	3.8	3.8	4.5	8.7	18.5	16.5	20.1	15.3	9.9	6.6	7,247	10,007
70 and over	5.7	5.8	5.4	12.4	28.2	19.7	15.5	10.3	4.9	3.5	5,361	7,586
White: 1970	63.0	58.4	17.8	6.7	12.2	13.4	21.4	18.8	7.4	2.5	7,011	7,840
1978 [2]	71.3	67.3	10.0	4.7	9.1	8.3	11.8	18.5	25.6	11.9	11,453	13,609
Black: 1970	6.8	5.8	28.6	8.9	20.2	17.2	16.9	6.8	1.2	.2	4,159	4,683
1978 [2]	8.1	7.0	15.6	10.0	13.1	12.2	13.4	16.8	16.2	2.8	6,861	8,541
FEMALE												
1950	56.9	24.7	75.5	18.1	5.7	.4	.2	.2			953	1,296
1960	65.3	36.5	62.8	14.0	17.7	4.3	.9	.2	-	-	1,261	1,861
1970	77.6	51.6	46.7	11.8	19.1	11.8	7.5	2.4	.5	.2	2,237	3,138
1975 [2]	85.0	60.8	31.9	13.5	18.8	13.2	12.5	7.8	2.1	.3	3,385	4,513
1978 [2]	88.6	71.9	27.7	11.9	17.2	12.1	13.5	11.8	5.1	.8	4,068	5,599
14–19 yr	12.2	7.2	66.9	11.9	13.2	4.8	2.4	.5	.1	-	1,118	1,769
20–24 yr	10.1	8.9	24.3	11.1	17.7	17.2	18.7	9.4	1.4	.2	4,588	5,104
25–34 yr	17.3	14.3	24.3	6.9	13.9	12.0	17.7	18.0	6.5	.7	5,839	6,557
35–44 yr	12.7	10.2	23.2	7.4	13.8	13.5	16.0	16.1	8.5	1.5	5,804	6,936
45–54 yr	11.8	9.3	23.6	8.4	13.4	12.7	15.8	16.7	8.2	1.2	5,672	6,806
55–64 yr	10.9	8.8	26.1	12.2	15.1	11.7	13.7	13.2	6.5	1.4	4,473	6,237
65–69 yr	4.7	4.6	23.7	21.3	23.3	11.7	9.7	6.1	3.7	.5	3,322	4,818
70 and over	8.9	8.6	17.5	24.3	32.1	11.2	7.0	4.6	2.4	.8	3,374	4,585
White: 1970	68.8	45.3	46.5	11.5	18.9	12.1	7.8	2.5	.5	.2	2,266	3,185
1978 [2]	77.1	62.7	28.2	11.2	16.9	12.1	13.6	12.0	5.1	.9	4,117	5,631
Black: 1970	8.0	5.8	48.9	14.2	20.7	9.4	4.9	1.8	.1	-	2,063	2,743
1978 [2]	9.9	8.0	23.9	17.2	19.2	11.9	13.1	9.9	4.6	.2	3,707	5,212

- Represents zero or rounds to zero.   [1] Includes persons with income deficit.   [2] Not strictly comparable with earlier years due to revised procedures; see text, p. 436.

Source: Statistical Abstracts of the United States (Washington, D.C.: U.S. Department of Commerce, Bureau of Census, 1980), p. 462

POVERTY

How many elderly actually live in poverty? The number is estimated at approximately 4.3 million, or approximately one-fifth; however, there is hidden poverty among the elderly. An additional two million elderly have no money and must live with their families. They do not live in actual poverty, but they have chosen to live as dependents of their children.[18]

The number of elderly actually living in poverty is decreasing annually, and at a faster rate than the general population.[19,20] The entire population's income is increasing, and fewer people are living in poverty. This sounds good, but it masks the problem of many elderly poor who became poor only after they became old and retired. Butler cautions the reader who interprets the statistics at face value in view of the elderly.[21] He asserts that the official statistics are being grossly conservative in their estimate of aged poor, and that the government definition of poverty is inadequate.

The problem to date has focused more on raising the economic deficits than the social and emotional deficits. The "poverty index" used by the Social Security Administration was based on the Economic Food Plan of the Department of Agriculture. "Until 1969, annual revisions of levels were based on price changes of items in the economy food plan."[22] After 1969, annual adjustments were based on the Consumer Price Index, not the food costs.[23]

A comprehensive concept of an "adequate" level must include all facets of a person's existence. Poverty is more than economic deprivation. It is loss of self-esteem, self-worth, and social and educational opportunity.[24] It "is above all a comparative concept that refers to a relative quality."[25] This concept must recognize the change in needs of advancing age; psychological needs related to working and income; a person's previous standard of living; the cost of leisure activities; and status maintenance.[26]

Several people have attempted to define what is meant by poverty, adequate income, subsistence income, or an adequate standard of living. Walther maintains they are all arbitrary, subjective terms, with intangible meanings.[27] Poverty was once assessed as having less than a standard level of income. The level changes with the cost of living and is influenced by inflation. Subsistence income is that amount necessary for food and cost of living. It is based on a food budget multiplied by a fixed factor. It has been used to assess the extent of poverty in the U.S., not the welfare of individuals. However, an arbitrary fixed measure of subsistence income does not correspond to "adequacy," which is an approximate and fluid concept.

Walther suggests that an evaluation of poverty might be more realistic if the extent to which the needs of the family are satisfied is examined.

The focus would then be on potential consumption, not current income. This approach also runs into problems including the barriers of calculating potential earnings, consumption, cost of living in individual areas, receipt of transfer funds, and reduction of earnings taxes and discounts.[28]

So attempts have been made to stabilize the concept of poverty both as an absolute and as a relative measure of deprivation, but an absolute standard implies a fixed quantity and a relative standard must establish what proportion of an income is "poverty." Orshansky, an employee with the Social Security Administration, developed poverty definitions based on the cost of a minimum basket of goods plus services needed, and determined that any income below what was necessary to purchase that was "poverty."[29] But there is no equivalence "between money and the personal value of what it buys."[30] This is the thrust of the problems involved in defining poverty.

Some people decry the deprivation of the elderly. They point to growth away from poverty for the general population in the last two or three decades. Still others more adamantly state that poverty among the elderly is a myth.[31] This author contends that it exists among the elderly beyond just economic deprivation. "The essence of poverty is inequality. . . . The poor are deprived in comparison with the comfortable, the affluent, and the opulent."[32] In the United States, the poor are disadvantaged in power, politics, and prestige. This is far greater than mere economic deprivation. What gives the inequality value and transmits a negative connotation to its bearers is the high status accorded to the philosophy of quality.[33]

SOCIAL SECURITY CONCEPT

In 1935, a retirement income program was instituted.[34] The Social Security Act was passed. It has been hailed as the most significant legislation to emerge from the United States Congress to date, and it has had a major impact on every citizen since that time. Considered an innovative measure and a significant break with earlier means of support after retirement, this Act contained the potential to make life financially more secure for the elderly. Until 1935, parents were cared for by their children as a matter of tradition. Social Security would now place the onus for support on the federal government as a managing agent for invested savings.

Social Security is uniform throughout the United States. Deductions are made from the worker's salary according to a scale of earnings and deposited into a federal fund to be returned monthly after that person's retirement, thereby constituting a pension. This is not considered welfare or public assistance, but the benefits from a retirement insurance program. The family is spared direct financial stress in part at least.[35]

The plan, however, was not intended to give everyone 100 percent protection against the hazards of life, but to provide at least a modest insurance against a poverty-stricken old-age, measured according to the average earnings over a period of years.[36]

The Social Security concept was predicated on the basic agreement that no one in the United States should suffer economic distress.[37] "The evolution of the Social Security Act represents a concern and commitment at the federal level to [ensure] domestic tranquility among our elder citizens."[38] It upheld the national philosophy that every person should earn a pension,[39] giving every person the dignity to grow old secure in the knowledge that his or her financial support during retirement had been planned.

Historically there were only a few rich people who could look forward to retirement with such assurance. In the past it had not been a problem in the majority of cases because people did not live as long, and those who did worked until they died. As longevity increased and the numbers increased who faced financially nonproductive years in later life, the need to find resolution for economic devastation became more immediate. For many, the matter of livelihood became the responsibility and moral obligation of the family. For others, the remaining options were to go to the "poor farm," to be taken in by "good-hearted" citizens, to panhandle, or to starve.

The final stimulus for passage of the Act was the Great Depression, which illuminated the glaring inadequacies of the average American's financial base.[40] It was a dynamic concept, based on the realization that growth, modification, and expansion would parallel the nation's population. It has been modified in some way on more than 15 occasions, and will continue to be changed to match the needs of those it serves. The major changes since its inception were to convert it from individual to family security in 1939; to extend the coverage to all families and to the self-employed in 1950; and to add medical insurance for those over 65 years of age, through Medicare, in 1965.[41]

Financing retirement needs is difficult and complex. The final Social Security plan was purposely left incomplete and open-ended, drafted with the intent of modification and extension as needs were identified in the populace. It was never intended to be a complete source of anyone's support, but a moderate assistance by average American standards.[42] The concept assumes that a person is able to save for retirement through Social Security, but pensions and other assets would be the primary source of retirement support.[43]

In 1965, there was a major increase in benefits, and from 1970 to 1977 alone the benefits increased nearly 100 percent.[44] The average monthly benefits for men increased from $131 in 1970 to $268 in 1977, and for women during the same time period from $101 to $213. These figures are further detailed in Table 5–2.

These increases are more readily evident in Figure 5–1.

Problems with the Social Security Concept

For its purpose, Social Security has been relatively successful. It has assisted millions in staying out of poverty, and it has encouraged and allowed people to plan ahead. For other hurdles yet to overcome, it has a long hard road to travel. Inflation and increased life expectancy have complicated the basic plan, although the concept remains constant. The challenges of continued increase of minimum benefits, earnings ceiling, household employment coverage, and increased standard of living are ahead. All have been debated in the past and will require resolution in the future. Women still feel the pangs of unequal recognition for work as homemakers and childbearers, where they produced no tangible income, even though the value of their contribution is recognized.[45] Spouse benefits are an implicit payment to wives for their time spent as housewives, but are based on the level of earnings of their husbands, not on the market value of housework.[46] Many wives did not work enough to accumulate the minimum number of quarters of employment subject to Social Security to draw benefits at 62 or 65. Now, after 65, some women are participating in programs such as "Rent-A-Granny," where women are working to accumulate the requisite number of quarters and become eligible for Social Security.

Another common attack on the concept of Social Security is that benefits are figured on wages earned over several back years, and that these wages have not kept pace with present-day costs of living. Salaries were lower, and opportunities were limited. Moreover, "workers who have low earnings, or who suffer disability, unemployment, or other adversity during the last decade of worklife, will face retirement with little or no savings, and with less than the maximum OASDHI benefit. . . ."[47]

In addition to the effects of inflation on those deductions, refined technology allows many workers today to command much higher salaries. They pay more into Social Security and can expect greater benefits at 65. In addition, automatic increases in the benefits attached to the present cost of living will be more equitable.[48] However, today's retiree earns inadequate benefits because of circumstances of the past. These arguments have not fallen on deaf ears.

In July 1979, Social Security payments were increased 9.8 percent. Some hailed this as a notable gain that would allow a more humane existence,

Table 5–2 Social Security Retirement Benefits by Sex: 1960–1978

SOCIAL SECURITY (OASDHI)—RETIREMENT BENEFITS, BY SEX: 1960 TO 1979

[As of end of year. Benefits in current-payment status. OASDHI = Old-age, survivors, disability, and health insurance. Full benefits begin at age 65; reduced benefits at age 62. The latter began in 1956 for women and in 1961 for men. See also Appendix III and *Historical Statistics, Colonial Times to 1970,* series H 245–259]

ITEM	Unit	1960	1965	1970	1973	1974	1975	1976	1977	1978	1979
MALE											
Number receiving benefits [1]	1,000	5,217	6,825	7,688	8,610	8,832	9,164	9,420	9,714	9,928	10,192
Full benefits	1,000	5,217	5,389	4,930	4,817	4,737	4,699	4,633	4,583	4,536	4,607
Reduced benefits	1,000	(X)	1,436	2,758	3,793	4,095	4,465	4,787	5,131	5,392	5,586
Average age	Years	73.2	72.9	72.6	72.3	72.3	72.3	72.2	72.2	72.2	(NA)
Percent aged:											
62–64 years	Percent	(X)	6.9	7.5	8.7	8.9	9.3	9.4	9.5	9.2	9.2
65–69 years	Percent	33.8	29.7	30.1	31.9	32.2	32.2	32.3	32.3	32.4	32.3
70–74 years	Percent	33.1	29.5	26.9	25.7	25.9	25.6	25.8	25.8	25.9	26.0
75 years and over	Percent	33.2	33.9	35.5	33.7	33.0	32.9	32.5	32.4	32.5	32.5
Avg. monthly benefits, total	Dol	82	93	131	183	207	228	248	268	292	327
Full	Dol	82	96	139	197	224	247	270	293	320	359
Reduced:											
Before reduction	Dol	(X)	90	129	181	206	228	250	272	297	334
After reduction	Dol	(X)	79	115	164	187	207	226	246	268	300
Minimum monthly benefits: [2]											
Full	Dol	33	44	64	85	85	94	101	108	114	122
Reduced	Dol	(X)	35	51	68	68	75	81	86	92	98
Maximum monthly benefits: [2]											
Full	Dol	119	132	190	266	275	316	364	413	460	503
Reduced	Dol	(X)	103	147	208	217	253	286	319	355	389
FEMALE											
Number receiving benefits [1]	1,000	2,845	4,276	5,661	6,754	7,126	7,424	7,744	8,106	8,430	8,778
Full benefits	1,000	1,896	2,192	2,352	2,527	2,526	2,521	2,670	2,669	2,684	2,772
Reduced benefits	1,000	949	2,083	3,309	4,227	4,601	4,903	5,074	5,438	5,745	6,006
Average age	Years	71.0	71.8	72.0	72.0	72.1	72.2	72.3	72.4	72.5	(NA)
Percent aged:											
62–64 years	Percent	12.6	12.2	11.5	11.9	11.8	11.8	11.6	11.6	11.3	11.2
65–69 years	Percent	36.3	31.6	30.1	30.7	30.6	30.4	30.2	30.0	29.8	29.5
70–74 years	Percent	29.0	28.1	25.4	24.2	24.2	24.2	24.4	24.3	24.4	24.3
75 years and over	Percent	22.2	28.1	33.1	33.1	33.4	33.6	33.8	34.1	34.5	35.0
Avg. monthly benefits, total	Dol	60	70	101	146	165	182	197	213	230	257
Full	Dol	62	75	112	164	186	206	224	243	265	298
Reduced:											
Before reduction	Dol	64	74	106	144	163	180	(NA)	(NA)	(NA)	(NA)
After reduction	Dol	56	65	94	135	154	169	183	198	214	238
Minimum monthly benefits: [2]											
Full	Dol	33	44	64	85	85	94	101	108	114	122
Reduced	Dol	26	35	51	68	68	75	81	86	92	98
Maximum monthly benefits: [2]											
Full	Dol	119	136	196	276	285	334	379	422	460	503
Reduced	Dol	95	105	152	213	220	253	286	319	355	389

NA Not available.   X Not applicable.   [1] Includes disability beneficiaries who attained age 65.   [2] Assumes retirement at beginning of year.

Source: Statistical Abstracts of the United States (Washington, D.C.: U.S. Department of Commerce, Bureau of Census, 1979), p. 338

Figure 5–1 Social Security—Selected Average Monthly Benefit Payments: 1960–1978

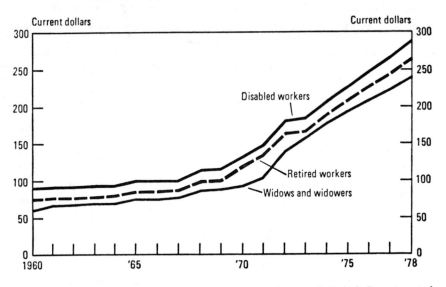

Source: Statistical Abstracts of the United States (Washington, D.C.: U.S. Department of Commerce, Bureau of Census, 1979), p. 324

that is, "lower the morbidity and mortality rate for [the elderly] . . . buy food for an adequate diet, warmth for protection from the winter cold and, perhaps, some little entertainment for the depressed."[49] Others rebutted that this increase was outstripped by inflation. Moreover, it was a double-edged sword for some. Increases in income reduced eligibility for other benefits. Instances were cited of reduced food stamps and Medicaid eligibility, and increased rent and loss of payment for transportation due to Social Security increases. "Gain adds up to spending even more money for food, medical services, rent and transportation."[50]

Another of the injustices in the Social Security Act that is frequently debated is the ceiling on earnings a person may accrue without jeopardizing benefits. A person cannot depend on work as a source of additional income unless it is below the accepted limit determined by the Social Security Administration. In 1978, the earnings ceiling was $3,000 a year for any Social Security beneficiary, and it has gradually been raised until it is now $5,500. The National Council of Senior Citizens wanted the ceiling liberalized, but not removed, so the option to work at least part-time after 65 was feasible. Some type of ceiling is necessary, it was argued, "so that the rich so-called retired do not draw money out of the pockets of the elderly Americans who need their Social Security checks just to maintain life itself."[51] In 1978, the ceiling was lifted for those over 70 years of age.

Social Security affords coverage to about 90 percent of all persons over 65, and 95 percent of all women and children will receive benefits if the husband dies. A worker can receive full retirement benefits at 65 years of age or reduced benefits beginning at 62. A widow gains full benefits at 62 or reduced benefits at 60. A severely disabled person is eligible to receive full benefits at 50, and a dependent parent has full benefits at 62. All must apply however; it is not automatic.[52]

Between 1958 and 1977, the Social Security rolls doubled, and yet there are more potential recipients who are not aware of their eligibility. It is a confusing and complex system, and for this reason anyone applying for the first time should go to the local Social Security Administration Office for assistance.

Other Federal Benefits

In addition to Social Security, federal benefits paid to the elderly take many forms. Benefits in dollars have increased steadily in annual total outlay, but there has been a shift in percentages where the money has been applied. Cash benefits have doubled between 1971 and 1978, while in-kind benefits have tripled. This is reflected in the 1979 Census Bureau report in Table 5–3. In 1979, Estes identified more than 80 federal programs in all, many of which negate benefits received in another program, or at least complicate the recipient's quest for benefits and confuse the issue of eligibility.[53] One effect of the Social Security Act was to encourage involvement in pension plans that augment total retirement income. The increases in private and government pension funds in billions of dollars are shown in Table 5–4.

It is in implementing various sources of income that the problems begin. About 35 percent of Social Security recipients also receive some type of pension, but pensions also have problems, which prevent total dependence on them for income.[54] The median pension payment for most older people is $99 a month. Many pension plans are unstable. They have many limiting provisions, often allowing no survivors benefits or having no money to pay legitimate benefits. Others disintegrate before the retiree can reap benefits. It has become such a problem that the Pension Reform Act was passed in 1974 as a basis for negotiating complaints against pension plans.[55]

Most of the programs are designed for specific target populations. For example, the Black Lung Benefit provides benefits to underground coal miners totally disabled by pneumoconiosis and to their dependents and

Table 5–3 Federal Benefits for the Aged, by Type of Benefit: 1971 to 1978

FEDERAL BENEFITS FOR THE AGED, BY TYPE OF BENEFIT: 1971 TO 1979

[For years ending June 30 except, beginning 1977, ending Sept. 30]

TYPE OF BENEFIT	BENEFITS (bil. dol.)								PERCENT		
	1971	1973	1974	1975	1976	1977	1978	1979	1971	1975	1979
Total outlays...................	44.0	56.9	65.7	81.3	92.0	95.7	103.9	116.4	100.0	100.0	100.0
Cash benefits............................	34.2	46.0	53.2	64.7	73.0	72.8	76.9	85.2	77.7	79.6	73.2
Social security......................	27.1	37.1	42.8	51.8	58.6	56.6	62.9	69.0	61.6	63.7	59.3
Railroad employees................	1.7	2.1	2.3	2.8	3.2	3.5	3.0	3.2	3.9	3.4	2.7
Federal civilian employees.....	2.3	3.3	4.3	5.5	6.4	7.1	5.0	6.2	5.2	6.8	5.3
Military retirement...................	.7	.7	.8	1.1	1.2	1.8	2.0	.8	1.6	1.4	.7
Coal miners ¹ ....,.,.,..........	.1	.2	.2	.2	.2	.3	.3	1.1	.2	.2	.9
Supplemental security											
income ²	1.4	1.1	1.4	1.8	1.8	1.7	1.9	1.7	3.2	2.2	1.5
Veterans pensions.................	.9	1.4	1.4	1.5	1.6	1.8	1.8	³ 3.2	2.0	1.8	2.7
In-kind benefits..........................	9.8	11.0	12.5	16.6	19.0	22.9	27.0	31.2	22.3	20.4	26.8
Medicare...	7.5	9.0	9.9	12.8	15.0	18.3	21.5	24.6	17.0	15.7	21.1
Medicaid .:............................	1.9	1.5	2.2	2.6	3.0	3.3	3.8	4.3	4.3	3.2	3.7
Food stamps........................	.2	.1	.1	1.0	.6	.6	.5	.5	.5	1.2	.4
Subsidized public housing.....	.2	.3	.2	.4	.4	.8	1.1	1.6	.5	.5	1.4

¹ Prior to 1979, represents benefit for coal miners' widows only.   ² Prior to 1974, represents Federal grants to States for aid to the aged, blind, and disabled.   ³ Includes other veterans' compensation for aged.

Source: *Statistical Abstracts of the United States* (Washington, D.C.: U.S. Department of Commerce, Bureau of Census, 1979), p. 334

survivors. In 1978, for example, only 139,000 miners and 301,000 dependents and widows received benefits.[56]

The majority of the elderly receive most of their income from Social Security benefits. Three-quarters of those over 65 receive no salary from employment. In 1981, the maximum benefit paid to a retired worker at 65 is $658.80, and the minimum is $153.10. A surviving widow receives what her husband had been eligible for. A couple will receive the worker's eligible amount, plus half-again that much for the spouse. Hence, a worker eligible for $653.80 would receive an additional $326.90 for the spouse, giving the couple a total income of $980.70 a month. For a retired worker and spouse receiving the minimum benefits, the total would be $229.65. The range is obviously great, and the average of $403.45 for a single retired worker carries various hidden implications when individually analyzed. Few will be receiving the maximum benefit, while the great majority will be closer to the average. Also, 30 percent will still be below the poverty level. For those who chose to receive benefits at age 62, affluence will be even less accessible.[57,58]

Table 5–4 Distributing Private and Public Pension Funds: 1950–1958

	1950	*1960*	*1970*	*1975*	*1978*
Private Funds	12.1	52.0	138.2	216.9	321.3
Public Funds	25.8	56.3	125.8	190.8	243.6
Total All Types	37.9	108.3	264.0	407.7	564.9

Source: Statistical Abstracts of the United States (Washington, D.C.: U.S. Department of Commerce, Bureau of Census, 1979), p. 340

SUPPLEMENTARY SECURITY INCOME

One important program that provides cash transfer of income directly to elderly persons over 65 is the Supplementary Security Income (SSI). This program was originally the separate programs for Old Age Assistance, Aid to the Blind, and Aid to the Permanently and Totally Disabled, which were combined in 1974.[59] By 1977, SSI guaranteed an individual $177.80 a month. If the income fell below that, the person was eligible for the difference. The SSI attempted to establish an income floor for the very poor, blind, or disabled.[60,61]

Supplementary Security Income is also managed by the Social Security Administration, but SSI payments are regulated by individual states. Social Security payments are federally established, and the scale is constant across the United States. Supplementary Security Income is based on a person's need for assistance. Receiving money from one program does not negate eligibility for the other; both can be awarded simultaneously.[62] Some states do hold adult children responsible for care of the parents, and this may influence whether or not a parent is deemed eligible for SSI.[63]

MEDICARE

The Medicare section of the Social Security Act (Title 18) is the most constantly debated and abused of the Social Security programs. Doctors, lawyers, nurses, hospitals, the American Medical Association (AMA), patients, and others run the gamut of confusion, use, abuse, support, and opposition. Some of this stems from the wide extent of the program's application and the precedent it sets for health care in the United States. When the original Social Security Act was written, the medical coverage was omitted because of heavy pressure from the AMA and the reaction to national fear of socialization implied in federally sponsored medical care.[64] Thirty years later, on July 30, 1965, Congress added the hospital and medical insurance provision to the original Act. It is Medicare, or Title 18, of the Social Security Act.

At the time of its inception, the plan was to offer hospital care to the elderly, but after congressional debate, coverage of medical expenses was also added.[65] Many see the plan as a compromise between the proponents of the bill and the powerful AMA. It focused on the elderly instead of the entire population, and it was agreed that the government would not interfere with the medical care delivery system.[66,67]

The basic goal of Medicare was to provide older adults with federal financial protection against heavy medical costs.[68] There are two sections of the program, the first for hospital insurance and the second for medical insurance:[69,70] It opened a new era in health care, a new spectrum of paid care through insurance regardless of an individual's financial background. It was not a simple health care bill.

There were some biases. The program forced inpatient utilization of medical facilities. Originally a patient had to be admitted to a hospital to have reimbursed care.[71] Only ten percent sought care in a doctor's office, even though 86 percent had abnormalities that could have been properly treated there. The unmet need of the elderly was to have accessible, reimbursible outpatient services.

Medicare is neither automatic nor free. Membership must be requested.[72] "Medicare does not cover all medical expenses, nor does it move in immediately to cover expenses that are allowed. Every recipient is responsible for a deductible amount."[73] The government reimburses a percentage of charges, but the patient is left to cover the remainder of the cost.

Expenses not paid by Medicare and other sources are often covered by Medicaid, a jointly administered health care program by state and federal governments, provided the patient can demonstrate indigency.[74] Medicaid is Title 19 of the Social Security Act. "Each state designs its own individual program within the broad framework of federal regulations, so there is great state-to-state variation."[75] Where Medicare ensures a health program for everyone over 65, Medicaid assists the needy of all ages who meet eligibility standards, that is, one is an insurance program for health care and the other an assistance program for health care.[76] The number of needy elderly receiving assistance through Medicaid has increased every year, as have the payments for their care as shown in Table 5–5.

> Coverage under Medicare is limited by time and type of care There are also deductibles, so that beneficiaries have to pay for the first $160 in costs themselves and $40 per day for each day over 60. . . . Patients with protracted and terminal illnesses often

Table 5–5 Monthly Medicaid Payments: 1970 to 1978

MEDICAL ASSISTANCE (MEDICAID)—UNDUPLICATED RECIPIENTS AND PAYMENTS: 1972 TO 1979

[For years ending **June 30** except, beginning **1977**, ending **September 30**]

BASIS OF ELIGIBILITY	RECIPIENTS (1,000)					PAYMENTS (mil. dol.)					
	1972	1975	1976	1977	1978	1972	1975	1976	1977 [1]	1978 [1]	1979 [1]
Total	18,312	22,413	24,666	23,833	22,946	6,299	12,292	14,135	15,847	17,805	16,879
Age 65 and over	3,417	3,699	3,808	3,619	3,786	1,925	4,649	5,192	5,758	6,727	6,264
Blindness	109	107	98	95	79	45	83	86	96	114	102
Disabled [2]	1,673	2,308	2,664	2,731	2,900	1,354	2,874	3,550	4,266	5,010	5,141
AFDC [3] program	11,373	14,438	15,882	15,099	14,066	2,101	4,063	4,598	4,789	4,914	4,622
Children	8,177	9,776	10,644	10,071	9,129	1,139	2,050	2,353	2,393	2,422	4,622
Adults	3,196	4,662	5,238	5,028	4,937	962	2,013	2,245	2,396	2,492	
Other	1,740	1,861	2,214	2,289	2,115	875	623	710	939	1.040	749

[1] Preliminary.   [2] Permanently and totally.   [3] Aid to families with dependent children.

Source: Statistical Abstracts of the United States (Washington, D.C.: U.S. Department of Commerce, Bureau of Census, 1979), p. 348

exhaust their Medicare benefits. When this occurs, recipients must use their own funds to continue care.[77]

In 1973, Medicare covered less than 50 percent of personal health costs of individuals who are old and poor.[78] In 1976, Medicare paid only $463 on an average yearly medical bill of $1,218 (still less than 50 percent), leaving the elderly client to deal with the balance through personal savings, loans, welfare, or default.[79] Because of Medicare older people are now able to have more medical care, but they also have more bills that are not paid by the program. It was expensive to be ill, but now it is even more expensive to get well.[80] The situation is a circular trap, referred to by Carl Eisdorfer of the University of Washington as the "Medicaid Waltz," wherein the needy may be refused care because of their need.

Medicare has funneled greater and greater amounts of money into the health care community.[81] The continued exponential increase in quantities of money is reflected in Table 5–6. The patients and the government are left in the quandary of weighing new expenses against old health deficits. Many of the costs are for vital health care needs. Many of the unpaid costs that patients want covered accrue because they are classified as health maintenance and primary prevention, such things as glasses, hearing aids, various prescriptions, routine physical examinations, and dental care. Medicare was designed to eradicate physical illness of the elderly, not to pro-

Table 5–6 Health Insurance Under the Medicare Program: 1970 to 1977

MEDICARE PROGRAM CLAIMS AND REIMBURSEMENTS: 1970 TO 1978

[Data reflect date claims approved for payment and cover only claims approved and recorded in the Health Care Financing Administration central records before Dec. 29, 1979. See text, p. 327 for explanation of coverage]

ITEM	Unit	PERSONS 65 YEARS OLD AND OVER					DISABLED [1]			
		1970	1975	1976	1977	1978	1975	1976	1977	1978
HOSPITAL INSURANCE										
Claims approved	**1,000**	**7,501**	**9,389**	**10,084**	**10,529**	**10,902**	**929**	**1,083**	**1,209**	**1,311**
Reimbursements [2]	**Mil. dol**	**4,844**	**9,430**	**11,489**	**13,095**	**14,851**	**984**	**1,299**	**1,604**	**1,908**
Inpatients:										
Claims approved	1,000	6,306	7,844	8,268	8,493	8,733	842	974	1,079	1,166
Admissions	1,000	6,139	7,405	7,796	8,132	8,410	849	970	1,088	1,178
Annual rate [3]	Rate	304	332	343	350	354	393	407	417	423
Covered days of care	Millions	80	84	88	88	89	9	10	11	12
Annual rate [3]	Rate	3,943	3,786	3,873	3,798	3,759	4,136	4,247	4,202	4,183
Per admission	Days	13.0	11.4	11.3	10.9	10.6	10.5	10.4	10.1	9.9
Hospital charges	Mil. dol	5,931	12,021	14,755	17,128	19,766	1,320	1,757	2,195	2,649
Per day	Dollars	74	142	168	194	221	148	174	200	228
Reimbursements [2]	Mil. dol	4,569	9,041	11,013	12,559	14,272	965	1,274	1,573	1,873
Percent of charges	Percent	77.0	75.2	74.6	73.3	72.2	73.1	72.5	71.7	70.7
Per claim	Dollars	725	1,153	1,332	1,479	1,634	1,146	1,308	1,458	1,606
Home health:										
Claims approved	1,000	571	1,009	1,237	1,472	1,655	70	91	111	127
Reimbursements [2]	Mil. dol	47	136	185	235	284	10	14	19	23
Per claim	Dollars	82	135	150	160	172	142	160	168	182
Skilled nursing facility:										
Claims approved	1,000	624	536	578	565	514	17	19	19	18
Reimbursements [2]	Mil. dol	229	253	290	301	295	9	11	12	12
Per claim	Dollars	366	472	502	533	574	556	571	622	673
MEDICAL INSURANCE										
Total bills	**1,000**	**[4] 39,695**	**73,235**	**82,654**	**94,790**	**106,346**	**6,658**	**8,570**	**10,786**	**12,829**
Physicians:										
Bills approved	1,000	32,850	57,209	64,268	73,573	82,132	4,597	5,868	7,427	8,908
Total charges	Mil. dol	2,157	3,907	4,471	5,349	6,156	344	440	572	698
Per bill	Dollars	66	68	70	73	75	75	75	77	78
Percent reimbursed	Percent	72.9	74.1	75.5	76.2	76.8	75.6	76.9	77.4	77.7
Surgical	Percent	75.5	75.8	77.2	77.6	78.0	76.5	77.8	78.2	78.4
Medical	Percent	71.5	72.8	74.4	75.3	76.0	75.0	76.4	77.0	77.3
Outpatient hospital:										
Bills approved	1,000	4,031	8,985	10,446	11,684	13,038	1,344	1,753	2,108	2,436
Reimbursements [2]	Mil. dol	85	315	420	526	645	143	196	235	272
Per bill	Dollars	21	35	40	45	49	106	112	111	112
Home health:										
Bills approved	1,000	430	544	645	739	805	44	55	64	72
Reimbursements [2]	Mil. dol	23	55	74	90	105	5	7	9	10
Per bill	Dollars	53	101	114	122	131	116	129	137	145
Other:										
Bills approved	1,000	2,380	6,498	7,296	8,795	10,372	673	895	1,188	1,414
Reimbursements [2]	Mil. dol	70	212	258	345	445	100	144	202	260
Per bill	Dollars	30	33	35	39	43	148	161	170	184

[1] Coverage not limited with respect to age.   [2] Amounts paid to providers for covered services; excludes deductibles, coinsurance amounts, and noncovered services as specified by law.   [3] Per 1,000 enrollees; enrollment as of July 1.   [4] Data reflect date paid claims were recorded in Health Care Financing Administration records.

Source: *Statistical Abstracts of the United States* (Washington D.C.: U.S. Department of Commerce, Bureau of Census, 1979), p. 348

mote health. Nor was it designed to serve the elderly in areas deemed "unreasonable and unnecessary."

The older person cannot afford to be ill long, and yet that person is incapacitated on the average about five weeks a year, two of those in bed, often-times hospitalized. The bill will be twice that of a younger person, because it takes twice as long to heal and requires more medication and treatment.[82] Some weigh the cost and go without care by preference. Moreover, in all diseases, costs have both direct and indirect financial impact. For example, heart disease has an indirect cost estimated to be 4.5 times greater than direct costs and strokes 1.7 times greater. The factors producing this involve the length of disability, aside from reduction of productivity, the disability due to pain, rehabilitation, and emotional depression.[83]

It would be ideal if Medicare payments corresponded to hospital and physician costs, but that is not the case. If the patient is going to gain the benefits intended by the Medicare program, then certain responsibilities are necessarily assumed by both the physician and the patient. It behooves patients to inquire into the best approach to their care, to counsel with the physician at the beginning of care, and to practice preventive medicine between visits to the physician. On the other hand, Freedman of the Connecticut State Medical Society also reminds physicians of their duty to counsel patients, being sure that the counsel is comprehended. Physicians and patients need to increase the communication between them for increased continuity of quality care.

There are many claims of praise and condemnation surrounding the success of federally funded health care. To determine the validity and extent of them is impossible, but they do not invalidate the intent of the program.

> Medicare has not failed to fulfill its legislative promise; rather it has failed to tackle the problems that fulfillment has raised. The lesson of Medicare is that a bureaucracy charged with and experienced in the payment of claims will have limited interest in confronting the health cost and quality problems to which third party claims payment leads.[84]

NOTES

1. Juanita Kreps, "The Economics of Aging," in R. Gross, B. Gross, and S. Seidman, eds., *The New Old: Struggling for Decent Aging* (Garden City, N.Y.: Anchor Books, 1978), pp. 66–73.
2. Ibid., p. 68.
3. Ibid., pp. 66–69.

4. J. A. Peterson and B. Payne, *Love in the Later Years* (New York, N.Y.: Association Press, 1975), p. 106.

5. *Statistical Abstract of the United States* (Washington, D.C.: U.S. Department of Commerce, Bureau of Census, 1980), p. 466.

6. Ibid., p. 456.

7. Peterson and Payne, pp. 103–4.

8. Ibid., p. 107.

9. Ibid., p. 115.

10. Ibid., p. 116.

11. Juanita Kreps, "Economic Growth and Income Through The Life Cycle," in M. Seltzer, S. Corbett, and R. Atchley, eds., *Social Problems of the Aging* (Belmont, Cal.: Wadsworth Publishing Co., 1978), p. 182.

12. J. Liang, E. Kahana, and E. Doherty, "Financial Well-Being Among the Aged: A Further Elaboration," *Journal of Gerontology* 35, no. 4 (1980):409–20.

13. Kreps, "The Economics of Aging," p. 71.

14. Kreps, "Economic Growth and Income through the Life Cycle."

15. Ibid., p. 185.

16. Ibid.

17. Ibid., p. 186.

18. Juanita Kreps, "Intergenerational Transfers and the Bureaucracy," in E. Shanas and M. Sussman, eds., *Family, Bureaucracy and the Elderly* (Durham, N.C.: Duke University Press, 1977), pp. 21–34.

19. Robin Walther, "Economics and the Older Population," in D. Woodruff and J. Birren, eds., *Aging* (New York, N.Y.: D. Van Nostrand Co., 1975), pp. 336–351.

20. Erdman Palmore, "The Future Status of the Aged," *The Gerontologist* 16, no. 3 (1976):301.

21. Robert Butler, "How to Grow Old and Poor in an Affluent Society," *International Journal of Aging and Human Development* 4, no. 3 (1973):277–9.

22. *Statistical Abstract*, p. 434.

23. Ibid.

24. Peterson and Payne, p. 112.

25. Charles Valentine, *Culture and Poverty* (Chicago: University of Chicago Press, 1968), p. 13.

26. H. Brotman and P. Paillat, "Income," *The Gerontologist*, no. 3 (Summer 1972): Part II:17–20.

27. Walther, pp. 339–41.

28. Ibid., pp. 342–8.

29. Kreps, "Economic Growth and Income," p. 187.

30. Linda George and Lucille Bearon, *Quality of Life in Older Persons* (New York, N.Y.: Human Sciences Press, 1980), p. 162.

31. Jerry Flint, "The Old Folks," *Forbes* 125, no. 4 (February 18, 1980): 51–56.

32. Valentine, p. 13.

33. Ibid., pp. 12–15.

34. R. M. Ball, "The Fortieth Year of Social Security in America," in Charlotte L. Sebastian, ed., *Papers From the Economics of Aging: Toward 2001* (Ann Arbor, Mich.: Institute of Gerontology, 1976), p. 11.

35. Jennings Randolph, "Social Security Strengthens America," in Charlotte L. Sebastian, ed., *Papers From the Economics of Aging: Toward 2001* (Ann Arbor, Mich.: Institute of Gerontology, 1976), pp. 197–8.

36. Barbara Silverstone and Helen Hyman, *You and Your Aging Parent* (New York, N.Y.: Pantheon Books, 1976), p. 158.

37. Walther, p. 336.

38. Randolph, p. 112.

39. Tish Sommers, "Social Security—A Feminist Critique," in Charlotte L. Sebastian, ed., *Papers From The Economics of Aging: Toward 2001* (Ann Arbor, Mich.: Institute of Gerontology, 1976), p. 57.

40. Walther, p. 336.

41. William Haber, "The Economics of Aging," in Charlotte L. Sebastian, ed., *Papers From The Economics of Aging: Toward 2001* (Ann Arbor, Mich.: Institute of Gerontology, 1976), pp. 3–4.

42. Wilbur Cohen, "Social Security: 1935–1975," in Charlotte L. Sebastian, ed., *Papers From The Economics of Aging: Toward 2001* (Ann Arbor, Mich.: Institute of Gerontology, 1976), pp. 185–94.

43. Paul Kerschner and Ira Hirschfield, "Public Policy and Aging: Analytic Approaches," in D. Woodruff and J. Birren, eds., *Aging* (New York, N.Y.: D. Van Nostrand Co., 1975), p. 368.

44. Carroll Estes, *The Aging Enterprise* (San Francisco, Cal.: Jossey-Bass Publishers, 1979), p. 86.

45. Sommers, p. 60.

46. Karen Holden, "The Inequitable Distribution of OASI Benefits Among Homemakers," *The Gerontologist* 19, no. 3 (1979):250–6.

47. Kreps, "Economic Growth and Income," p. 182.

48. Ball, p. 12.

49. Richard Neiman, "Social Security Increase Therapeutic," *New England Journal of Medicine*, no. 7 (August 16, 1979):390.

50. Michael Glenn, "Social Security Increases a Mirage?" *New England Journal of Medicine*, no. 21 (November 29, 1979):1242.

51. "Change Looms for Social Security," *Geriatrics*, no. 1 (January 1978) :15–16.

52. Cohen, pp. 194–5.

53. Estes, pp. 76–117.

54. Estes, p. 86.

55. Silverstone and Hyman, p. 158.

56. *Statistical Abstract*, p. 341.

57. Estes, p. 87.

58. Kerschner and Hirschfield, pp. 365–6.

59. Estes, p. 87.

60. Kerschner and Hirschfield, p. 369.

61. Silverstone and Hyman, p. 158.
62. Ibid., pp. 158–60.
63. Ibid., p. 166.
64. Judith M. Feder, *Medicare: The Politics of Federal Hospital Insurance* (Lexington, Mass.: Lexington Books, 1977), p. 1.
65. Erwin Wilkin, *The Impact of Medicare* (Springfield, Ill.: Charles C. Thomas, 1971), pp. 3–50.
66. Kerschner and Hirschfield, p. 359.
67. Feder, p. 1.
68. Kerschner and Hirschfield, pp. 358–9.
69. Silverstone and Hyman, pp. 162–3.
70. Marguerite Mancini, "Medicare: Health Rights of the Elderly," *American Journal of Nursing* 79, no. 10 (October 1979):1810.
71. Kerschner and Hirschfield, pp. 359–60.
72. Silverstone and Hyman, p. 162.
73. Ibid.
74. Mancini, p. 1810.
75. Silverstone and Hyman, p. 165.
76. Ibid., p. 166.
77. Mancini, p. 1810.
78. Kerschner and Hirschfield, p. 359.
79. Silverstone and Hyman, p. 163.
80. Wilkin, pp. 40–53, 127–9.
81. Ibid., pp. 127–9.
82. A. J. Celebrezze, *The Older American* (Washington, D.C.: U.S. Government Printing Office, 1963), pp. 14–15.
83. N. S. Hartunian, C. N. Smart, and M. S. Thompson, "The Incidence and Economic Costs of Cancer, Motor Vehicle Injuries, Coronary Heart Disease and Stroke: A Comparative Analysis," *American Journal of Public Health* 70, no. 12 (1980):1249.
84. Feder, p. 156.

Part II

Management of the Health Promotion and Maintenance Service

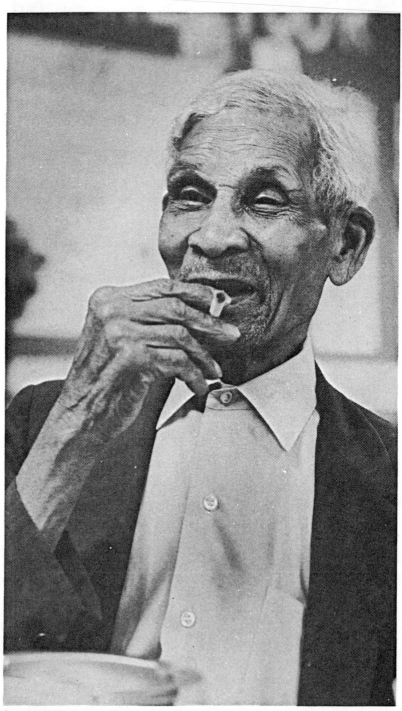

Courtesy Albuquerque News

Chapter 6

Ambivalence: The Stigma of Aging, The Crippler of Attitudes

Dianna Shomaker

HISTORICAL DEVELOPMENT

International

Several consequences of aging have been recognized, and its victims have been subjected to denunciation throughout history. Some of these consequences include physical deterioration, with its loss of youthful beauty and vigor; mental deterioration, which robs a person of memory and reasoning acuity, and thus of autonomy; and social deterioration, which creates a change in position and status in family and society. There is ample evidence that growing old has been distasteful to many people, but not always consistently. Reactions to the deterioration vary according to legal and cultural rules and rituals.

A circularity exists among the mental constructs of prejudice, attitude, ambivalence, and stereotyping, regardless of the subject. The effect of this tendency may be either positive or negative,[1] but in all cases the way a person, group, or object is perceived influences subsequent behavior in relationship to it.[2] Ambivalence and stereotyping pervade all aspects of living and are usually integral parts of attitudes.

The ambivalence springs from lack of clarity in feelings toward old people. Widespread misinformation gives rise to support of erroneous attitudes based on half-truths and prejudices.[3] These are learned early in life, are subject to secular influences, and change throughout history.[4,5]

Attitudes are "predispositions to respond toward a person . . . in either a positive or negative way."[6] On the other hand, a stereotype is "a set of beliefs which purport to describe typical members of a category of people, objects or ideas. These beliefs are then acted upon as if they were true, regardless of the empirical facts."[7]

In 1979, Crockett, Press, and Osterkamp reported that in today's society age is a deciding factor in how a person's behavior is perceived. That is, "an older person who is alert, interesting, and involved is perceived as deviating from stereotyped expectations and is evaluated more positively than a younger person who exhibits these same characteristics."[8] Many report that elderly who are friends, relatives, or acquaintances are often seen as exceptions to the stereotypic norm society has projected upon the older population.[9] This willingness to accept tacitly stereotypes of the elderly is far from being a modern result of urbanization and industrialization. However, for those viewing aging today, it appears to have intensified, largely because there is a greater elderly population in which to observe the aging phenomena.

Philosophies of the past included the older person, but there were so few elderly that it was seldom necessary for philosophy to be manifested in everyday life. Population was held in check by famine, wars, and disease so that older people were simply an occasional byproduct of the times.[10] The ambivalence toward growing older varies within cultures and across time. It is never static or consistent. In ancient history, for example, the aged seemed to maintain an important place in Chinese, Indian, and Chaldean cultures, but those were culturally stable, unadaptable societies. As they changed, so did the position of the elderly.[11]

The concept of humanism developed in Greece, and aging was one of the basic factors within it. It was also in Greece where the hiatus between youth and aging was identified as the difference of acme and nadir, contrasting the two extremes of a continuum. Greek literature presents an idealistic image of the older person, as modeled by Nestor in Homer's *Iliad:* wise and noble, distinguished among chiefs.[12] Sparta was ruled by a council of men over 60 who held their posts until death. It was termed the *gerusia.*[13] This image of the wise elder was defended and dramatized by authors and poets such as Plato and his followers, but then rejected by the Aristotelian thinkers who succeeded them. Traits such as wisdom and usefulness were countered with those of cynicism and hesitation. Even Plato advanced some qualifications on the tenure of ruling groups, perhaps because of abuses of the *gerusia.*[14] So the ambivalence continued. "The plays of Sophocles, Euripides and Aeschylus firmly support the notion that there existed in Greece a genuine and wholesome relationship between aging men and youths."[15] But Aristotle countered with the pessimistic notion that many old people were not sure of anything, and they added qualifiers to their decisions and made emotional responses that diluted their strength.[16] "Greek comedy offers a ruthless exposure to the unpleasant physical symptoms of old age . . . and a calculated disregard of those aspects . . . which are honored, exalted and glorified."[17] On the other hand, Cicero, a Roman, praised the attributes of growing older if individuals were willing to groom their growth and not lament lost youth.

This series of contradictions further demonstrates the historic precedents of ambivalence toward aging and the aged. "Bacon and Shakespeare followed Aristotle in disparaging old age and their near contemporaries in the 17th century America followed Cicero in their veneration of old age."[18] Aging seems to assume a dialectic quality. Authors and citizens spoke of the need for experience and knowledge, which the mind of the elderly could provide, and at the same time scientists were searching for means of rejuvenating youthful beauty and physical vigor. There was a burgeoning of scientific curiosity about the ambivalence regarding aging. People had both the urge to live and the fear of death, a desire for wisdom without relinquishing youth and vigor.

In the early nineteenth century, Jean Jacques Fazy coined the word "gerontocracy" to describe the French government in a political critique of the aging parliament with a negatively described age-related set of behaviors.[19] The position of the elderly in the esteem of others has continued its decline until today it is crippled by the acceptance of stereotypes and public ambivalence.

National

By 1890, the hiring practices in the industrialized United States had turned a cool shoulder to virtually everyone over 40 years of age. Children filled jobs in the cities that once employed their fathers. In 1905, the prominent physician William Osler publicly declared his disdain for the older population by elaborating on the comparative uselessness of people over 40, and the absolute uselessness of people over 60. He maintained that the greatest mental creativity was accomplished between the time a person turned 25 and 40. Anything and anyone beyond that demarcation were not particularly noteworthy. The loss of esteem for the older person received even greater perpetuation when Teddy Roosevelt removed all older men from the Navy and the Rough Riders, replacing them with younger men, who were often naive and ill-equipped by comparison.[20]

This national image of uselessness of the aged was reflected in U.S. international policy as well. The immigrant policy was reinterpreted to exclude those people of marginal use, as Roosevelt planned "a resurgence of national strength and productivity"[21] that required strong young workers. Older immigrants were refused passage from foreign countries by U.S. directive or were turned back at Ellis Island. The mechanism for such a policy "surfaced in 'tests' of literacy, work skills, health and employability."[22] Many immigrants were unable to meet such standards, and by 1927 persons over 45 years of age seeking entry to the U.S. had dropped to nine percent of the total.

The foreign elderly were not the only population that felt the sting of ambivalence and stereotypic rebuke. It was internally directed at elderly U.S. citizens as well. Tibbits maintains that this declining esteem progressed to derogatory stereotypes that influenced legislation, housing policy, and many programs funded through the government.[23] By 1971, the White House Conference on Aging mounted an attack against damaging stereotypes and called for recognition of physical and cognitive capacities among the elderly. In 1977, according to Tibbits, there was a request to accord the older citizens a place in a new value system with a functional relationship internalized in support systems, leisure, education, and work.[24] This followed the work of Butler in which he identified the theme of bigotry against the older population as comparable with those of racism and sexism in potency. He termed it "age-ism."[25] Age-ism is discrimination against people because they have survived to old age. It transcends ethnic boundaries and sex, and is incorporated into housing policy, hiring practices, forced retirement, and economic accessibility, which creates an inhuman limbo perpetuated by the folklore of fearful propagators.[26] It is inculcated in hostile humor and derogatory labels, reinforced by cultural attitudes and stereotypes. It appears to stem from younger people's insecurity when confronted with persons or groups who, to them, symbolize powerlessness, disability, and deterioration.[27] It creates the greatest loss of all for the aged by stripping them of their freedom of choice.[28]

MECHANISM OF DEVELOPMENT OF AMBIVALENCE

The fear engendered in the concept perpetuates itself in what Meyerhoff describes as "insidious circularity" through a cycle of ignorance, denial, fear, rejection, guilt, avoidance, and ignorance.[29] The anxiety is built on the concern for quality, or lack of quality, in the future. A person may wonder if the pattern of care given to the preceding generation will become the standard offered to him or her.

Once the old have been identified in a negative profile, the message seems to become internalized and nationalized, and both young and old seem to accept it. Even the advocates of the elderly, who are usually younger and who set up programs to help them, accept large portions of it. Their public spokespersons usually arise among the young, preretirement population. Although they are linked with the elderly by a common cause and possess the facts to destroy the negative profile and stereotypes, the spokespersons often subtly accept the proposition that the elderly are "least capable, least healthy, and least alert." They explain a seeming paradox by insisting the elderly are also a heterogeneous population and that the majority of those known to the advocate are exceptions to the image.[30] Further, it has been suggested that these very advocates unwittingly use negative stereotypes for their cause in developing programs for the elderly, representing them as helpless and dependent, with little concern for damage that might be done to their own constituents' freedom and autonomy or for older persons' need to choose their course of living.[31] This same author postulates two failure models that grow out of this pattern of ignoring others' right to individuality.

The first is the "incompetence model" in which the older citizens are referred to as a homogeneous group of helpless individuals. This model is often the basis for funding of programs and research. The plea is for money to correct the deficiencies in and improve the quality of life for the elderly, and hence the basic tenor of society. This approach is not unique to those seeking funds for the elderly. Statistical objectivity for accounts of famine, deaths, resources, and so on are often clouded with subjectivity. People seem more willing to accept negative "facts" than positive ones, especially where funding is in competition. Funding is offered to study, correct, or abate the travail of the miserable, oppressed, poor, disadvantaged, and declining, but organizations simply do not fund those causes that already have been resolved.

Negative stories are believable and tragic. People want disservice and injustice corrected. Moreover, it appears that

> "many people have a propensity to compare the present and the future with an ideal state of affairs rather than with the past or with some other feasible state; the present and the future inevitably look bad in such a comparison. . . ."[32]

Even though advocates using the incompetence model produce resources and programs useful to a portion of the elderly, their words are often as damaging to self-esteem as "those who damn with benign neglect" and ageism, creating a sense of failure among the elderly.[33]

The second model, the "geriactivist model," posits rigid standards that also are often unattainable, leaving the elderly in a position of not being able to win as individuals. Proponents of this philosophy see little reasonable purpose in sitting quietly enjoying only conversation and television; they maintain that quality is only given to retirement years through activity and involvement in the community. If such a challenge is rejected, a person is a failure at growing old. This extremist model ignores personal choices and internal control of self, ultimately increasing powerlessness and anger, and minimizing self-esteem.

The negative consequences of inertia are minimized by exposing older people to increased stimulation. To increase self-sufficiency while preventing excessive disability and infantilism among sedentary elderly seems to be a worthy goal, but the approach may be excessively harsh and critical. There are elderly who have internalized the message that they are ill and have extended the concept to all manner of activity. They have created disability where none actually exists.

It is this disservice that needs the attention, not that of the quiet satisfaction of leisure. Sorting the two sedentary extremes has been the difficulty. For those who have created excessive disability through withdrawal, isolation, and inactivity, a more demanding and stimulating environment will negate some of the consequences established, create less helplessness, and increase conscious awareness of physical needs and capabilities.[34] To those who have achieved this level of awareness and who maintain autonomy, the ultimate implementation of a geriactivist approach has the potential to damage a person's self-esteem. The geriactivist argues that inertia is a consequence of the aging process. Decline and improvement are possible but tend to follow previously established patterns; people do not fall into inert states because they pass a prescribed number of years.

Palmore's study in 1963 concluded that there is a high positive correlation between the attitudes and activities of older people.[35] That is, decrease in activities is reflected in decreased satisfaction. He demonstrated a definitive tendency for persistence of life-long behavior patterns of activities and attitudes, finding no evidence of increasing rigidity or differentiation. The concept and process of ageism harbors a deeply embedded thorn of ambivalence.

Who should care for older persons? Moreover, how should others interact with them? Inhibition of open honesty and feelings preserves the ambivalence. There is an admonition to "honor thy father and mother," and to show respect, love, and compassion, but personalities are not always honorable or lovable, and relationships are not always the result of compatible unions. Also, skill in communication is not always at the fingertips of those involved. The experience of living should allow resolution, but ironically often bars a person from that very goal. The fact that people are biologically linked often does nothing but compound the problem with guilt. Even when persons' universal imperfections are recognized, speaking honestly of feelings about those imperfections brings about personal and cultural implications of failure to care for and love the elderly. "It is fairly easy to talk about aging and older people, but it is more difficult to talk about aging with older people . . . the discussion gets bogged down in explanations, and . . . communication is . . . stopped before it begins."[36] Epstein maintains that patterns of interaction based on these fears and guilt can only be polemic. That is, "while we lack the skill we need to talk to each other, listen to each other, learn to know each other, we are doomed to veer from love to anger, tenderness to hostility, caring to confusion and frustration in our relationships."[37]

The ambivalence, then, is most pointedly demonstrated in the ambiguity of a person's communication skills. Unfortunately this is not unique to a specific group of people. It is seen between all age groups. When continuously practiced, it is difficult to eradicate.[38] Also, with the elderly, there are often more roles between young and old, operating in tandem to confuse the paths of communication.

Humor

One obvious area of ambivalence in communication is the use of humor and joking where the elderly or the aging process may be the butt of the jest. Not only is ambivalence the essence of a joke, but the interpretation of humor as it reflects attitudes about the older age group has been fraught with conflict. The plasticity of humor requires a person to be aware of many levels of meaning, and it has been from this perspective that authors have attacked one another's interpretations of humor and the value of humor in society.

"It is difficult to decide on the social attitude which a joke is conveying."[39] Palmore, Davies, and Richman analyzed large amounts of humor in an attempt to determine attitudes toward the elderly.[40,41,42] Weber and Cameron attacked those analyses in 1978.[43] Then *The Gerontologist* printed a series of rebuttals surrounding the debate. Although these researchers did not agree on methodology or the interpretation and categorization of the humor, there did seem to be consensus that there are many jokes in which the elderly are the brunt. The disagreement arose after attempts to interpret the impact of such jokes. Certainly the motivation for relating such jokes is not to be confused with their cultural value. Davies contended that humor was a form of aggression against a group of outsiders.[44] Palmore supported Davies' position and maintained that prejudice was perpetrated against the elderly through a mask of humor, just as it is against ethnic groups and females.[45] Richman observed that the major value of humor in this instance was not to express negative or positive attitudes, but to express complex attitudes toward complex issues.[46]

The attitude from which a joke issues is a function of a great number of variables that range widely from one person to another. It appears that the interpretation of the joke in relation to the elderly still has need of study. The major question is whether a person's interpretations reflect social implications toward the position of the elderly in society.

While debates continue to rage, positive functions of negative jokes can be found upon which a person can act in advocacy toward the elderly. The subject matter of the jokes can serve a positive purpose. Experience has shown that humor combined with love is often received positively regardless of the message, while humor devoid of love and warmth is sarcastic and negative. It is this double-edged message of ambivalence that turns humor either therapeutic or destructive. Negative jokes can convey malice and negative attitudes, but they can also become a vehicle for social change pointing out areas of injustice and insensitivity that cultural patterns have imposed on the elderly.[47] They can be barometers of the discrepancy between the cultural expectations of elderly behavior and those of the elderly individual. On the other hand, they can serve as reminders that all people must be aware of self-acceptance of age-appropriate tasks, and must recognize potential areas of personal growth.

Further, jokes can point out misplaced values in society. In addition, as with ethnic and religious groups for example, persons within the group often initiate negative humor as a self-critical tool.

Research

Research into empirical documentation of various attitudes toward aging began to evolve in the late 1940s and early 1950s. Findings demonstrated an association between aging and the decline of, and disrespect for, the elderly. Research results of the 1960s concluded that certain "social and psychological events became viewed as precursors of aging attitudes . . . and these attitudes assumed a dominant role in the behavior of the elderly."[48] By 1970, attitudinal research instruments were refined to delve further into generalized negative views toward the aged.

Contributions of the older person accomplished in the past were not accorded the same degree of attention and influence as were the prospective contributions of the young today.[49] There are quantifiable differences between attitudes of young and old people. Data of one study presented evidence of a "significant lack of awareness in younger people of potential satisfaction in middle and later years".[50,51] This contrast of age-related attitudes toward what getting old might be like and what it really is like is the basis for many of youth's attitudes toward the older person, and an underestimation of what maturity entails. The older person generally was optimistic toward the years ahead, and perceptions of needs and values took on new interpretations not readily apparent to the younger and less experienced person. This dynamic and positive process is available at any age, but is defined and interpreted by the situation and is difficult to anticipate or project into the future.[52]

The myth that assumes that older people are less open to change than younger people has been empirically denied by Herzog, who concluded that older women do not change their attitudes less than younger women.[53] She studied women of above-average education and found that normally older women were more apt to change their attitudes than were younger women. This coincides with Riegel, whom Herzog reported found "that old people who survive longer are more able, less rigid, less dogmatic, and less negative toward life than are people who die earlier."[54]

The most poignant demonstration of the conflict between age-related attitudes about the older person was in 1962 when Kogan and Shelton identified opposing attitudes between young and old in relation to each other.[55] The older age group strove to maintain independence, but the younger age group assumed their parents would some day become dependent upon them. Additionally, the young felt rejected by the older persons, and the older feared rejection by the younger persons.

Ambivalent attitudes in society-at-large pervade the nature of care provided for the elderly by the professional service providers. Age is a major influence in predicting the attitude a person holds toward working with the elderly. Wolk and Wolk studied professional workers' attitudes toward the aged, and determined that the older worker has a more positive attitude than does the young.[56] That is, the older professional working with older clients holds more positive and fewer negative attitudes than does the younger professional. They tested social workers, medical and nursing students, graduate students, licensed practical and registered nurses, and psychologists. Among most of the participants, experience correlated with attitudes, contrary to the expectations of the investigators. Those service providers who had had positive experiences in their early primary contacts with the elderly demonstrated a more positive attitude toward them. The attitudes of student nurses either improved or remained positive if they worked with "well-elderly" first and later with "ill-elderly," giving them the opportunity to learn and understand healthy elderly before encountering those with deprivation.[57] Overall, both young and old professionals accepted the negative stereotype of senility and physical deterioration, but the older professional emphasized the need for physical independence, which the younger did not.[58]

In contrast, Gillis rejected the tested hypothesis that nurses over 45 years of age who had had more than nine years of experience as RNs in a hospital would have more positive attitudes toward aging.[59] In fact, this was initially true but declined after two years of experience with the elderly. Many people have noted problems among service providers that make adequate care for the elderly increasingly difficult to obtain. Studies have shown that nurses hold negative attitudes toward the elderly, even though they may accept fewer stereotypes about them.[60] In addition, they prefer not to work with the elderly even when offered a pay differential.[61]

Change of attitude is not seen in all professional settings. "When the relationship with the aged is satisfying to the younger workers' needs, we may expect attitudes to shift in a more positive direction."[62] Wilhite and Johnson found that the attitude of nursing students and the degree of change was "functionally related to faculty [members'] attitude toward aged."[63] In contrast, Spence et al., tested first- and fourth-year medical students and discovered that the two classes shared the same conceptions and misconceptions of stereotypes and prejudices against aging.[64] There was a major lack of difference between the two groups. Medical education failed "to mitigate factors injurious to . . . aged patients."[65]

Tuckman and Lorge began a series of studies in 1952 analyzing the degree to which people accepted stereotypes regarding the capabilities of the elderly. In 1959, Solomon and Vickers studied the attitudes of medical students and physicians using the questionnaire developed by Tuckman and Lorge.[66] As with the study by Spence, the attitudes of medical students did not change significantly during their clinical experiences.[67] Another conclusion was that "little change appears to have taken place in attitudes toward the aging over the past 25–30 years since the first publication by Tuckman and Lorge, despite a growth in the volume of literature and personnel devoted to study of aging."[68] Even so, the staff of the geriatric facility that they studied accepted fewer stereotypes, had a greater understanding of elderly persons' needs, and offered greater quality of care. The outstanding finding of the study was in the attitudes of the female housestaff, where the differences were noticeably significant. These women demonstrated an "unusually depersonalizing attitude toward older persons," especially when compared to the female medical students and the female geriatric staff and all male respondents.[69]

Along this same line, Epstein reports that at the National Institute of Mental Health (NIMH) over one-half of the psychiatrists never see aged patients, and those who do spend less than four percent of their available time with them.[70] This is not because the elderly don't need more attention, but because the psychiatrists think nothing can be done for them. Therefore, these stereotyped attitudes perpetuate ambivalent, discriminatory treatment toward the elderly.

Hatton challenges such a conclusion, pointing out the lack of agreement in society as to the nature of barriers to health care for the elderly.[71] Nobody really knows what a desirable attitude toward aging is. On the other hand, it is known that the elderly population is heterogeneous, not homogeneous, with each person needing respect for his or her individual self-esteem and uniqueness.

As with every period of living, this period also has potential for personal growth commensurate with individual resources, limitations, and interests. The task is to facilitate personal growth and that requires improving discretionary attitudes toward the elderly. However, in many schools such as medicine and nursing, the gerontology curriculum content is fragmentary. This is tragic, since students enter school with prejudices and attitudes learned over the years of growing in a particular society. If these students have an insensitive mindset toward the dynamics of aging, their attitudes will trigger poor quality care and support for the client.[72] That is, care will be characterized by such condescending patterns as shouting at those who are not deaf, failing to give adequate time for responses, giving hurried and vague directions, making superficial inquiries into problems, expecting inappropriate responses from clients, interacting with punitive predilections, or not attempting to develop the skill to know the client as a unique human being.[73]

Alberta Hospital in Canada found that if staff members allowed "an old man to hesitate a few moments before answering a question, he received personal validation from his reply."[74] If no time was allowed, the staff felt frustration was precipitated in the old man. Given less-than-effective attitudes toward the elderly, what is required to improve them? Hugh Downs maintains ". . . the motivation lies in realizing who the aging are. And they are *us*, all of us. Short-change the old today, and you short-change yourself tomorrow. There lies the nub of it."[75]

POTENTIAL FOR CHANGE

Fortunately a trend is beginning toward positive change in behavior and attitudes toward services and attention offered the elderly. Progress is slow, and the transition is incomplete as yet. In May 1975, the National League for Nursing (NLN) encouraged increasing gerontological content in basic curriculums and continuing education programs for nurses. This was reinforced by the American Nurses Association (ANA) directive to provide curriculums that will prepare nurses for care of the elderly on the premise that more sensitive attitudes are achieved through increased knowledge and experience.[76]

Ambivalence has pervaded attitudes toward the elderly for centuries, and has been acknowledged and perpetuated by all age groups. Communication between and among age groups is complicated even today by that ambivalence. It is a two-fold problem for both groups to surmount. In the past, refusal to accept the challenge to rise above such obstacles has resulted in lower self-esteem of the older person and has compromised communication between age groups, because "any factor or group of factors that adversely affect the self-concept can have far-reaching effects upon communication."[77] Communication is hampered by conflicting differences in individual estimates of worth, moral code, values, productive power, common interests, sensory capacities, decision making, and education.[78] Because of this, most communication takes place between people who are very close in age, who know each other, and who are in face-to-face contact. There is an inverse ratio between age and communication. The greater the discrepancy, the less conversation.[79] Yet communication is the glue that unifies a society. It is necessary for continuation of a culture. If there is a problem with communication, the continuity of society in its present state of unity is in jeopardy.[80]

If communication between age groups is difficult, it is not surprising that communication between professional service providers and the elderly is difficult. To test the ability of student nurses to communicate with the elderly, a person only needs to restrict conversation based on nursing skills. The difficulty is demonstrated in exponential proportions.

The author imposed this task on junior and senior nursing students during one semester. The ability to draw out sullen, depressed, indifferent clients was more evident when not masked by discussions surrounding nursing tasks. Even with older adults who had little or no health impairment, there was stress that seemed to result from inability to converse because of the vast age separation. Students expressed a feeling of powerlessness in trying to get a conversation moving among clients in nursing homes and at senior citizens' centers. They didn't know what to talk about or how to increase the clients' self-esteem. There often seemed to be an inability to understand how it might be to be older, and that created a communication barrier. The students asked questions, and, once any sort of reply had been received, they would bring the conversation back to themselves, where they felt more secure. The message for self-esteem was "I don't want to talk about you, let's talk about me;" "I am afraid of you;" "I don't understand you;" and "You are different from me." Reciprocal discomfort seemed apparent from the older persons as well, but it was more painful with the students because they were ostensibly training themselves to bridge that communication gap.

Communication between service providers and older clients needs to exist. It needs to be free from stereotypes and negative attitudes, sensitive to needs and worth. "Through belongingness, or being valued, we develop a feeling of self-esteem. We must all justify our existence somehow in order to find meaning in our lives."[81] Older persons have the basic right to ask relevant questions that will allow protection of self and development of new roles.[82] Such questions allow people freedom to be responsible for control and planning of their use of time and potential. But often, elders declare, no one listens to them or cares about their questions. This isolation of the elderly can create stimulus deprivation of all age groups, minimizing even greater sources of communication. Interpersonal interactions increase in proportion to contact with other people, radio, newspaper, and television.[83] Hartford astutely observed that "some disorientation is due to no orientation, that is, lack of stimulating contacts and communication with other people."[84]

Everyone has greater potential than will ever be realized in a lifetime. The secret of maximizing more of that potential through time is to continue learning and interpersonal contacts. However, to avoid the extreme philosophy of the geriactivists, individuals need to recognize that maximizing personal potential is an equally personal philosophy and a pattern of choices made by the client, not by the care provider.[85] Regardless of the depth of such commitment, survival at any level requires meaningful communication, as minimally clouded by stereotypes and negative attitudes as possible within a close circle of friends of varying ages, interests, and backgrounds.[86]

How does a person demonstrate sensitivity for a client's worth and self-esteem? The guidelines are not age-specific, but often fear and ambivalence block application during interaction with the elderly. Most people feel a certain degree of elation when offered praise and recognition. Such interaction, when sincerely offered, increases not only self-esteem but a sense of trust and confidence in a relationship.[87] Opening the channel to share with another is often successful if initiated by sharing things about one's self, followed by questions on the same issues directed to the client. Sharing takes many forms: sharing food, surprises, losses, pain, happiness, humor, and more. All these items are important, and effective interaction requires both parties to recognize and discuss them.

Opening the flow and pace of conversations to greater depth sometimes starts with superficiality but is built on individuality, attention, profuse use of the other person's name, realistic promises, meticulous anticipation of needs that are not verbalized, and clearly defined limits of a relationship. Discussion and closeness are enhanced by emphasis on the importance of birthdays, holidays, and major events, and are assisted by touch, honesty, tact, and predictability.[88] To assert these qualities is not an innate talent. It is a talent to be consciously groomed and perfected throughout each interpersonal contact over time, so that a person learns to deal with sadness and joy, recognize and validate assumptions before acting, and identify realistic assets and liabilities.[89] Implicit in this is a growth in awareness of stereotypes and attitudes. Some people can accomplish this informally; others might prefer using tools such as those Epstein and others have developed, which assist in identifying attitudes and behavior patterns.[90]

For all it should culminate in the rejection of the perjorative word *senility*, which is used by many to refer to the natural common denominator of the aging process.[91] This awakening will also require not only knowledge of the normal but the pathological processes of aging, and the skill to handle dependency, directness, and criticism.[92]

Regardless of the pace and depth of conversation with older clients, there is often a feeling of powerlessness when they lapse into long periods of reminiscence. Current events and news items of the present world are also commonly avoided, thereby dismissing the older persons' opinions as well as experiences as valueless. For many, once this misconception is removed, conversation tends to flow more freely. It can add new dimensions to reminiscing. According to Burnside, reminiscing is not negative in and of itself; it can become a means of improving self-esteem by recognizing accomplishments of the past.[93] It allows an individual to face changing status and physical capacity. It often brings a person up-to-date, and opens thought in a direction aligned with present-day activities. It allows opportunity for order and organization in life, past and present.

Humor is also all too often missing in dealing with older adults. Humor's negative aspects were discussed earlier; it needs recognition for its valuable positive attributes as well. Laughing and joking can either keep people at a distance or encourage closeness and warmth. Older human beings are just that, *older human beings*. They need pleasure in interaction and incidents just as young human beings do. Pleasure is a major need in existing, regardless of age. It is valuable in both praise and criticism.[94] But fear, boredom, and insensitivity often weigh more, keeping humor suppressed. "Sometimes it takes an old person to teach the value of joy and humor."[95] If a person is to find rewards in working with the elderly or anyone else, it is necessary to instill pleasure and humor in work and interaction.

Not only is humor valuable for increasing self-esteem, it is physiologically important for exercise and deeper respiration. Why should good laughs cease to be when a person becomes older; what can bring pleasure in their stead? Why should it be an age-specific deprivation?

In summary, history has carried with it negative and positive attitudes in conflict with one another for the position of the elderly in society. The conflict demonstrates itself not so much in distaste for aging and the problems incumbent upon those enmeshed in that process of longevity, but in the ambivalence people have not been able to rise above. The attitudes have invaded and garbled the communication process both between the elderly and intergenerationally. The results have been ineffective development of people's potential after they reach that vague area termed "old age."

NOTES

1. B. Devine, "Old Age Stereotyping: A Comparison of Nursing Staff Toward the Elderly," *Journal of Gerontological Nursing* 6, no. 6 (1980):26.

2. M. Seltzer and R. Atchley, "The Concept of Old: Changing Attitudes and Stereotypes," Bill Bell, ed., *Contemporary Social Gerontology* (Springfield, Mass.: Charles C. Thomas, 1976), p. 203.

3. C. Epstein, *Learning to Care for the Aged* (Reston, Va.: Reston Publishing Co., 1977), pp. 47–101.

4. Seltzer and Atchley, 1976, p. 203.

5. B. Bell and G. Stanfield, "Chronological Age in Relation to Attitudinal Judgments," Bill Bell, ed., *Contemporary Social Gerontology* (Springfield, Mass.: Charles C. Thomas, 1976), p. 224.

6. Seltzer and Atchley, 1976, p. 203.

7. Ibid.

8. W. Crockett, A. Press, and M. Osterkamp, "The Effect of Deviation from Stereotyped Expectations Upon Attitudes Toward Older Persons," *Journal of Gerontology* 34, no. 3 (1979):368.

9. Ibid.

10. J. Freeman, "Medical Perspectives in Aging (12th to 19th Century)," *The Gerontologist* 5, no. 3 (1965):1–7.

11. Ibid.

12. M. Haynes, "The Supposedly Golden Age for the Aged in Ancient Greece," *The Gerontologist* 2, no. 1 (1962):93.

13. F. Eisele, "Origin of Gerontocracy," *The Gerontologist* 19, no.1 (1979):406.

14. Ibid.

15. Haynes, 1962, p. 94.

16. Ibid.; H. J. Oyer and E. J. Oyer, *Aging and Communication*, (Baltimore, Md.: University Park Press, 1976), p. 4.

17. Haynes, 1962, p. 95.

18. Eisele, 1979, p. 406.

19. Ibid., p. 403.

20. G. Gruman, "Cultural Origins of Present-Day 'Age-ism': The Modernization of the Life Cycle," in S. Spicker, K. Woodward, and D. Van Tassel, eds., *Aging and the Elderly* (Atlantic Highlands, New Jersey: Humanities Press, 1978), pp. 366–9.

21. Ibid., p. 366.

22. Ibid.

23. C. Tibbets, "Can We Invalidate Negative Stereotypes of Aging?" *The Gerontologist* 19, no. 1 (1979):10–20.

24. Ibid.

25. R. Butler, "Age-ism: Another Form of Bigotry," *The Gerontologist* 9, no. 3 (1969):243–6.

26. A. Comfort, *A Good Age* (New York, N.Y.: Simon and Schuster, 1976), p. 35; R. Kalish, "The New Ageism and the Failure Models: A Polemic," *The Gerontologist* 19, no. 4 (1979):398; Butler, 1969:243–6.

27. Epstein, 1977, p. 7; Butler, 1969, p. 243.

28. Butler, 1969, p. 246.

29. B. Meyerhoff, *Number Our Days* (New York, N.Y.: Simon and Schuster, 1978), p. 19.

30. Kalish, 1979, p. 398.

31. Ibid., pp. 398–402.

32. J. Simon, "Resources, Population, Environment: An Oversupply of False Bad News," *Science* 208, no. 4450 (1980):1437.

33. Kalish, 1979, p. 399.

34. Epstein, 1977, p. 13.

35. E. Palmore, "The Effects of Aging on Activities and Attitudes," in V. Brantl and Sr. M. Brown, eds., *Readings in Gerontology* (St. Louis: C. V. Mosby, 1973), pp. 66–69.

36. L. Haak, "A Retiree's Perspective on Communication," in H. Oyer and E. Oyer, eds., *Aging in Aging* (Baltimore, Md.: University Park Press, 1976), p. 19.

37. Epstein, 1977, p. 10.

38. Ibid., p. 8.

39. T. Weber and P. Cameron, "Comment: Humor and Aging—A Response," *The Gerontologist* 18, no. 1 (1978):75.

40. E. Palmore, "Attitudes Toward Aging As Shown by Humor," *The Gerontologist* 11, no. 2 (1971):181–7.

41. L. Davies, "Attitudes Toward Old Age and Aging As Shown by Humor," *The Gerontologist* 17, no. 3 (1977):220–6.

42. J. Richman, "The Foolishness and Wisdom of Age: Attitudes Toward the Elderly as Reflected in Jokes," *The Gerontologist* 17, no. 3 (1977):210–9.

43. Weber and Cameron, 1978, pp. 73–79.

44. L. Davies, "Humor and Aging Restated," *The Gerontologist* 18, no. 1 (1978):76.

45. E. Palmore, "Replies," *The Gerontologist* 18, no. 1 (1978):76.

46. J. Richman, "Replies," *The Gerontologist* 18, no. 1 (1978):77–8.

47. Weber and Cameron, 1978, p. 74.

48. B. Bell, ed., *Contemporary Social Gerontology* (Springfield, Ill.: Charles C. Thomas, 1978), p. 198.

49. Seltzer and Atchley, 1976, pp. 203–4.

50. M. Borges and L. Dutton, "Attitudes Toward Aging," *The Gerontologist* 16, no. 3 (1976):220–4.

51. Ibid., p. 220.

52. Ibid., pp. 221–3.

53. A. Herzog, "Attitude Change in Older Age," *Journal of Gerontology* 34, no. 5 (1979):697–703.

54. Ibid., p. 702.

55. N. Kogan and F. C. Shelton, "Beliefs About Old People," *Journal of Genetic Psychology* 100 (1962):93–111.

56. R. L. Wolk and R. B. Wolk, "Professional Worker's Attitude Toward the Aged," *Journal of the American Geriatric Society* 19, no. 7 (1971):624–39.

57. S. Tobiason, F. Knudsen, J. Stengel, and M. Giss, "Positive Attitudes Toward Aging: The Aged Teach the Young," *Journal of Gerontological Nursing* 5, no. 1 (1979):18–23.

58. Wolk and Wolk, 1971, p. 638.

59. Sr. M. Gillis, "Attitudes of Nursing Personnel Toward the Aged," *Nursing Research* 22 (1973):517–20.

60. N. Kogan, "Attitudes Toward Old People: The Development of a Scale and an Examination of Correlates," *Journal of Abnormal and Social Psychology* 36, no. 1 (1961):44–54; M. Brown, "Nurses' Attitudes Toward the Aged and Their Care," Annual Report to Gerontological Branch, USPHS, Contract No. PH 108–64–122; J. Tuckman and I. Lorge, "Attitudes Toward Old People," *Journal of Social Psychology* 37 (1953):249–60.

61. M. Campbell, "Study of the Attitudes of Nursing Personnel Toward the Geriatric Patient," *Nursing Research* 20, no. 2 (1971):147–51.

62. Wolk and Wolk, 1971, p. 638.

63. M. Wilhite and D. Johnson, "Change in Nursing Students' Stereotypic Attitudes Toward Old People," *Nursing Research* 25, no. 6 (1976):430.

64. D. Spence et al., "Medical Student Attitudes Toward the Geriatric Patient," *Journal of the American Geriatric Society* 16, no. 9 (1968):976–83.

65. Ibid., p. 976.

66. K. Solomon and R. Vickers, "Attitudes of Health Workers Toward Old People," *Journal of the American Geriatric Society* 28, no. 4 (1979):186–91.

67. Spence et al., p. 197.

68. Solomon and Vickers, 1979, p. 190.

69. Ibid., p. 189.

70. Epstein, 1977, pp. 115–44.

71. J. Hatton, "Nurses' Attitudes Toward the Aged: Relationship to Nursing Care," *Journal of Gerontological Nursing*, no. 3 (1977):21–6.

72. C. White, "The Nurse-Patient Encounter: Attitudes and Behaviors in Action," *Journal of Gerontological Nursing* 3, no. 3 (1977):16–20.

73. Epstein, 1977, p. 107.

74. D. Scott and J. Crowhurst, "Reawakening Senses in the Elderly," *Canadian Nurse* 71, no. 10 (1975):21.

75. H. Downs, "Thirty Dirty Lies About Old" (Niles, Ill.: Argus Communication, 1979), p. 158.

76. Tobiason et al., 1979, pp. 18–23.

77. Oyer and Oyer, 1976, pp. 11–12.

78. Ibid.

79. J. Woelfel, "Communication Across Age Levels," in H. Oyer and E. Oyer, eds., *Aging and Communication* (Baltimore, Md.: University Park Press, 1976), p. 68.

80. Ibid., pp. 64–74.

81. J. Ellis and E. Nowlis, *Nursing, A Human Needs Approach* (Boston, Mass.: Houghton Mifflin Co., 1977), p. 36.

82. Haak, 1976, p. 31.

83. Oyer and Oyer, 1976, pp. 6–8.
84. M. Hartford, "Maximizing Your Potential in Aging," *Aging: Today's Research and You* (Los Angeles: USC Press, 1978), p. 57. Lecture series.
85. Ibid., pp. 59–64.
86. Ibid., p. 57.
87. I. Burnside, *Working With the Elderly Group Processes and Techniques* (North Scituate, Mass.: Duxbury Press, 1978), pp. 8, 84, 377.
88. Ibid., pp. 82–4.
89. Ibid.
90. Epstein, 1977, pp. 47–101.
91. Burnside, 1978, p. 95.
92. Ibid., p. 85.
93. Ibid., p. 135.
94. Ibid., p. 90.
95. Ibid.

Chapter 7

Normal Aging: A Challenge to Adaptation

Dianna Shomaker

The concern of this chapter is not with pathology and death, but with living and the normal process of aging. Many articles have expounded on the negative aspects of aging, describing the older population in general as a problem. Recently, there has been a rebuttal that is based on the positive aspects of aging. Each argument has to some degree denied the existence of the other, often in extreme terms, yet the processes they describe operate intertwined in the same organism throughout life, compensating and adapting in myriad means for survival. The decline in certain physiological parameters is inevitable. However, if mental and cultural values are deliberately developed to capacity, reality more and more represents the clarification of past distortions, and a closer examination of the use of compensation and adaptation to emphasize positive potentials.

What follows is an examination and description of normal aging in relationship with psychological, social, and cultural challenges facing the elderly, and the normal changes in the physiology of a person as aging continues. The emphasis will, in all areas discussed, be toward means of adaptation and compensation, because energy is better spent concentrating on those areas of aging in which potential for positive development exists. Where negative change is inevitable it must be recognized, but full importance must be given to areas in which positive change is within an individual's capability.

PHYSIOLOGICAL AGING

Longevity varies among species, and there is a range unique to each species, which suggests genetic control as a major factor.[1] Biological processes that appear to play major roles in determining longevity are those related to progressive accumulations of mutations in the DNA of cells, decline in immune surveillance, increase in free radicals, and crystallization of collagen fibrils, along with the life-long functional structure of the cells' mechanism.[2,3] The implication is that biological influence for change takes place over time as a gradual and multifaceted complex. Many of the changes are predictable, and new norms of stability are established, and then passed, as an individual ages. These are predictable through laboratory tests of blood sugar, hormone levels, blood protein, pH, blood volume and pressure, heart rate, and more.[4] All values are influenced by stress and disease, and may be inaccurately measured for old persons. Other physical changes are readily observable, for example, wrinkles, graying, balding, slowing gait, voice change, posture change, physical redistribution of fat, and muscle changes. Attempts have been made to quantify physical changes as a measure of the rate of aging, but the task is far more complex in mature than in younger people. Borkan and Norris report the possibility that many "biological ages" may be manifest in one individual, and suggest that even those persons who look older than their chronological age might very well have a wide range of physiological measures.[5]

"Aging is expressed not in individual cells but in cell lineages."[6] It is the function within the cell and the sequence of cells that influences the efficiency of the body in relationship to aging. For example, a red blood cell has a life span of about 120 days. The cell acts as an energy factory, which is a key role in the life process of the organism, and maintains oxygen transfer and hydration. These cells, through the proteo-glycan protein molecules contained in them, bind water in the body, which prevents drying or dehydration. All such molecules are constantly being replaced, but the rate of replacement slows with age. This slower turnover rate results in a reduced ability to bind water, causing drying of the cells.[7]

The homeostatic balance of the body is maintained by compensating changes in structure and demands. Many gerontologists postulate the aging mechanism is genetically controlled, and this has been the basis for theories about faulty enzyme support of cell ability, "aging genes" that slow biochemical pathways, and accumulation of genetic errors and subsequent physiologic changes that have come to represent aging.[8] However, the body's water content changes throughout life, and it is not clear how significant that fact is in comparing young and older persons. Goldstein and Reichel report that deviation from norms based on young adults is much less marked when allowances are made for "the relative gain in adipose tissue, with its low water content and relatively inert metabolism."[9] Reviewing this literature does not clarify the hazards of using standards of laboratory tests across age groups, but it does suggest some degree of inaccuracy that needs to be understood and corrected. Age-corrected standards in many laboratory tests of body function will have to be established before normalcy itself is established or deviation can be declared in any interpretation.[10]

Aging is accompanied by bone loss that creates thinner-walled but larger bones. The loss can be as great as 20 percent in postmenopausal women, but this loss is an orderly parallel with other changes in the rest of the body. Cardiac output, muscle mass, and body weight also decline in about the same proportion. Why would a person need constant bone mass when there is decreasing muscle mass? Problems arise when people abuse their bodies rather than recognize a need for adaptation to a new norm. The reaction to lessened muscle mass often appears to be denial, in which the body is forced to perform at the level the person expected when much younger. Another segment of this advanced age population recognizes such changes and interprets them as a signal of the end of life. These persons give up and hasten the decline toward death. Another problem arises when older people are overweight, and rely on thinner bones with smaller, weaker muscles than before.[11]

Bad nutritional habits and poor exercise patterns can jeopardize not only posture but the efficiency of other body systems. These two major areas need to be understood by both the elderly and by service providers if the dangers of fad diets and inactive or sporadic activity patterns are to be avoided. To exchange strength for another ability is the positive message an individual must understand, and the course that person must pursue. The past can be effectively used to prepare for and enlarge the present. It is worthless for a person to pine for what was and thereby hinder development of new skills. Such activity is not only inconvenient and destructive, it is a shortsighted expression of work. ". . . 'tis neither by bodily strength, nor swiftness, nor agility, that momentous affairs are carried on, but by judgement, counsel and authority; the abilities for which are so far from failing in old age, that they truly increase with it."[12]

Over time, height has been influenced both by the aging process and by the increases whereby a person can gain "fuller achievement of one's genetic potential."[13] The average height of humans has increased during the twentieth century primarily due to better nutrition. However, this influence is minimized by the time an individual reaches middle age. Older persons most often decline two to four inches in height. Body height and arm span are nearly equal in younger adults, but after about the fifth decade of life, a person's span measurement remains relatively constant while the height declines. This is due to bone loss in the matrix, decline in size of fibroelastic disks between the vertebrae, erosion of the articular processes of the bones, and decrease in muscle mass and elasticity, which allows some stooping or bowing of postural attitude.[14,15]

There is also a decrease in respiratory capacity with aging—approximately 30 percent—paralleling the decrease in other systems. This is partly due to normal decrease in muscle strength.[16] Involution of other tissues in the body is similar to that seen in muscles, and often these changes are associated with a decrement in protoplasmic mass and an increment in connective tissue and fat deposits.[17]

The body gives messages of the need for role change as it ages. In some ways the involutionary messages of some systems come much later in life than those of the senses. The renal, cardiovascular, and respiratory systems in normal healthy adults are examples of such delay, and any failure in capacity is not evident until stress is introduced beyond maximum endurance. In many instances it is a multifaceted process whereby decreasing muscle strength and circulation compromise the body reserves of the elderly.

If body functions are analyzed during exercise, it is evident that there is need for additional oxygen, nutrients, and elimination of metabolic waste. These are obtained through increase in flow of respiration and blood. Among the elderly, these demands often result in higher blood pressure, heart rate, and lung function. Decreased muscle strength minimizes the body responses and results in restricted muscular work. "For the older individuals to provide enough oxygen to sustain the increased activity of exercising muscles, they must move 50 percent more air in and out of the lungs than their younger counterparts."[18]

The eye and ear involute early and decline rapidly, requiring compensation for speed of accommodation, dark adaptation, critical flicker, and auditory function.[19] For many, this entails use of greater wattage and diffusion in lighting, allowing longer time to adjust to change in lighting, and change in distance and depth. For others, compensation comes from reading glasses. Hearing is often impaired in the higher frequencies by the age of 50, especially in the ability to discern consonants. The most satisfactory method for dealing with this problem, aside from hearing aids, is for persons to lower their voices and face the impaired with lips in clear view in a good light, and to speak slowly and clearly.

To many the ultimate indicators of aging are the skin and hair, that is, the degree of gray hair, absence of hair, or the number of wrinkles. Alteration in appearance is due to subcutaneous fat loss, decreased pigmentation, and lessened blood supply to the skin. Many older persons are believed erroneously to display pallor due to these factors. Most age-associated skin changes are not life threatening, but the damage is mainly to the self-esteem of the older person. In this youth-beautiful society, many fear the outward signs of aging demonstrated in the skin. Older persons also have pride and are concerned about their appearance, and changes in interaction are noted when less touch is offered to wrinkled persons than to younger persons. Sublimation often comes through grandchildren. With the attention and criticism our youth orientation has generated, wrinkles may some day be considered beautiful in their own right.

Changes in the structural function of the skin create a need for creams to alleviate itching due to decreased oil glands and massage to prevent pressure sores that often occur with less fat and peripheral circulation. Clothing has to be more consciously selected to compensate for changes in peripheral circulation, insulation, and the number of sweat glands, all of which cause greater sensitivity to cold.

If and when there is physiological decline, it is often not the direct result of age change. Moderate exercise improves the functioning of the body and often reverses physiological decline that accompanies disuse or sedentary life style.[20] Deterioration need not be fixed and irreversible. So convincing was the statement that aging constituted deterioration that until recently no one challenged the permanency of such changes. Two areas in which the conventional opinions have been challenged are EEG alpha rhythm changes and reaction time. Two of the exciting prospects in the literature are Woodruff's query into the reversibility of certain physiological age-related EEG changes, and others' attempts to study reaction time.[21,22] With biofeedback, positive improvements have occurred in alpha rhythms of brain activity. Reaction time can be increased, although its decline from the levels of youth cannot be fully eradicated. DeVries maintains that in certain situations the older person's percentage of improvement is roughly equivalent to that of the young, although the older person starts from lower achievement levels.[23]

A message that recurs throughout Woodruff and Birren's work is that stimulation or lack of a necessary level of it might well account for diminishing levels of physiological function and related behavior changes.[24] The question they ask is whether these changes are inevitable, and if so, is the rate of decline hastened by the assumption of such inevitability? In some areas they have demonstrated diminution or reversal of such decline. One manner of improving physiological change is through improving the psycho-socio-cultural aspects of the older adult.

AGING IN PSYCHOLOGICAL AND SOCIAL CONTEXT

There may be no such thing as normal aging. Perhaps those elderly who are happy and achieve greater longevity are merely exceptions to a widely-held concept of aging. The literature describes the aging process primarily in negative terms: decrement, decline, decay, and deterioration, and this negativity becomes a stereotype from which death appears the only escape. Is that the process authors refer to as "normal aging?" The implication is that there are no positive changes, functions, or forward movement.

However, there is little biological basis to indicate a general and inexorable loss of competence. Negative periods in other phases of growth, development, and maintenance not only allow for change to a more positive norm, but are not viewed as negating immediate competence. So often is this negative finality expressed that it is difficult to separate the results of the normal process of aging from pathologic effects.

Moreover, the validity of the collective concept of aging is confounded by the use of norms established to determine the capacity to function that are appropriate only for younger people, and that leave no meaningful criteria for "old-age."[25] For example, drug dosages and their elimination rates are established for persons who are younger and have different patterns of adaptation. Further, laboratory tests, until recently, were almost entirely measured against younger age cohort results. Probably most significantly, working ability and beauty standards are also measured against a norm established during youth.

It is difficult to dissociate normal aging and pathology. Experts are not certain whether the progress of natural aging processes or of disease are being measured when categorizations of "aging" are attempted, and the pathology of aging has received the lion's share of recognition in the literature. It is equally difficult to determine the onset of "aging." In attempting to determine the boundaries of shared traits among older adults, a person runs the risk of stereotyping, as well as of overgeneralizing the onset and rate of the aging process. Unfortunately, the genetic, sexual, and cultural differences among people are commonly minimized, and the effects of these influences are not fully taken into account in descriptions of the aging process. In spite of these problems, investigators have continued to attempt the definition of aging.

Aging is a natural process that brings changes in physiology at the level of molecules and cells, as well as in the psychological and sociocultural parameters of an individual's existence. Aging is a passage of time, which, though described in chronological terms, is a process involving time, the application of stress, and continuous drain on an organism's resources. Implied in these factors is continuous change in function of the organism in response to stress and the availability of resources.

Physiologists maintain that aging is part of a growth, development, and aging continuum. These events have their onset with fertilization and their termination with death. Chronological age and physiological age rarely seem to coincide because of the constant, dynamic interaction of genetic composition and environmental impact. Biologists, similarly, adduce that biological aging is the sum total of all changes in the living organism through time and leads inevitably to functional impairment and death. Both definitions insist on a beginning and end of the process regardless of how the stages are defined in sequence or in terms of time.[26]

The core of the problem appears to be this: how may that aging process beyond the end of procreative functioning be defined in such a way as to recognize decreasing ability to survive stress, and to measure against appropriate norms of functioning, not the norms of disuse and inability?

Even in light of the numerous theories of aging, there is a positive, holistic potential for creativity and development. This fact is commonly overlooked. The second half of life has not been expanded merely to wait out death with a sense of doom and uselessness. Both definitions of aging, that is, that of growth cessation posited by physiologists and the other of declining functional ability advanced by biologists, assume aging has its genesis in the developmental stage of life. That in turn suggests if quality and quantity are to be added to longevity, it is advisable to start early. It also suggests that uselessness can be avoided to some degree if talents are developed during the life-sequence. In this context, aging is inseparable from the developmental processes of life and, in the absence of disease, is imperceptibly imposed upon the individual.[27]

In the past, when life spans were short, the purpose and pattern of existence were concentrated upon the procreative function. Increasing longevity has given rise to pondering the use of years beyond perpetuation of genes. The first 20 years of life are given to growth and development of the body and preparing the individual for survival. The next 20 years are spent developing and reflecting upon new ideas and raising children. What lies beyond these four decades?

It seems logical that this becomes a new stage of growth where other potentials should be mastered, realized, and developed. This concept is not new. Many seem reluctant to attempt it however. Cicero, in his discourse on old age, urged his readers to recognize change and encourage the talents of the new prospects offered. In a positive reflection, he developed an argument for those old who are willing and able to develop abilities and skills of the mind. For this there is little need for muscle strength as much as there is a call for the prudence of age to counsel and temper the rashness of youth.

If only strength is valued, then the whole of humankind is gone, and there is little left but to await death. However, those who age successfully are those who are active; who continue to apply abilities; who continue to improve through taking every opportunity to improve the self.[28] In short, in the words of Cicero:

> . . . while you have strength, use it; when it leaves you, no more repine for want of it, than you did when lads, that your childhood was past; or at the years of manhood, that you were no longer boys . . . old age in its maturity, has something natural to itself, that ought particularly to recommend it.[29]

Centuries later, the literature reflects similar admonitions to society to allow the elderly options and support as they approach old age. Where the elderly will accept it, there is a definite need for life-long education as a deterrent to obsolesence, as a preparation for other careers, and for greater use of the elders' full intellectual potential.[30]

According to many psychological studies, the pattern established in early years reflects the pattern followed in later years. That is, a person who is unmotivated, dependent, negative, wishful, or habitually dissatisfied will continue those traits into old age. A dependent child will be more satisfied if married to someone on whom he or she can depend and, upon reaching maturation or old age, will expect others to take responsibility for his or her care. In contrast, an innovative "maverick" child will probably be difficult to hold down during the future stages of living. Cicero observed that a person's internal or psychological composition developed during youth is the servant to old age. Those who have not cultivated a means of easing stress will find life irksome and happiness elusive regardless of age.[31] The studies of personality and its relationship to longevity and the quality of life in those postprocreative years suggest that an element of Darwinism can be recognized among older survivors. Not only is it more likely that the fittest will survive the longest, but this dyad of fitness and longevity is correlative with role flexibility and the creativity implied by the concept.[32]

Adaptation

Adaptation is the major mechanism for survival. Some demands for adaptation accrue over generations, while others are merely the result of stress in a single lifetime.[33] The desired norm is to maintain a homeostatic balance within the mechanisms for adaptation, while courting the needs and purposes of the body over time. According to Timiras: "In the final analysis, the continuing ability to adapt depends more on the individual's capacity to reappraise and readjust the hierarchy of steering and self-regulatory mechanisms in response to stress than on the fixed and unchanging efficiency of any single organ or system."[34] Functional competence is, then, the ability of the dynamic organism to interact with its environment for the success of the total being, requiring continual adaptation and resolution of stresses.

Change is inevitable, but it is unique to every individual in both degree and rate. Not only are there organ changes over time, there are changes in performance that are not always consistent or uniform. Not all tissue begins to involute at the same time. These changes increase the challenge of successful adaptation. Physiological reserves are reduced in the cell capacity. It is a differential rate of change in organs that reduces their earlier coordination and precision in interrelated functions.[35] Reduced reserves often are only evident when an individual experiences severe stress. Often the adaptation creates a new norm in functioning ability, which is misconstrued as decline or inability rather than change to a new norm and need.

Change is not necessarily fatal. Timiras asserts that stress may not "fatally challenge the body's tolerance, but functional decrements of old age may increase the frequency with which stresses are experienced."[36] However, there is an exponential increase in the probability that the capacity of the body will be exceeded. Death is not due to old age, but to the failure to meet the challenge of stress as it increases with longevity.[37]

Spirituality

Greater depth can be added to a person's existence through consideration and development of the individual's philosophy of life. A person finds a basis for evaluation of self-worth, significance of life, and means of coping from personal philosophy, and it is necessary to sense dignity and quality in life as daily change in society and self are confronted. Old age of itself is not especially honorable.[38] In fact, the value of life in Western civilization is often validated through theosophy and the tenets of religion. This approach helps people recognize their worth as beings. Western religion is a strand of philosophy that might be analyzed in this context. According to the Judeo-Christian principles, a human "is more than what he [or she] does."[39] That is, "one's worth transcends accomplishments."[40] In a society based on consumerism and the work ethic, a person's worth tends to be measured by production, achievement, and upward mobility, implying an economic basis for a perception of aging.[41] On the other hand, a positive religious philosophy offers a means by which this economic, work-oriented aspect can be expanded to recognize the value of the lives of those who are no longer financially productive.

Religion emphasizes dynamic change and growth for all age groups, including those beyond significant economic contribution.[42] Time is spent reflecting on the significance of the past as a guide to the future of life.

There is a need for living fully in the present, without irrevocably giving up the past. Acceptance of things past as having been necessary allows for successful coping to maintain integrity in planning today and tomorrow. Through religious philosophy ". . . the particularity and peculiarity of one's own life can be undertaken with an added measure of hope."[43] As in the discussion of other sociocultural influences, religious philosophy suggests ". . . the appreciation of the open-endedness of both personal and social development . . . toward full human maturity."[44] That is, practical religion today reflects upon truth, relevance, and the meaning of life, and so offers guidance for everyday practical actions. It thus offers a counteraction to the stagnation of older lives created by social forces in Western society.[45]

There is conflict in reports about the importance of religion in later years. Moberg maintains that those who have religion praise it and attest to its increased value parallel to aging.[46] Those who do not consider themselves religious deny any positive effects from its consideration. However, older people are more apt to belong to a church than any other type of organization. Religious values, as with all other cultural and social values, vary from one individual to another. For some, religion will enhance their lives, while for others it will not only offer little strength for coping, it will serve as a distraction.[47] But for both, in some ways, it is a demonstration of a means by which "Western civilization has attempted to give expression to its awareness of the potentially positive dimension of aging."[48]

Larue emphasizes the effect of religious concepts on patterns and attitudes of daily living.[49] The importance and emphasis of religion in a person's life can often change as readily as with those people who have other values, and they also vary among individuals and religious philosophies. Those in good health and who have already achieved considerable longevity often claim it is a reward for their faith, while others in pain and agony may grieve over past misdeeds and the resultant punishment. For some, religious belief in life after death offers solace and assurance; for others it invokes fear. Still others see it as an escape from misery.

The practical problems of the older person in organized religion also vary. Church activities are often segregated by age and sex where common interests and attitudes prevail, and often the groups are for younger adults with little regard for the needs of the elderly. Although churches appear to be reawakening to the needs of older parishioners, for those who have found religion a sustaining force throughout their entire lives, the needs have not diminished, and there is often no older age group in which to share concerns. Attempts to cross age boundaries to join a younger group are not always comfortable for the elderly. Where groups have been formed, there is not always a concerted effort to focus on the positive and on improving individuals' potential. Instead the focus is often on their debilities, an action that is "demoralizing and downright poisonous."[50]

In the present context, religion should be considered in broader terms than that of organized denominations. The concept of religious belief is important in every known society,[51] and the religious network is made up of many elements: economic, political, social, physical, and cultural. Extradomiciliary activity surrounding religion decreases as people age and lose the ability to be mobile. Moberg has observed that this creates difficulty in carrying out participation in religion, but a compensating factor is demonstrated in a more devout and intense spirit of religious philosophy.[52] Berghorn et al. support this theory, with speculation that loss of spouse and money, which so often accompany aging, are compensated for by religiosity. That is, the extent of religious belief increases with social isolation.[53] In turn, if aging people are religious ". . . the faith that sustained them in dark moments of the past, perhaps defensively, is now an enjoyable cosmology that beautifies and validates their present days."[54]

NOTES

1. Samuel Goldstein and William Reichel, "Physiological and Biological Aspects of Aging," W. Reichel, ed., in *Clinical Aspects of Aging* (Baltimore, Md.: Williams & Wilkins, 1978), pp. 430–1.
2. Ibid., pp. 430–3; Paola S. Timiras, "Biological Perspectives on Aging," *American Scientist* 66, no. 5 (1978): 608–12.
3. Seong S. Han and Jan Holmstedt, *Cell Biology* (New York, N.Y.: McGraw-Hill, 1979), p. 179.
4. Patricia Hess and Candra Day, *Understanding the Aging Patient* (Bowie, Md.: Robert J. Brady, 1977), p. 35.
5. G. A. Borkan and A. H. Norris, "Assessment of Biological Age Using a Profile of Physical Parameters," *Journal of Gerontology* 35, no. 2 (1980):177–84.
6. Leonard Hayflick, "The Cell Biology of Human Aging," *Scientific American* 1, no. 1 (1980):58.
7. Seong Han, lecture. "Biology of Aging," Institute of Geontology, University of Michigan, June 4–8, 1979.
8. Hayflick, pp. 64–5.
9. Goldstein and Reichel, p. 429.
10. Ibid.
11. Han, lecture, 1979.
12. M. T. Cicero, *Cato Major, or His Discourse of Old Age* (New York, N.Y.: Arno Press, 1979), p. 37. Reprint of 1744 ed. by Ben Franklin.
13. I. Rossman, "Human Aging Changes," in I. Burnside, ed., *Nursing and the Aged* (New York, N.Y.: McGraw-Hill, 1976), p. 82.

14. Han, lecture, 1979.
15. George Adams, *Essentials of Geriatric Medicine* (New York, N.Y.: Oxford University Press, 1977), p. 7.
16. Ibid.
17. Timiras, "Biological Perspectives," p. 607.
18. Ibid., p. 608.
19. Ibid., p. 607.
20. Diana Woodruff, "A Physiological Perspective of the Psychology of Aging," in D. Woodruff and J. Birren, eds., *Aging* (New York, N.Y.: D. Van Nostrand Co., 1975), pp. 181–2.
21. Ibid., pp. 184–9.
22. Herbert deVries, "Physiology of Exercise and Aging," in D. Woodruff and J. Birren, eds., *Aging* (New York, N.Y.: D. Van Nostrand Co., 1975), pp. 257–6.
23. Ibid., p. 272.
24. Diana Woodruff and James Birren, eds., *Aging* (New York, N.Y.: D. Van Nostrand Co., 1975), pp. 201–78.
25. Timiras, "Biological Perspectives," pp. 605–13.
26. Ibid.; Adams, pp. 1–11.
27. P. S. Timiras, *Developmental Physiology and Aging* (New York, N.Y.: Macmillan, 1972), p. 408.
28. Cicero, pp. 43–61.
29. Ibid., pp. 70–1.
30. Timiras, "Biological Perspectives," p. 613; Matilda W. Riley, "Aging, Social Change and the Power of Ideas," *Daedalus* 107, no. 4 (1978): 49.
31. Cicero, pp. 6–21.
32. Jan Dynda Sinnott, "Sex-Role Inconstancy, Biology and Successful Aging," *The Gerontologist* 17, no. 5 (1977): 461.
33. Timiras, "Biological Perspectives," p. 606.
34. Timiras, *Developmental Physiology*, p. 556.
35. Adams, pp. 10–11.
36. Timiras, *Developmental Physiology*, pp. 414–5.
37. Paul M. Spiegel, "Theories of Aging," in P. S. Timiras, ed., *Developmental Physiology and Aging* (New York, N.Y.: Macmillan, 1972), p. 566.
38. R. L. Katz, "Jewish Values and Sociopsychological Perspective on Aging," in S. Hiltner, ed., *Toward a Theology of Aging* (New York, N.Y.: Human Sciences Press, 1975), p. 136.
39. Evelyn E. Whitehead, "Religious Images of Aging: An Examination of Themes in Contemporary Christian Thought," in S. Spicker, K. Woodward, and D. Van Tassel, eds., *Aging and the Elderly* (Atlantic Highlands, New Jersey: Humanities Press, Inc., 1978), p. 39.
40. Ibid., p. 46.
41. Katz, p. 143.
42. Whitehead, p. 43.
43. Ibid., p. 42.

44. Ibid., p. 44.
45. D. S. Browning, "Preface to a Practical Theology of Aging," in S. Hiltner, ed., *Toward a Theology of Aging* (New York, N.Y.: Human Sciences Press, 1975), pp. 152–64.
46. D. O. Moberg, "Religiosity in Old Age," in B. Neutgarten, ed., *Middle Age and Aging* (Chicago: U. of Chicago Press, 1968), p. 497.
47. Whitehead, p. 46.
48. Ibid.
49. Gerald Larue, "Religion and the Aged," in I. Burnside, ed., *Nursing and the Aged* (New York, N.Y.: McGraw-Hill, 1976), pp. 573–83.
50. Ibid., pp. 578–9.
51. Forrest J. Berghorn et al., *The Urban Elderly* (New York, N.Y.: Allanheld, Osmun and Co.), p. 111.
52. Moberg, p. 508.
53. Berghorn et al., p. 111.
54. P. W. Pruyser, "Aging: Downward, Upward, or Forward?" in S. Hiltner, ed., *Toward a Theology of Aging* (New York, N.Y.: Human Sciences Press, 1975), pp. 114–5.

Chapter 8

Planning for Retirement

Dianna Shomaker and Joann Buck

REVIEW OF THE DILEMMA

Almost everyone experiences some sort of retirement in later life. The definitions of that experience vary, and its success is influenced by health, financial resources, social resources, and the retiree's own subjective assessment of the status acquired before and associated with the retired condition.[1,2]

Review of the authors' experience and the literature from others' observations suggests little emphasis has been placed on improving happiness and effectiveness during the steadily increasing number of years that younger persons may experience in retirement.

Retirement has been described as an informal rite of passage. For some it is the demarcation between production and nonproduction. For others it is the transition from work to leisure. It has been heralded with ceremony and obscured in indifference. It varies with the social context and the personal biographies of the individuals involved. For all it is a sociological variable within the lifespace of an individual, "denoting a transition, separating the older person from his or her previous roles and initiating another phase of the life cycle."[3] It is a social process that requires careful attention to the attitudes of retirees and those in the networks of their support systems; openness of the channels of communication; and the flexible preplanning that will augment life satisfaction in later years through the best use of a person's skills, experience, resources, and potential.[4,5] It encompasses both overt and subtle changes: a person's goals, motivations, roles, and sexual and emotional needs. Each individual has developed a specific style of adult life by retirement age. That style will continue to influence aging experiences and decisions throughout the balance of life.

People retire for many reasons and in a variety of ways. Some adapt more successfully than others. Most people now retire some time during their sixties. Retirement has mostly been involuntary, but voluntary retirement is becoming more common. Only 28 percent of the wage and salaried workers who retired in 1960 did so voluntarily, but there has been a growth in the number of those who now do so. Many prefer leisure time rather than working. Moreover, off-time leisure has gained greater respect than it was accorded at the turn of the century.[6,7] Laws that require retirement motivate most people; some are willing, some are not. Others retire because of poor health, unemployment, or simply because it is financially feasible. In general, the timing of the occasion is influenced by a person's desired goals, new opportunities, financial resources, or expected rewards in retirement—or the reverse of any of those items. Age is a poor criterion for retirement regardless of a person's potential.[8]

There is little evidence to support the popular notion that development of a negative attitude toward retirement stems from no longer being employed. Rather, it has been found that such an attitude arises from the conditions of retirement itself, including chronic illness, feelings of uselessness, and reduced income.[9] There is mixed sentiment regarding retirement, however. Some people look forward to developing repressed pursuits or to a change of focus. Some have never been able to afford leisure time, and given the opportunity for ample leisure, do not know what to do with it. Some "fail" in retirement and return to work. Others sit down to rest, calling an end to their activity. Often there is an awesome disparity between what was envisioned for retirement and the realities of daily living after work has ceased. Many couples, who years ago thought that they had arranged for ample financial support through their retirement, have found that the highly inflationary economy has reduced their income to subsistence level. Lack of preparation has left this group without the skills or motivation to produce additional income. Often the small wages that are available to the retired alter their income enough to reduce their eligibility for valuable medical and assistance programs. It is often counterproductive for these elders to work for a wage.

Catastrophic illness or accident can render a longtime friend or marriage partner incapable of communication, self-care, or any kind of adult expression of life other than basic functions. Care for such an individual can be accomplished in a variety of ways, but at what expense to the partner who has survived in good health? Personal needs may be set aside in order to provide care for a spouse or sibling. Sexual and emotional needs of the healthy partners are often frustrated when patterns of a lifetime are broken and social mores deny the adaptations that might otherwise seem natural. These more basic changes are accompanied by other subtle and far-reaching changes that continuously evolve. For the male who has always been the breadwinner, the loss of meaningful daily work might result in a threat to self-esteem and sense of self-worth, while his spouse continues with valuable contributions toward maintenance and supervision of the home. Moreover, many older women have adjusted to life style changes of increased freedom and free time ahead of the men. For both, their emotional needs and desires are subjected to new evaluations. Their satisfaction and maintenance depends on the ability to adjust to change.

Relationships with grown children are affected by the retirement of the parents. Often children sense a new responsibility for the parents. In some instances siblings have the first shared meaningful responsibility since they left home. Retirement often changes income and thus reverses roles: the dependent children become heads of households; the family leaders become dependent; grandmothers raise second generation children; daughters mother their parents. The wide variety of personalities and circumstances make the prediction of an individual's behavior under the stress of these changes difficult.

There are economic fantasies in which no one is financially secure. There are catastrophic illnesses and accidents that seem entirely unprovoked. Well-intentioned behaviors evaluated on unspoken assumptions create misery between parents and children who try to assist one another; for example, a widow, secure in the knowledge that she has her own home in which to live out her life is moved by her children to their home where she will be secure and safe. As a result, she loses purpose, self-motivation, and independence. Hence the security desired by the widow in her own home was taken from her for the very reason she wanted it.

> To most older Americans, a high degree of independence is almost as valuable as life itself. It is their touchstone for self-respect and dignity. It is the measure they use to decide their importance to others, and it is their source of strength for helping those around them.
>
> Whether they enjoy the degree of independence they desire depends partly on the role they play in the community, partly on the condition of their health, and partly on the adequacy of their incomes, housing, medical care, and other essentials.[10]

Success in retirement has been attributed to various approaches; while there seems to be no correlation between peoples' commitments to work and their attitudes toward retirement, better adaptation to retirement is demonstrated by those who had an optimistic attitude toward the process before retiring.[11] These persons advance in accordance with the plan for using their potential to make their later years full.[12,13] Those who retire voluntarily are shown to have more positive attitudes and higher satisfaction in retirement.[14] Others stand still as though immobilized, neither re-treating nor advancing, complacently marking time.[15] Those who were absorbed in their earlier work often verbalize feelings of being an "empty vessel" upon retiring; those who devoted their energies to vigorous pursuit of a goal often experience some level of depression when the pace slows. For both extremes and for those in between, marshaling interests and resources in detailed planning far in advance of retirement have resulted in expressions of success after retirement.[16] "The retired exhibited lower morale than the employed principally because they had more negative evaluations of their health, were more functionally disabled, were poorer and were older and *not* simply because they were retired."[17]

Success requires that a person maintain a satisfactory self-identity and adequate social interaction with both family and peers in a flexible process unique to that individual's needs, choices, resources, and constraints.[18] Failure of a retirement plan, as in the research that studies it, lies in the inability to confront the variables of a person's experiences and potential, as well as the opportunities and limitations of "the specific social milieu into which an individual retires."[19]

There are new dilemmas surfacing as longevity increases and populations expand. In society, people interact daily with family, friends, and others. Parents and children are influenced by the actions, plans, and values of one another, and even though at least half of the persons over 65 years of age live alone, their lives continue to be influenced by their families.[20] Despite the separation from children, there is often an unplanned and unforeseen need to rely on them as aging places limitations on physical and material resources. Often children who are raising families of their own also assist their parents. Today, more than in the past, there are many "children" of retirement age themselves supporting three generations: themselves, their parents, and their own children. The potential exhaustion, frustration, hostility, guilt, and resentment due to emotional and material strain will compound itself if there has been little or no preplanning and communication about decisions and disposition of goods, goals, and alternate goals, and flexibility in means of implementation.[21]

Another problem is that of the older person who has no spouse or children, is suffering diminishing resources, and has no preretirement plan. Attempts to create a plan of action when already in the vortex of a crisis are often met with failure, and result in resigned despair.

> Without the often tempering effect of loving concern from a close family member, the single older person faces the hazard of enlarging on his [or her] negative emotions and of dwelling on his [or her] hurts. Without the tugging of others to reach out or react

or respond or love, a single person growing old may turn . . . inward, contemplating his [or her] own hurts and angers and pains.[22]

Many of the agonies of retirement need not exist, but people approach the process in some degree of naiveté. Barfield and Morgan found not only a large degree of random variance in people's plans for how and when to retire, but also an overwhelming number of people who professed ignorance of such a fundamental matter as the amount of retirement pension they could expect to receive.[23]

For many, retirement is an event yet to come. The actuality of the state of retirement in the present, rather than in the future, robs the retiree of a visible future. It is difficult to continue projecting to the future that which is now present. Thinking should be reoriented to consider retirement a process, a long-term series of adjustments and planning beginning many years before elimination from the work force and ahead of any potential crisis. This does not preclude a need to adapt. Rather it assumes the constancy of adaptation throughout life and incorporates the process of retirement into the planning that made adaptation successful at earlier stages of challenge and change. Effective use of "resources maximize[s] the probability that an individual will develop a satisfying self-image and that he [or she] will be able to maintain a satisfying conception of himself [or herself] even in the event of change."[24]

The quality of life in the future necessitates planning and action on all levels. That is, people retiring must establish what is desired after retirement and who will accompany them, and they must assess limitations, resources, capabilities, needs, and desires. At the same time, they should clarify expectations, share concerns, and create a sequence of flexible goals to be initiated at the proper time.

The person must not undertake these considerations alone, however. The process must incorporate open communication with spouse, children, lawyers, physicians, and business partners, perhaps using group meetings or some type of minimal counseling where appropriate. "Pre-retirement planning programs go a long way toward identifying alternate roles, activities and strategies that will be rewarding in their own right."[25] Planning can be successful if the universally important issues of health, finance, environment, and law are holistically approached, and the planning is balanced in emphasis and scope, fully utilizing the uniqueness of the individual. However, the process is not always objective or simple.

The natural conclusion of the retirement phase of life is death or loss so severe that the person is no longer referred to as retired, but rather in terms that describe a more dependent condition. This fact is unpleasant to many older people and their families, so discussion of planning for later life—closer to death—is only partially accomplished, if at all. Family relationships and communication skills are an important factor in this situation. If there is an openness and a desire to express expectations and fears, as difficult as the subject matter may be, some progress will be made. If there is immature development of interrelationships among the adult members and a lack of trust and communication, then the planning will proceed without the full participation of the remainder of the family. This is not necessarily disastrous when the nonparticipant is only superficially involved, but is critical when the nonparticipant is the elder.

PLANNING FOR RETIREMENT

The concept of planning for retirement and aging can provide a format for a positive and constructive approach to some of the more pressing problems of the aging process for all members of the family. The plan includes not only material affairs, but also mental and emotional issues. It is, specifically, a family effort to assess their resources, understand the probabilities for the aging individuals, and prepare in appropriate measure to meet the probable needs. Indeed, where the options are limited, this kind of foresight and planning can surmount tremendous problems.

The planning process should begin as soon as there is a desire to do so on the part of the family or anyone in the family. Planning will obviously be done for and around the family elder, regardless of chronological age. In many cases open discussion and mutual decisions are possible. However, in some cases the quality of mental health within the family will impede this kind of honesty. Many families are ruled by autocrats who do not believe in participatory planning, but will hand down their wishes and instructions. If they do this, the family legacy may be in good shape, and the children will know what is desired and expected of them. However, if there is no planning and there are no instructions, other arrangements for decision making will take precedence during times of crisis, manipulating whatever time and resources are available for immediate action. The prime concern is that the basic plans should be made before a catastrophic illness or accident makes communication of desires and wishes impossible. If the father is the only one with access to funds and he has a stroke and cannot communicate, his financial resources will not be available to the family to use until legal proceedings are completed. If he did not inventory his estate, including insurance, bank accounts, locations of assets, documents, and will, then there could be confusion and delay or even loss of assets and resources. Consequently, planning should start as soon as possible.

The planning process is just that, a process. It requires updating, reworking, and a continuous effort as the aging experiences unfold. Once the family has established the process and seen it work, it is easy to keep in place to meet the future needs of succeeding older people in the family.

Planning for the experience of aging and retirement involves everyone in contact with the adult who constitutes the support system. Those who are obligated to care for the family member are considered "family" even though they are not always biologically related. Some individuals within a family may not want to participate in the process. They should not be allowed to disrupt the process. Even the elder who refuses to participate should not be allowed to dictate that the children suffer the results of failure to plan. The elder can be kept informed of the prevailing plans and may realize their worth at a later date. Regardless of involvement, everyone should be kept informed of the plans and made to feel that participating is welcome.

Every family is always involved in negotiating roles, relationships, and growth. The development of a plan is not always accomplished by calm, straightforward discussions. The expectations and emotions of the past influence the level of willingness within the family to help, to support, and even to agree. Conflict among family members is not necessarily negative. It can be an outlet for interpersonal exchanges that are much needed for the members of the family to understand each other.

Planning Process

Of what exactly does the process of planning consist? The process is basically a three-stage cycle: (1) the assessment and evaluation of the family and the estate; (2) the development of options for action (solutions); and (3) the arrival at a mutual understanding regarding commitments and expectations.

During the planning process the family will examine the seven basic areas of concern enumerated in Chapter 1, and incorporate solutions that take into account not only these individual issues but also the interrelationships between these issues.

Assessment

Any plan of care must begin with an assessment of present resources. First, resources are taken to mean finances. How much, what kind, where, under what restraints, if any? The extent of financial resources of the entire family should be assessed. Second, resources should include all other appropriate kinds of assistance; for example, elders need drivers, companions, assistance with chores and housework, meals, housing, and other types of in-kind support. Then the issue of how to plan around resources available must be addressed. For example, if there is no money available, what services are available to older citizens? Are public and private programs the same in each of the towns where the children live? If not, relocation before a crisis is a possibility.

Assessment of the emotional health and climate of the entire family is necessary. The degree to which family members are able to express themselves is crucial to both the decision making and implementation of the estate plan.

In addition, assessment should include taking into account the elder's future physical health. Diminished eyesight often limits the ability to drive; poor hearing inhibits satisfying socialization; and physical immobility compounds the ease with which a person performs daily living tasks. These often jeopardize independent living arrangements. Not only does physical constraint in the future require awareness in planning; so do emotional needs and personality traits developed throughout a lifetime. People who got along well with others and need socializing may prefer residing in a senior community; others may prefer more privacy.

Once the information is gathered, some possible plans can be projected. The family as a group needs to evaluate the situation based on the information now available. Strengths and weaknesses can now be identified, and solutions can be determined that best reflect the family assets and philosophy. A family that believes in providing the care has to weigh this against probable health and physical needs. It would be unrealistic to keep a parent at home if the daily medical requirements exceed the capabilities of an average household without medical experience, equipment, or the finances to set up a mini-hospital in the home.

Parent participation in this phase provides a supportive context in which their wishes may be made known. Most persons have thought about what types of care are emotionally suitable for them, what type of arrangements they prefer after death, and what legacy they are leaving. But few people ask parents about these issues, afraid to bring up the subject lest the mere mention of problems should create a new reality. The final picture of desires, needs, and resources may not coincide with what was assumed, but it is better to work from this known assessment than from a vague, unvalidated assumption.

Development

Following assessment and evaluation, the family needs to develop options or solutions to problems made apparent in the preceding stages.

Ideally, each problem should have more than one alternative solution. Some problems will appear to defy resolution and will require more time, cooperation, and creativity to develop alternatives. In addition, the family should develop plans for at least two potential futures. Depending on a single expectation defeats the purpose of planning. Flexibility is crucial; those who were not flexible enough have often been heard to utter over and over, "I never thought it would be this way," or "I didn't plan for this disease." Inflexibility and rigid expectations prevent and hamper truly creative problem solving. However, it is important not to take this process beyond the reasonable. It is just as dangerous to try to plan for every possible future as it is to plan for none of them. The goal is a process or system of problem solving that the family can implement with an air of awareness and readiness.

Many families will need outside help in developing their options, gathering information about resources and programs available, and arriving at solutions. Help is available from physicians, lawyers, counselors, community health nurses, mental health workers, senior citizen centers, area agencies on aging, nursing homes, day care centers, hospices, and hospital discharge planners. Once the options are understood, the family, as a group, should review the resource information and the options, and arrive at a mutual understanding regarding the state of affairs. The group needs to support a united plan of action whether that be the further development of alternatives and solutions, or acceptance of available options. The aim is to express love and support to the family members in the experiences that lie ahead, assuring them the freedom to age and die as they choose and establishing a base from which assistance can be offered if needed. The goals do not include manipulative planning of the lives of others, dictatorial influencing of another life, or denying a person the right to direct his or her own affairs as long as possible in life.

The environment in which family discussion takes place is important. It should occur in a place where the family is comfortable, both physically and emotionally. The environment should be private, the process dignified and respectful. Children who are too young to understand and who might interrupt should not be included. This family discussion will be important, but it need not be dreary or conclude with decrees. Appropriateness is the key concept here. A sincere and clear discussion in relaxed circumstances has great impact and vitality. The discussion should be an offering of data gleaned from assessment of family and community. Through this process of simple review, the group can mutually accept the development of specific information toward solutions. Everyone can, to some level, be informed and alert to the context in which the specifics are developed. Information should be organized to avoid confusion, but an attitude of cooperation is more important than perfection of detail. As the discussion progresses, the consensus will become clear and similarities and differences will become apparent. However, the family does need to reach a mutual understanding. It does not require total agreement or unanimity, but all positions must be revealed, explored, and understood.

Agreement

Completing the process or cycle requires an agreement. If the best accomplished is an agreement that there are problems (that the family cannot agree), but that a commitment will be made to work at resolving differences so that the family legacy can be supported, then that is the level at which agreement must be reached. For some families, this change in relationships is far more than had been previously developed and will in itself be a positive contribution to the family legacy.

The commitments to the plans will vary, even as the individual family members vary. It is important that commitments blend support and assistance together.

Now the plan is put into motion. Changes are implemented as needed. The plan can be updated and reviewed as is necessary. Changes in health, finances, or other relevant areas should stimulate a reassessment of the whole situation to ensure that the issues are still balanced. The parents can continue to do as they will, free to enjoy the retirement and aging experience with a minimum of anxiety and fear of the future. The children and potential care providers are in the best possible position: they know what is expected of them; they know what to expect from others; and they have time if they need it to prepare for the future.

The following case study is hypothetical and based on the experiences of many elders and their families. It illustrates both the development of a specific plan for retirement and aging, and the implementation of the planning process through the aging experience. Their level of resources is plotted on Figure 8–1.

Case Study

The Martin family has tremendous human resources. John and Louise have six children. Four are grown and have families of their own, and two young adults are just entering their own independence. In addition to this large nuclear group, John and Louise have brothers and sisters who are close, both emotionally and geographically, and so represent a resource for their aging experience.

Figure 8–1 The Martins: Evaluation

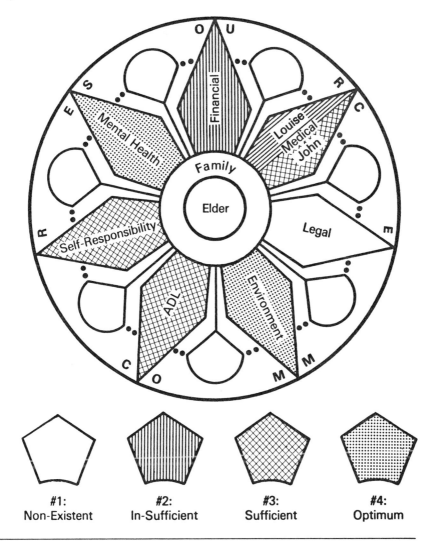

#1: Non-Existent

#2: In-Sufficient

#3: Sufficient

#4: Optimum

The strength of this family is challenged by their minimal level of financial resources. Though they live in their own home, it is mortgaged to pay for the children's education. Savings are non-existent. Their modest income represents the maximum of John's earning power. While Louise has worked most of her life, she is not presently working because of health problems that are steadily increasing. They are both 61 years old. Their modest income is sufficiently high to deny them access to subsidized medical care available to the destitute, but inadequate to begin to cover minimal preventive medical care. For financial reasons, they avoid going to the doctor.

The independent children are in much the same financial situation. They can only give minimal financial aid to their parents. Those children still living at home will soon be gone, relieving John and Louise of the cost of their care. John and Louise's financial resources are just adequate to cover their present life style, but it is unlikely that they will be able to keep pace with added expenses should major problems develop.

Neck injuries from an automobile accident have incapacitated Louise. Being involuntarily confined to bed or her recliner, her digestion and strength have declined. John is apparently in good health, although his hearing has been gradually declining for many years. He is fully employed, and the demands of his job are sufficient to provide daily exercise and stimulation. He has not had a medical checkup for 14 years, and he calls the physician only when occasional bouts with the flu or a cold keep him from work.

Legally John and Louise Martin are unprepared for retirement or the possibility of any catastrophic illness. There are no inventory of affairs, will, or instructions as to their wishes. There is no clear-cut, concise picture of the pattern of insurance and pension support that John and Louise have accumulated. They are not familiar with exactly what insurance will and will not cover.

John and Louise have maintained the same residence for most of their adult lives, and in their younger years had remodeled and improved the house to meet their needs and desires. They looked forward to living there, comfortable and safe, for their remaining years. The home is single-level and presents no immediate problems of access or maintenance. Their social environment has been equally suitable and secure. They are familiar with their community, active in church groups, and involved in the lives of their children and neighbors.

The mental health rating for the Martins is optimum. While they as individuals have no interests or hobbies, their lives have been so active and productive that this itself has been their interest and hobby. Both individuals are positive and confident of their future. They communicate well with each other and the children. While they are not afraid of conflict and emotional interchange, the basic understanding and support are there and are reaffirmed mutually on a regular basis. Both John and Louise have a talent for problem solving, one sharpened by the experiences of their lives. Louise is presently experiencing some problems with her lack of activity and stimulation, but is good-natured and willing to explore positive outlets for her energy. She is aware that she will need to make an effort and accomplish a recuperation to her previously-held state of good health.

The ADL rating for the Martins is less than perfect. Louise is hampered in housekeeping tasks. John has taken over the cleaning, and one of their daughters is doing the laundry. Louise can still manage the tasks of cooking, but she cannot drive the car. The rest of the family is helping her with errands, and John co-ordinates these.

The doctor foresees a time when Louise's neck brace will be unnecessary and the side effects of the neck injury, dizzyness and headaches, will subside. Louise is fairly assertive in finding assistance for her needs.

Case Study Analysis

By using the holistic approach to elder care and representing the Martins' strengths and weaknesses on the basic model, it can be seen that they are weak legally, strong in terms of their mental health and environment, and have sufficient resources in the other areas, except that Louise is considered to be at an insufficient level of physical health because she is partially dependent as a result of the neck injury.

The Martin family decided to use the concept of planning for retirement to solve some of the immediate problems as well as to prepare for the care of the elders in their family. Interest in the project ranged from enthusiastic to merely "interested." While John and Louise were good problem solvers and confident in their own capacity to survive, they were also astute enough to realize that a united family effort was going to be required. At the family gathering the system was explained, and the tasks for gathering information allotted.

Both Louise and John needed complete physical examinations and medical consultation regarding possible strengths and weaknesses in their future. A lawyer was required to analyze the papers and documents that did exist and to begin preparing those instruments that did not exist: a power of attorney to be used in case of catastrophic illness; a will, instructions regarding care, and post-death arrangements; and an inventory of affairs and locations of documents. Community resources were investigated, and eligibility criteria were obtained for a wide variety of services, both in-home and institutional. The state and city social service offices were contacted for information and referral to any and all potentially appropriate agencies and services.

During this same period, John and Louise and two of their children worked out three possible futures for the purpose of preparing for what might reasonably be expected to happen. The possible futures outlined were based on their mutual survival as a couple and one for each case in which one survived the other. Throughout this period John and Louise began to see the support system that they had developed through the years. Their abilities as parents brought them warm and enthusiastic support. Understanding and respect were returned. This experience of seeing their family united to assist them was one of the highlights of their family life and was a fulfillment of some of their hopes and dreams.

When all the information was gathered and the leads pursued, the family once again came together to examine the plan. They spent an evening reviewing the information and expressing their reactions. The possible futures were presented and substantially agreed upon as to their likelihood. The Martins found that in the evaluation of their situation, some members of the family felt more at ease than others about being open and candid regarding expectations, but the general attitude was good, and the evening closed with a mutual understanding of the state of affairs.

The family agreed on several points. John and Louise were in no immediate danger. Barring an immediate catastrophe, they would survive as things were until they reached the mandatory retirement age. At that time their financial situation would be worse because of the loss of John's wages. They would then need additional income, from a source as yet unidentified. No one member of the family had resources adequate to cover all the needs, but several members would be able to help with small amounts.

Their medical situation was weak. Louise was in need of regular medical attention, and John needed to institute regular checkups to maximize his present state of good health. The finances for some of this would have to be developed: the health insurance from John's job would help with Louise's immediate needs. The mental and emotional health of John and Louise was excellent.

Family members combined the information available with their own needs and realities and came to an understanding of appropriate and realistic commitments. A voluntary system of contributions began to clarify itself as family members talked and thought about not only their present situation, but also their goals and ideals.

The solutions formulated were as follows:

- Care for one or both parents subsequent to a debilitating crisis would require placement in a state-supported nursing home. Their eligibility for this program had been determined by the state social service office. Because the Martins had a small income, they would be required to make a monthly payment. This payment would be less than the daily cost of care, and the family felt that a united effort would ensure its payment. Nursing home care would be supplemented by family members, who would maintain a regular visitation program. They could provide outside activities, mental and physical stimulation, companionship, and the continuance of their family relationships.

  If the crisis left the parents in need of nonmedical care, it was agreed that this would be provided for by the family themselves, in their homes, rotating among those capable of helping. Louise's younger sister, a recent widow, offered to join the household if and when it was deemed appropriate to assist in housekeeping or offer personal care in exchange for a rent-free place to live.

- The plan for a second sort of future was to extend the availability of living quarters with family members to either or both parents. It was felt that if and when one died, the other would most assuredly be welcome and useful in the homes of their children. Some family members lived alone, and it was agreed that these separate households could be consolidated should there be that demand.

- The third plan was more complex and was based on the possibility that both parents would live quite a few years in a healthy state, lucid and active but unable to be financially self-sufficient. Negotiations and arrangements for the consolidation of households were initiated. Emphasis was put on establishing arrangements that were realistic and workable for all parties, allowing each participant maximum freedom and independence. The arrangements would more than likely change with time. The in-home services in the community, where appropriate, would be used to the fullest, for example, nursing and chore services, meals, and transportation available to the homebound. It was agreed that the children would help their parents seek and develop activities and interests that would sufficiently motivate active interest and learning.

The search for medical information had brought to light the existence of an HMO (Health Maintenance Organization) in the community. For a sum, neither small nor completely out of reach, this service could be available to John and Louise. The decision was made that this would represent the best medical service for the money for both parents.

Since the preretirement planning session of the family, many changes are apparent. When the basic model, as shown in Figure 8–1, is compared with present plans, the strengths and weaknesses of the Martin family plan demonstrate that the legal weaknesses have been eliminated. During the planning period, resources and desires were clarified. That in itself organizes the situation enough to rate legal issues sufficiently developed. If within the next year the necessary legal instruments are prepared, the issue can be rated optimum.

Strengths of mental health, self-responsibility, and environment continue at optimum levels, and ADL skills continue at a sufficient level. Financially, the rating has continued to be "insufficient," but several options have been discussed that will allow the family as a unit to cope with financial constraints.

The results of this series of interactions among the Martins were positive and more successful than had the process not been conducted. The family continued to meet periodically to update plans. The future did not conform to their plans, however. John suffered a major debilitating crisis almost immediately after retirement and required more medical attention than was feasible at home, but less than required a stay in a state-supported, full-care nursing home. He was placed in an intermediate-care facility, and a portion of his expenses was subsidized. The HMO program paid many of his medical expenses. John died after three years of institutionalization.

Louise was able to recover most of her physical health, mobility, and independence. Soon after John's placement in the care facility, she gave up her home and relocated with a sister in a location closer to John. A larger and younger branch of the family bought her house, and the arrangements provided the younger adults with an opportunity to own a home and kept this resource within the family. Sufficient financing was arranged for Louise through the family.

Initially Louise was an asset to her new companion. She was good-natured and sensible. She was a willing and capable babysitter and continued to be active in her family involvement. Participation in a Senior Citizens Club, church group, family, and friends made her feel valid and self-confident. With the passage of time, however, Louise's siblings and companions died or became ill. Louise's ability to greet change with enthusiasm began to fade, and her tolerance for the social and moral changes of her world began to lessen. Louise lost her desire to participate in all of the previously satisfying activities and chose instead to be alone and introspective. A family conference led to decisions to change Louise's living environment to include someone who could motivate her to a greater level of activity and to involve her in the local day care program for the elderly. She found the new program satisfying. The staff at the day care center was able to ensure appropriateness of her activities, give assistance, offer transportation and meals, and provide a therapeutic program that improved her mental and physical health. In addition, it was a source of new friendships.

Louise died of pneumonia while living with a daughter's family. She had been ambulatory all of her life and was never strictly homebound. Her children had always included her in the family get-togethers, and she had maintained a modest ability for participation. The family had committed itself to care for her in turn, making sure that care providers had vacations and evenings and weekends off, and that respite care for them was available whenever they needed it.

The plans did not really end when both John and Louise were dead. Their family, once involved as care providers, were in various states of their own aging experiences and needed this systematic approach to their needs. That is the legacy at its best, supporting each in turn and changing to meet circumstantial change and the specific needs of each individual.

CONCLUSION

Any group that identifies itself as a family can make this work. Success depends on the accurate understanding of the context in which the aging experience will take place, that is, the truth about possibilities, the openness of expression of wishes and needs, and the strength of commitment in the care providers.

Retirement planning provides a family format that is supportive of the elder. Support of the elders validates their worth visibly for all to see, and so fosters confidence and a freedom from fear of aging as an example for the young. This is positive, a gift from the old to the young, and the reward for the toil of the care provider. Large families work well, but so do small ones. Two people are enough. One of the basic truths about aging is that few people can do it alone.

It is a mistake to believe that because a person looks at the future, it will be predictable and acceptable. Many people possess unrealistic expectations of tomorrow. The costs are frequently high both financially and emotionally. Perhaps that price can only be paid in the aging experience of the younger generation. The degree to which the issue of attitudes toward a person's own death can be expressed will dictate the degree to which anxiety about the topic can be reduced. Most say that they would rather be dead than severely incapacitated. If so, this should be expressed to family members who may need help voicing that decision. The resources have to be measured against the needs.

How does an individual retire with dignity? It can happen only if that person goes to something more interesting and satisfying. Retiring to the sidelines of life, a person drops the participant status and becomes a spectator. Not to play the game is to invite forgetfulness and loss of skill, which leads to a sense of slipping away.

One of the central issues of preretirement planning is that the level of personal commitment of those involved dictates the level of care given. If family members are at low levels of acceptance and understanding, then fear, revulsion, guilt, and a host of real and imagined problems become part of daily living. This can debilitate elders' attitudes to the degree that they become overinvolved in negative reflections.

A system can be developed that will not ruin the succeeding generations financially or emotionally. The consequences are both freedom and support for parents. They are offered the option of moving into their aging experiences with the possibility maximized for successful attainment of their goals. A renewal of faith and a growth of confidence in the future result.

NOTES

1. Robert Atchley, "Issues in Retirement Research," *The Gerontologist* 19, no. 1 (1979): 44–54.

2. Jon Hendricks and C. Davis Hendricks, *Aging in Mass Society* (Cambridge, Mass.: Winthrop Publishers, 1977), p. 256.

3. Ibid.

4. E. Palmore, "Compulsory vs. Flexible Retirement: Issues and Facts," in B. Bell, ed., *Contemporary Social Gerontology* (Springfield, Ill.: Charles C. Thomas, 1976), pp. 172–7.

5. Bill Bell, ed., *Contemporary Social Gerontology* (Springfield, Ill.: Charles C. Thomas, 1976), pp. 151–8.

6. G. L. Maddox, "Retirement as a Social Event in the U.S." in B. Neugarten, ed., *Middle Age and Aging* (Chicago: University Chicago Press, 1968), p. 361.

7. L. A. Epstein and J. H. Murray, "Employment and Retirement," in B. Neugarten, ed., *Middle Age and Aging* (Chicago: University of Chicago Press, 1968), pp. 354–6.

8. Atchley, pp. 44–54.

9. Hendricks and Hendricks, pp. 255–6.

10. A. Celebrezze, chrm. *Older American*; President's Council on Aging (Washington, D.C.: U.S. Government Printing Office, 1963), p. 7.

11. J. Poitrenaud et al., "Factors Related to Attitude Towards Retirement Among French Pre-retired Managers and Top Executives," *Journal of Gerontology* 34, no. 5 (1979): 723–7.

12. B. Smith, *Aging in America* (Boston: Beacon Press, 1973), p. 132.
13. R. Havighurst, et al., "Male Social Scientists: Lives After Sixty," *The Gerontologist* 19, no. 1 (1979):55–60.
14. Douglas Kimmel, K. F. Price, and J. W. Walker, "Retirement Choice and Retirement Satisfaction," *Journal of Gerontology* 33, no. 4 (1978):575–85.
15. Smith, p. 133.
16. Ibid., pp. 124–33.
17. G. B. Thompson, "Work Versus Leisure Roles: An Investigation of Morale Among Employed and Retired Men," in B. Bell, ed., *Contemporary Social Gerontology* (Springfield, Ill.: Charles C. Thomas, 1976), p. 194.
18. Maddox, p. 359.
19. Ibid., p. 363.
20. Smith, pp. 145–8.
21. Ibid., pp. 107–9.
22. Ibid., p. 111.
23. R. Barfield, and J. Morgan, "Trends in Planned Early Retirement," in J. Hendricks and C. D. Hendricks, eds., *Dimensions in Aging* (Cambridge, Mass.: Winthrop Publishers, 1979), pp. 325–6.
24. Maddox, p. 362.
25. Hendricks and Hendricks, p. 249.

Chapter 9

Relationship with Aged Parents

Joann Buck, Chiyoko Furukawa and Dianna Shomaker

Almost everyone, regardless of age, is sustained emotionally and physically by the relationships formed with other people. These people are primarily family members, but friends, coworkers, and neighbors may also be considered among the relationships developed.

Relationships tend to be dynamic and influenced by the developmental stages of life span. Although relationships are important at every stage, they become especially vital to the elderly in coping with losses that occur more frequently. For example, death of a spouse, retirement, and decline in health status all contribute to emotional and financial problems. These events may also be responsible for relationship changes with others. The strength of family relationships contributes to the support and assistance the elderly person needs in coping with critical life changes.

Interpersonal relationships and their continuance or severence is dependent upon the behavior of the aged person in dealing with other types of losses. The loss of hearing and sight often prohibits full participation in social interaction. Behavioral changes may occur as the elder attempts to find adequate coping behaviors that can compensate for the loss. Often society is quick to notice this "unusual" or aberrant behavior in an elderly individual, while the same behavior in a younger person is acceptable and may even be viewed as interesting. Understanding the dynamics of relationships and behaviors of older persons is critical to health promotion and maintenance care.

POSITIVE IMPACTS UPON INTERPERSONAL RELATIONS

Relationships

Murray defines relationships as "an interpersonal process in which one person facilitates the personal development or growth of another over time by helping him [or her] to mature; become more adaptive, integrated, and open to his [or her] experiences; or to find meaning in his [or her] situation."[1] This definition seems especially suited to family situations in which parents are the facilitators for their offspring to grow and mature to adulthood. On the other hand, middle-aged children or younger offspring are also in a position to assume the facilitator role depending on the circumstances. An example might be preparing a frail elderly parent to adjust to an institutional setting when this is mutually decided to be the most appropriate plan of care.

In most instances, when relationships are established, the process is one of reciprocity. The parent may be the facilitator, even in the parent-younger child relationship, but the resultant growth and experience is shared, and both participants are likely to benefit from the effects of the relationship. This notion also applies to the middle-aged child who assists parents to accept institutional care. The opportunity to experience the elderly parent's adjustment to institutional care gives impetus for the offspring to think in terms of when they must face the same decision in the future.

Jourard contends that personal relationships are characterized by keen interest in the subjective and personal side of each other's lives. Intrinsic to the relationship is a personal interest in a person's health, well-being, happiness, and unique identity that goes beyond the role performance.[2] In other words, it is not an obligatory activity, but rather one in which the individual chooses to participate because of interest in the other person. There is evidence that suggests that most offspring of older people demonstrate these concerns of well-being for their aged parents. Studies related to affectional aspects of intergenerational relationships suggest that when the elderly parent becomes ill, an immediate response by most families is seen.[3]

Some characteristics that apply to healthy personal relationships with the elderly include the following:[4]

- knowing or having an accurate concept of the other's idiosyncrasies;

- liking more of the other person's traits than disliking;

- feeling concern for the growth and happiness of the other;

- behaving in ways that promote the growth and happiness of the other;

- communicating effectively and fully disclosing oneself to the other;

- imposing feasible demands and expectations on the other;

- respecting the autonomy and individuality of the other.

Since people change with the progression of developmental stages, healthy interpersonal relationships may become impaired or threatened unless appropriate adjustments are made. When the relationship is healthy, the demands that each person makes on the other are open, reasonable, and compatible with the well-being and happiness of the other. Respect for autonomy and individuality are demonstrated in a healthy association because the "real self" is known by each other.[5] These attributes prevent the deterioration of the established affiliation. When problems with relationships occur, it is due to overestimating or underestimating the necessary changes. To illustrate, a recent widow may try to keep up those relationships that require a spouse for participation, or a newly retired person may attempt to keep up the same contact and association with former coworkers. Often when relationship problems remain unresolved the result may be an excessive dependency and decreased self-esteem on the part of the elderly person.

Family Relationships

The primary function of the aged's family is to provide companionship among its members, physical necessities, maintenance of motivation and morale, and continuing communication and patterns of interactions.[6] How effectively these functions are executed determines the quality of support and continued survival for the older person. Family ties are vital to the emotional and economic functions of the older person.[7]

An organization unlike any other social establishment is required for the family to accomplish their relationship tasks. The economic, political, social, educational, and religious aspects of the family must be met satisfactorily to ensure the basic needs of life. This means that members must attend to the production and distribution of goods and services to family members, settle internal difficulties for maintenance of order, train individuals as necessary, and find ways to maintain a sense of purpose within the family unit.

Some of these family tasks become paramount when changes occur in an aged member's life style because of illness or other problems. Often the pooling of family resources is required to compensate for the changes. New or adjusted living arrangements may become necessary as well as determining which offspring is to be the primary caretaker. As aging progresses, the elderly individual may become more involved with the family rather than with nonkin relationships. If the aged person has no children, siblings can become the primary support system and provide emotional support and encouragement during a crisis.

As members of the older population increase and family units become smaller, the care of elderly parents must be assumed by fewer children. Thus, other alternatives of caring for the aged should be explored.[8] It is not unreasonable that family emotional ties are strained when the care needs are complex and long-term, when, for example, day-after-day supervision, personal maintenance, and other essential services are needed to sustain an elderly's activities of daily living.[9] When mutual affection or strong filial responsibility prevails, as in some family situations, the necessary care may continue without the consequence of alienation and disaffection for the aged parent. Treas proposes that society should assist the family in caring for the elderly parent by providing tax breaks, special allowances, and direct reimbursements to family caretakers to promote support for continuance of care.[10] Furthermore, other systems to relieve overburdened caretakers should be made available by developing additional day care centers, home aides, meal deliveries, and other supplemental services.

A basic understanding of the aging process is helpful for sustaining positive family relationships. It is necessary to view aging as an ongoing process that incorporates past experiences, life styles, patterns and personality traits, and individualized results influenced by cultural and other psychological differences.[11] The elderly are not apt to give up lifetime behaviors simply because they have become older. Persons who have always been meticulous about their grooming will continue to give priority to this trait. The caretaker of such elders must make special efforts to meet this need; otherwise, frustrations may be manifested through unusual behavior.

In fulfilling particular needs, family members must be cognizant of the role reversal that may add to an already difficult situation for the elderly to maintain independence. The parent becomes the child, and the situation results in psychological threat to both generations.[12] This role conflict occurs with the elderly person who tenaciously guards the status of parent and decision maker. Many are reluctant to relinquish authority to the offspring even if they are dependent financially, physically, and otherwise.[13] Frequently, family caretakers are placed in the parental role without any choices. A negative consequence in such cases may be a resentment of the obligation or the emergence of hostile behavior to ventilate long-standing suppressed feelings.

To resolve or prevent family difficulties, it is essential to create a positive familial interaction and relationship. Bengtson employs perceptions, problems, and processes to analyze interactions between generations for the assessment of family relationships.[14] These three factors are the necessary components of family membership for meeting the challenges of continuous changes for each generation.

Perceptions

Perceptions are the images that each generation has about the others within the family and within the context of the broader society. Differences in perception among family members are inevitable because individual developmental rates are not the same. However, grandparents and grandchildren show a degree of cohesion and acceptance. One explanation for this positive relationship is that they can enjoy each other because the role of grandparents excludes the power or authority over the grandchildren.

Bengtson contends there is a serious generation gap in American society, but the differences are not necessarily wide apart.[15] Some differences are unavoidable as consequences of generational development, and beliefs and values influenced by historical events. Each generation experiences issues different from those faced by others; thus, perception of the problems by each generation may be disparate. For example, individuals who grew up during the depression years tend to be more fiscally conservative than those people growing up in the decade of the 1960s.

Problems

There are four different problems related to interaction between generations that could affect relationships, namely, role transition, autonomy and dependency, equitable exchange, and continuity and disruption.[16] Role transition deals with the changing roles and expectations inherent in growing up and becoming older. The change in societal views affects roles, as demonstrated by the increase of women in the work force today compared to the previous 20 years. This status of working women has brought changes in the care of aging parents. In the past, when multigenerational households prevailed, elderly parents joined the younger family for care and to make contributions to the family function. This situation has become less likely as the women, who were the primary caretakers of elderly relatives, seek employment outside the home to supplement family income and pursue a career.

The issues concerned with autonomy and dependency can create difficulties for all family members. For the elders, to become dependent and lose control over their lives must be distressing. It should be a challenge to all family members to find a proper balance between dependency and autonomy for their aged parents. Since older people do not necessarily enjoy receiving without giving in return, the goal is to find equitable exchanges that allocate fair giving and receiving between the family and older parents. The giving may be a family legacy, tradition, or theme for continuity to prevent disruption of family characteristics, which is thought to be an important theme throughout the generations.[17] Disruptions to the family may occur from geographical mobility, divorce, changes in life styles, and death.

Processes

Processes refer to the methods used by families to work out problems using available resources. The effectiveness of family members to resolve problems concerning their elders depends on their abilities to negotiate, resolve conflict, and find a satisfactory solution. It is necessary to work toward the attainment of desired outcomes through negotiation, which must be a give and take process with everyone's contribution. Conflicts should be discussed openly to allow expressions of differing opinions and to ensure the autonomy of individuals with opposing viewpoints. Satisfactory solutions must be found for the family relationship to continue and for the interpersonal well-being of individuals as the parent becomes older. Sooner or later, the relationship between the parent and offspring will be tested as aging progresses and support from the children becomes necessary. Thus, family relationships are important to most people and can never be dissolved.[18]

Support Systems for the Elderly

When dealing with problems, most persons, even with extensive individual resources, are unable to single-handedly match the effectiveness of assistance from group efforts.[19] As a person becomes older and individual resources tend to decrease, required assistance comes from people in social networks and other support systems that the person has developed throughout life.

A network comprises a chain of persons with whom an individual has had contact and those who are potential candidates for relationships.[20] Generally, individuals choose a person for the network for egocentric purposes and may use the relationship as a building block for a social organization in their interest. Characteristics unique to the social network are that it lacks boundaries, is fluid in nature, and individuals in the network may be deleted or added as the need arises. The kinship network is an example in which changes occur because family size may vary throughout an older person's lifetime. Some older people relate closely to distant kin or adopt people as kin since this type of relationship is meaningful and important to them.[21] New family members are added through birth and marriage; loss of members occurs with death, separation, or divorce. The tenacity of kinship bonds continues despite wars, conquest, slavery, immigration, politics, and ideological and cultural changes, and leaves little doubt that there will be a demise of parent-child relationships.[22]

Support systems are similar to social networks, but have functions and attributes of their own. A support system is defined as "a set of persons consisting of focal or anchor person, all the family, all the friends, and all the relationships among these people."[23] Caplan, a community psychiatrist, coined the term "support system," which has the same implications as the social network described by anthropologists.[24] Support systems are characterized by enduring relationships over time, which have intermittent or continuing ties and possess a low degree of variance in sharing pertinent information. Also the type of support provided may be organized or spontaneous, and the services are given by either professionals or nonprofessionals. In most instances, organized support is vital to the well-being of the older individual to supplement sporadic and spontaneous assistance. An older person needs help with activities of daily living that is organized and continuous, while the need for major maintenance of the elder's dwelling may be on a sporadic basis.

Generally, the informal relationships come from kin, friends, neighbors, and acquaintances, and these relationships tend to be reciprocal in nature and benefit both participants. On the other hand, formal associations are with professionals who deliver specific services on a systematic basis, and the major objective is for the benefit of the client.

The need for support systems may be either on a short-term basis to deal with a crisis or on a continuous long-term relationship.[25] Regardless of short- or long-term relationships, the people who provide the support may assist by pooling an individual's psychological resources; sharing necessary tasks; and giving material goals, skills, and suggestions to improve the handling of the episode.[26] Thus, relationships tend to provide emotional support and assist with specific tasks that the individual is unable to perform. The availability of these supportive measures may be the difference between continued maintenance in the community or institutionalization for the elderly person.

The current relationship status between older parents and their offspring is one of support and care. According to Streib, there is evidence that suggests that most parent-child relationships remain intact.[27] A small percentage of older people reported that they had not seen their married children in the previous year.[28] Thus, some theorists' beliefs about the present and future status of the isolated nuclear family as a pattern do not seem to have support.[29] However, there is a need to be aware of the major variables that influence social relationships and of the changes in human behavior for the next generation. Factors such as ethnicity, religion, race, residence, occupation, and education will become significant to qualify, modify, and accentuate generalizations about the relationships between older people and their offspring.[30] The influence of these factors on the elder's support system will require further study. Nevertheless, Streib maintains that even if major changes in the restructuring of society occur, "the family as an institution and as an interacting group will tend to operate basically in ways which are familiar to contemporary Americans, with emotional and mutual help patterns of prime importance."[31]

This position is supported by Murray, who contends that most senior citizens are satisfied with their relationships with their offspring regardless of geographical separations.[32] Moreover, there is a positive feeling about the kinship affiliation, which is shown by mutual affection, ongoing communication, giving and receiving, and the elderly's feelings of financial assurance. Generally, the support systems from the adult children are direct or indirect, but all contribute to the optimal functioning of the older parent.

A divergent and less positive viewpoint about the future relationship of the aged and the family is forecasted based on emergence of alternative life styles. Somerville predicts that efforts to change the traditional family structure are likely to accelerate in the next decade or so.[33] She cites that significant societal forces like the women's movement, youth's quest for personal closeness, decreased commitment to the Protestant Ethic, and more emphasis on individualism all question the traditional family values. Moreover, when this generation of people becomes middle-aged or aged, they are likely to continue with the experimentation mode and alternative ways of family relationships. Undoubtedly, these changes will continue to be viewed negatively by those who subscribe to the traditional ways of family life.

Social changes are powerful events, as shown by changes in the attitude toward the aging since the Industrial Revolution. The agrarian, multi-generation family structure is now less evident, and this has created problems in the care of frail elderly parents. However, new social programs such as Medicare, Medicaid, elderly day care, home health services, homemaker services, and friendly visiting programs have emerged to provide health promotion and maintenance care for the older population. These experiences should ensure that future generations will continue to meet the challenge to augment the optimal level of wellness for the elderly group.

In summary, an individual's lifetime behavioral patterns usually continue until death. The ability to sustain these patterns is often contingent upon the relationship with the family and others. The formation of a support system and social network evolves from the relationships a person develops throughout life. A positive aging experience for the individual and family occurs when there is an open and supportive relationship. All persons involved must be able to express their desires and expectations so that conflict may be resolved. A successful aging experience benefits not only the elderly person, but also the family members and others. The benefits include continued positive relationship and insight into the aging process for the family members and others in preparation for their own aging experience.

NEGATIVE IMPACTS UPON INTERPERSONAL RELATIONS

Guilt

It would be absurd to assume that the relationships between grown children and their parents are without adversity or that the time spent in earlier interactions idyllic. Furthermore, guilt is not restricted to the feelings of children toward their parents; parents also express similar feelings when reflecting upon relationships with children and younger relatives.[34] Even beyond these complex feelings, statistical reporting may lead to the naive assumption that relationships are either guilt-ridden or free of guilt, but regardless of when the pattern was established, there is fluctuation reaching both ends of the continuum. For many, guilt is borne in preference to the potential pain of discussing conflicts. Frustration and unresolved conflict are of course damaging to positive relationships. For many people the relationship, regardless of its quality, is so vital to the individuals involved that great care is taken to avoid disrupting the status quo, even to the extreme of denying the existence of poor relationships.

Parent Abuse

Symptoms of conflict and various uses of power have been reported among all groups and persons where there is an inequality of some sort. When power is used to alleviate conflict, guilt, or ambivalence, aggression, exploitation, and hostility result. This use of power is not always detectable. Moreover, it is not isolated in one age group; there are many universal factors.

Since the early 1960s, there have been many accounts of child abuse. Spouses, usually wives, have been recognized as another abused group, but this has often been hidden. Recently, accounts of grandparent and parent abuse by grown children and spouses have also been reported. In reflection, this is not new to the older age group; they have always had much in common with the younger groups. Historically, "Parents were often abandoned to almshouses or asylums."[35]

The issue of parent abuse and its causes is complex. Most people do not neglect their parents when they become old and frail. Yet, studies demonstrate increasing incidences of neglect, abandonment, and conscious deprivation of the elderly by their grown children. In seeming contradiction, studies have published findings that assert that contact with at least one child is frequent. The difference between the reports is the evaluation of those contacts. The quality of the contacts is yet to be proven. The real nature of intergenerational relationships is not so simply defined, and distance between adults and their aging relatives is irrelevant to the quality of the contact. Separate households are no more of an indicator of disintegrating family ties than is living together a sign of family stability.[36]

Recently, Representative Claude Pepper (D.-Fla.) chaired hearings of the House-Senate Committee on Aging to investigate allegations that psychological and physical abuse toward the elderly is prevalent.[37] The hearings revealed that 2.5 million aged are psychologically or physically abused every year through beatings, robbery, and torture. The practice is speculated to be as widespread as child abuse. It is perpetrated by family members, children, and spouses, just as child abuse is inflicted by parents. The predominant pattern involves a history of violence in the family where the elder person, who was once an abuser, becomes dependent upon the children, who then in turn become abusers of their parent. The cycle seems to be self-perpetuating, with episodes triggered by economic factors that stress emotions. Problems based on poor health and economic stress are a major cause of family difficulty across the life cycle. Stress due to poor health often culminates in neglect or untimely admission to a nursing home.

Stress based on economic factors is a two fold dilemma. First, it has been found that children, in the guise of caretakers, have confiscated the monthly checks received by their parents. Then food, clothing, and shelter are provided by the children as they deem necessary. In many cases this has proven to be a benefit and a necessity for the parent. But there have been many more cases where the discretion and intentions of the children were not nearly adequate to justify confiscation of another's sole income. Parental welfare was impaired because funds were used for needs of the children in priority to needs of the parents.

Second, economic conflict arises because children must, at least in part, support their aging parents. In some cases younger family members must find employment to at least partially support the care of the older parent. There are few support services in the community to offer assistance or relief to the children. Economically these middle-aged children are caught in a double bind. They must care for their dependent children in addition to providing for their own care and needs. They must also care for many of the needs of their elderly parents. In the meantime, they are supposed to be planning for their own retirement. Moreover, as the parents grow older, the financial dependency seems to increase proportionately.

Money is not the entire issue. Most parents are cared for. They aren't physically abandoned. They have at least some modest Social Security, Medicare, or pension assistance. Kreps maintains that for the most part "These forms of income maintenance in old age have largely replaced intrafamily support in which the wage earners provide income for their own aged parents and have enabled most older people, having their own financial resources, to live apart from their children."[38]

Do the changes in financial issues decrease family conflict? Apparently conflict arises without heavy stress on economic dependencies. Alleviation of financial demands does not minimize the need for emotional attention and, in fact, can hamper the needs and rights beyond monetary security. O'Brien maintains that social and psychological abuse of the elderly is more damaging than the physical abuse that often accompanies it.[39] Pepper estimates that actual physical battering is only proven in one-third of the cases investigated.[40] What is reported by the elderly is exploitation, neglect, rejection, isolation, and other psychological mistreatment by relatives. The daughter or son who provides for physical care or financial coverage but avoids the sensitive contact prompted by love may be just as guilty of parent abuse as the child who inflicts physical punishment. The bruises are to the emotions in one situation and to the muscles and bones in the other.

Pepper describes the typical abused person as a 75-year-old woman from a middle-class background who has noticeable disabilities and is psychologically mistreated by her relatives.[41] In addition, she may be locked out of her house and poorly clothed, and suffer from bruises, malnutrition, lacerations, uncleanliness, and dehydration. There has been no attempt to describe the personality patterns of victim and aggressor, but a person might draw from the literature on child abuse. England succinctly delineates the victim to be hypersensitive, apathetic, unresponsive, rejecting or difficult when overtures are made, and a person who cries or whines persistently, taxing the efforts and patience of the care-giver.[42]

Abuse occurs in all social classes and is episodic. The family is often isolated without support from other family members. Most important, there are discrepancies in descriptions of the causes and sequence of events that are not only incompatible from one teller to the next, but with the injuries themselves. As with child abuse and spouse abuse, it is not always possible to find sole cause with one of the individuals in the dyad.

In these encounters, guilt is not difficult to identify. Not only is it evident as the prime mover of many of the past feelings, it is just as often present again as the product of the exploitation.[43] Guilt can be hidden or exposed, but is always the result and the signal of wrongdoings. It is coupled with lowered self-esteem and resentment, and appears just as often for omitted acts as for committed acts. Guilt is often disguised with polemic responses of withdrawal or oversolicitous behavior serving the same end.[44]

Feelings of guilt arise in grown children who feel they failed to do their best or neglected their obligation to repay parents for the time and money expended on them when they were younger. For the person with the emotionally difficult or ailing parent, it is often not possible for the guilt to be discharged and a feeling of emotional equilibrium established. Moreover, it is often unrelenting and emotionally draining. Feelings of both parents and children can stem from inability to cope adequately under stress. These tests of creativity, emotion, and resources are pushed to the limit every day by unplanned, often unforeseen demands of both the environment and the persons involved. Guilt may be triggered by outsiders as well as self-inflicted. In every occasion it is an emotion that is self-defeating if allowed to continue.[45]

Labeling

Behavior patterns are age-graded. There are ways for a child to act that are different from those of adults. Further, the ways that were acceptable for a productive adult may bring castigation to a retired citizen. If an individual persists in displaying inappropriate age-grade behaviors, family and friends are inclined to conclude that the older person is "slipping," "confused," or "senile." These ambiguous terms are predicated solely on the reinterpretation of behavior in light of age-grade change. The elderly as a population have become roleless. The performance of a task in a particular way has been disallowed. Critics are no longer willing to weigh the circumstances of the elderly person's behavior. That in turn legitimizes the argument of the critics. Yet what makes them roleless? Are they any different than when they were younger, under similar circumstances?

In many ways they are not. Behavior and demeanor are guided by social assumptions and expectations. In following the rules of these behavior pattern expectations, others judge the value of the person's contribution to the occasion. As persons age, it is more often the younger, productive person who assumes the role of "judge," and an infraction of societal rules is seen as an act of senility. If one examines behavior and demeanor displayed in public places, there is often little change from earlier years; the conflict comes in the reduction of their role to an ambiguous state, and it is this ambiguity rather than an absolute change that causes others to attach negative labels of deterioration.

Arguing against the use of such terms as "senile" and "confused" is not to imply such a condition does not exist. On the contrary, there is a set of behaviors that accompanies psychosis, organic disequilibrium, drug toxicity, malnutrition, and many other physical impositions that has been termed Organic Brain Syndrome and that internally controls behavior. This is what was originally referred to as "senile behavior" or "senility." It has a cause. However, there is another situation where a person's behavior does not conform to social norms, and there is no organic cause. These people are also referred to as "senile," and it is more often than not an unjust evaluation.

In these cases the tragedy is that observers fail to evaluate such behavior in light of lifelong personality and mannerisms. Many have been acting in the same way their entire lives, but it was camouflaged by other activities, that is, jobs, family, and hobbies. Encounters were shorter, interruptions more frequent, and occasions to observe them were less continuous. Now, as an older person, that is reversed. Intensity and frequency may remain the same, but be observed more often, although it is also reasonable to argue that some elderly increase the intensity and frequency in lieu of other pasttimes to while away increased dull moments. If the behavior was always "strange," it takes on new abnormal dimensions when a person becomes "old."

Those faced with what appears to be increased "strange" behavior in their parents or acquaintances often too willingly seek to resolve it by applying a label. When the behavior exceeds the boundaries of the tolerable in reality or visibility, others unthinkingly consider the diagnosis ("senile") as a "cure." "When people attach the label 'senility' to an older person, they stop looking for the cause."[46] In effect people say, "It's incurable, now I don't have to bother with it any longer."

Unfortunately norms from which labels evolve tell us little of individuality. "Appropriate responses" are often judged by the standards of the observer, not the actor, and the judgments are based on generalized, poorly substantiated myths and stereotypes taken out of the context of society— just like the elderly's behavior is taken out of the context of a total lifetime.[47] A behavior that is rationalized in youth is often labeled "senile" in a person's more mature years, regardless of the degree of difference in the behavior from youth to old age. Losing glasses frequently when young is thought to be due to forgetfulness, but as life progresses and the habit presents itself, it is recognized as a sign of "old age." If a young person is impaired by failing faculties and presents a sloppy or messy image, the behavior is referred to as just that, but at age 70 or 80 that same behavior brings a shake of the head and ruminations on the subject of mental decline.

An understanding of the concepts of deference and demeanor is a requisite for understanding the behavior often associated with nonphysiological senility. Deference, according to Goffman, is a component of a person's activity. The function of deference is to show, symbolically, how someone respects the "sacredness" of another. It is a means of confirming relations with another and of showing appreciation. It can take many forms, but two of the major ones are avoidance and presentation.

Avoidance includes not invading personal space, keeping ceremonial and physical distance, and protecting intellectual private property. It prevents threats to another's demeanor through use of tactful blindness, joking, diplomacy, and monitored and selected conversation topics.[48] Interactions are guided by symmetrical familiarity and ritual.[49] Avoidance allows people privacy and the freedom of letting down their facades.

Presentation, although the opposite of avoidance, still does not attack another's facade, though it does imply entrance into another's personal space. It is a ritualistic pattern that communicates respect for another's "sacredness;" it includes offering beneficial assistance, giving gifts and compliments, and giving applause to show approval.[50]

Demeanor, on the other hand, is the aggregate of the socialization traits a person displays. It includes the way an individual dresses and presents to others. There are various styles and degrees of demeanor, just as there are of the use of deference. It is also a type of communication, carrying a message of image and trust. "In our society, the 'well' or 'properly' demeaned individual displays . . . discretion . . . sincerity . . . modesty . . . command of speech . . . emotions . . . desires . . . and . . . poise."[51] The poorly demeaned person is more likely to be just the reverse: using loud, inappropriate talk; swearing; belching; being crude; or demonstrating inadequate discretion in manners and tone.[52]

Deference and demeanor are complementary to one another; both are necessary and equal to validate a person's image. It is the interaction of deference and demeanor that creates a unification between people. People rely on others for validation of their social image through feedback. They are graded by others according to the degree they violate ceremonial rules of social intercourse. Avoidance allows people to maintain some degree of demeanor through concealment of some indignities, but a person's response is preferably in accord with the respect for conscious ceremonial rules of socialization and value for others. Without attempts to present a groomed demeanor and deference, the price is often loss of relationship with self and society. Those who respond inappropriately are subject to isolation by others and pressured by constraint and coercion.[53] For the aged in particular, there is the constant threat from society and family that if elders are uncivil, they risk being institutionalized.[54] The message is that to retain independence, elders must keep social abilities current.

Failure to use deference and maintain demeanor when old has a different meaning than when young. Of the four women in the following examples, the argument persists that their behavior is comparable to that of younger people, but is seen differently because of their accumulated years.

Mrs. A and Mrs. B

These two women are almost inseparable friends. They are well-dressed, well-groomed, warm, friendly, social women. Their voices are animated, but modulated. When they are both at the senior center, they sit together and chat quietly. When activities are introduced, they participate freely but together. They eat lunch and snacks one beside the other and ask questions of concern to each other. They are physically very self-sufficient, needing neither help to ambulate nor reminders to adequately perform toilet functions. They never demonstrate hostile behavior. They are opinionated, but usually express opinions quietly to each other or to the staff. They seek out conversation with others.

An interesting part of their sociability is their conversation pattern. They sit together and converse for hours, commenting on scenes as if those scenes were "before their eyes." The two sides of their conversations, though integrated and modulated as though the women are interacting with each other in a dialogue, in fact have nothing in common. The sounds, gestures, and postures are within the boundaries of social regulation, and the women abide by cues for giving attention to one another, relinquishing the floor, and not interrupting. The betrayal of their effort is that the content is neither related to any particular topic before them nor to each other. There is interplay of sounds and behaviors, but disparity in content. It is a marvelously controlled series of interactions to observe; they ratify each other's existence and each other's social conduct, but not their individual secular orientation.

It appears that these women want to "act normally;" they work at it very hard. Their very presence in free society is threatened if they don't. These women are coherent in many areas and can carry on normal life, which allows them to stay with their families in the evenings and not be subjected to 24-hour nursing home care. If they lose this thread of "socialization," institutionalization will be a much greater likelihood.

Yet vacuous conversation is not restricted to the senile or the elderly. Children in play carry on separate conversations while seeming to socialize. Executives and politicians, intent on their own opposing aims and interests, often mask their divergent motivations and manipulate conversation processes so they will achieve some unstated goal in the guise of another person's ends. Their conversation, in pursuit of those ends, may be no more rational or coherent than that of Mrs. A and Mrs. B, but their age and status prevent them from being considered "confused" or "senile."

What all these people have in common are use of deference and establishment of demeanor. One defers to the other for a chance to speak. When that is accomplished, the second demonstrates good manners by responding, smiling, and looking at the other person. There is a shared intent of interaction, not necessarily of subject matter. This process is necessary because it gives value to the individual's historic accomplishments and demonstrates a present orientation of awareness; if a person shares with the world in conversation, that person is still a human being.

Mrs. C

Mrs. C is a study of dynamic contrasts with the two ladies in the previous example, with one major exception: her behavior also is not identifiably different from that when she was younger. She appears to have been a feisty woman who, upon occasion over her lifetime, embarrassed her family in antics devoid of much "polish." Her social graces waffle between polite conversation and acceptable manners to rejection of any activities or socialization offered to her. Her demeanor is characterized by good grooming, but otherwise she denounces others, rejects comments, and is occasionally rude and disruptive in group activities where she is a member. She has come to realize that such behavior will ensure a continuation of attention and a certain degree of civil inattention, where people will ignore her crude, abrasive behavior or laugh at it. A person will receive favorable attention or civil inattention only while remaining within the boundaries of propriety.[55]

Until recently, Mrs. C had not reached the boundaries of behavior that the group would tolerate, so the limits of her aggressive behavior continued to expand and intrude upon those around her. The group as a whole continued to ignore her behavior. The majority of the time she chose to be outside the activity pattern, but physically within the group. She sent distracting messages, refused to participate, and unfolded her demeanor outward in a scowling, hostile manner. The level of her distractions became intolerable and began to disrupt group activities.

One day when this was going on, the entire group got up without previous agreement and moved to a new spot across the room, leaving her alone, baffled, powerless, and reprimanded through nonverbal communication. She shouted at them to come back; they totally ignored her. She had refused to defer to the rules of respect that allowed participation within the bounded area of the group, and breach of the rules brought alienation. She attempted to act as though she were an island without need of others, but she soon realized they were her source of confirmation. She stopped her offensive behavior, resumed a well-demeaned facade, and quietly joined the relocated group. To be able to function at some level of acceptable socialization is the key measurement of independence.

Mrs. C chose to demonstrate her independence through negative socialization, or lack of deference and demeanor. She was not reverting to, but no doubt was continuing to use, her child-age rules. She seemed to be shocking people through poor manners and unrestrained behavior as she reportedly had in earlier times.

There is considerable speculation as to whether Mrs. C's behavior is conscious and controlled. Regardless, the social value of it is the same whether it is intentional or inadvertent, caused by psychological factors or physical factors. If people act "senile," they are treated as such whether they are "smart-alecks" caught in lifelong habits or victims of Alzheimer's Disease. Such dramatic behavior seems to be an attempt to continue to control environment and society, the assumption being that a person who can control self in relationship to control imposed on environment will also be able to avoid isolation and institutionalization.

Mrs. D

Mrs. D was attractive, poised, and extroverted. She had always been proud of her appearance and social graces. Her eyesight and hearing began to fail markedly and with it, inevitably, her demeanor. In several attempts to remain self-sufficient, she jeopardized her image by not deferring to others.

Her hair and her clothing became disheveled. Mrs. D's impaired hearing and vision jeopardized her social interactions in receiving feedback from others validating her image. She could neither see the revealing details of crowds, television, or facial expressions, nor hear auditory stimuli necessary for pleasing conversations, directions, and communication. In addition, her mobility slowed and was often seriously impaired. Mrs. D often could not move with the stimuli, and instead was left in sensory isolation. She became socially involuted, losing degrees of both deference and demeanor.

Without vision and hearing it is natural to lapse into reverie and reminiscence. This is precisely what happened to Mrs. D. Her impairment limited the ability to receive new information; therefore that which was known became more precious and was rehashed, retold, and rearranged *ad infinitum*, further reducing her capacity to fit in with the group socially.

Mrs. D was labeled by many as "senile." She was demonstrating behavior change due to physical impairment, a process that is not specifically age-related. Similar impairment among younger people has been demonstrated to have the same results, but without the negative labels.

It must be said as an addendum that Mrs. D's incapacities are also partly reversible, as they are among younger people. She cannot regain her eyesight, but she can begin to cope with the loss and find ways to present a better-demeaned person, as well as to defer to those who can assist her.

As people age it appears that they must demonstrate greater degrees of deference and demeanor to avoid being labeled as incompetent. People compensate for poor demeanor and deference by being capable and independent, but once physical capabilities begin to decline, there are not as many resources for compensation.

The cases analyzed according to deference and demeanor concepts show that, in conversation, deference and demeanor are more important than the content of the messages verbalized. This supports the old adage, "It's not what you say but how you say it that counts." In peer group activity, those who exceed the boundaries of the acceptable are reprimanded by the members. Excessive lack of deference will bring alienation from the group and negative feedback. Finally, physical decline requires a sharing process of the participant deferring to others for that period of compromised capability. As Frankfather asserts, it is possible to initiate "imaginative and resourceful survival strategies, as well as mental acuity for environmental contingencies" with the assistance of the society in which one interacts.[56] Such response organizes social experiences to counteract possibilities of devaluation.[57]

In conclusion, whether positive or negative, the family support system is the motivational factor in maintaining the elderly in the community. It provides a means of survival and continuity to their lives, and is crucial to the continuation of relationships with others. For many families, intergenerational behavior patterns function on a perfunctory level with little awareness of motivational factors. Awareness and understanding of such behavior can contribute considerably to the satisfaction of those involved in the interactions. Regardless of quality, all these relationships have a depth to them that should not be dismissed at face value and a potential for greater warmth and appreciation that should be developed.

In terms of positive relationships within the social network, it is important to have an understanding of the needs of the elderly and an ability to communicate openly and develop a sensitivity to individual differences. Moreover, negative relationships can be transformed into more positive behavior patterns by considering individual variability within the context of their life styles and environments.

NOTES

1. Ruth Murray, M. Marilyn Huelskoetter, and Dorothy O'Driscoll, *The Nursing Process in Later Maturity* (Englewood Cliffs, N.J.: Prentice-Hall, Inc., 1980), p. 52.
2. Sidney M. Jourard, *Personal Adjustment*, Second Edition (New York, N.Y.: The Macmillan Co., 1971), p. 310.
3. Vern L. Bengtson et al., "The Generation Gap and Aging Family Members," in Jaber F. Gubrium, ed., *Time, Roles, and Self in Old Age* (New York, N.Y.: Human Sciences Press, 1976), pp. 253–5.
4. S. Jourard, *Personal Adjustment*, p. 238.
5. Ibid., p. 358.
6. R. Murray, *The Nursing Process in Later Maturity*, p. 295.
7. Ibid., p. 296.
8. Judith Treas, "Family Support System for the Aged" in Abraham Monk, ed., *The Age of Aging* (Buffalo, N.Y.: Prometheus Books, 1979), p. 186.
9. Ibid., p. 191.

10. Ibid., p. 192.

11. Paulette Robischon and Alice M. Akan, "The Family and Its Role With the Elderly Parent," in Adina M. Reinhardt and Mildred D. Quinn, eds., *Current Practice in Gerontological Nursing* (St. Louis, Mo.: The C. V. Mosby Co., 1979), p. 161.

12. R. Murray, *The Nursing Process in Later Maturity*, p. 303.

13. Ibid., p. 303.

14. Vern L. Bengtson, "You, Your Children & Their Children," in Bernice O'Brien, ed., *Aging: Today's Research and You* (Los Angeles, Cal.: The University of Southern California Press, 1978), p. 19.

15. Ibid., p. 23.

16. Ibid., pp. 23–30.

17. Ibid., p. 27.

18. R. Murray, *The Nursing Process in Later Maturity*, p. 302.

19. Carol C. Hogue, "Support Systems for Health Promotion," in Joanne E. Hall and Barbara R. Weaver, eds., *Distributive Nursing Practice* (Philadelphia, Pa.: J. B. Lippincott Co., 1977), p. 67.

20. Elizabeth Bott, *Family and Social Network*, Second Edition (London, Eng: Tavistock Publication, 1971), pp. 248–330.

21. Robert N. Butler and Myrna I. Lewis, *Aging and Mental Health*, Second Edition (St. Louis, Mo.: The C.V. Mosby Co., 1977), p. 120.

22. Ibid., p. 119.

23. Carol C. Hogue, "Support Systems for Health Promotion," p. 68.

24. Gerald Caplan, *Support Systems and Community Mental Health* (New York, N.Y.: Behavioral Publications, 1974).

25. Carol C. Hogue, "Support Systems for Health Promotion," p. 68.

26. Gerald Caplan, *Support Systems and Community Mental Health*, pp. 1–40.

27. Gordon F. Streib, "Old Age and the Family," in Ethel Shanas, ed., *Aging in Contemporary Society* (Beverly Hills, Cal.: Sage Publications, 1970), p. 31.

28. Ibid., p. 31.

29. Ibid., p. 31.

30. Ibid., p. 33.

31. Ibid., p. 34.

32. R. Murray, *The Nursing Process in Later Maturity*, p. 303.

33. Rose M. Somerville, "The Future of Family Relationships," in Beth B Hess, ed., *Growing Old in America* (New Brunswick, N. J.: Transaction Books, 1976), p. 354.

34. Anita Harbert and Leon Ginsberg, *Human Services For Older Adults* (Belmont, Cal.: Wadsworth Publishing Co., 1979), p. 156.

35. Morton Puner, *To The Good Long Life* (New York, N.Y.: Universe Books, 1974), p. 127.

36. Ibid., p. 129.

37. "Elder Abuse in Homes," *Geriatric Nursing* 1, no. 3 (Sept./Oct. 1980):153–4.

38. J. Kreps, "Intergenerational Transfer and the Bureaucracy," in E. Shanas and M. Sussman, eds., *Family, Bureaucracy and the Elderly* (Durham, N.C.: Duke University Press, 1977), p. 33.

39. M. A. O'Brien, "Battered Grandparents": Does This Term Apply to Elderly People in New Zealand? *New Zealand Nursing Journal* 72, no. 3 (March 1979): 3.

40. "Elder Abuse in Homes," p. 153.

41. Ibid., pp. 153–4.

42. F. England, "Detection of Non-Accidental Injury," *Nursing Times* 75, no. 4 (1979): 1858.

43. B. Silverstone and H.K. Hyman, *You and Your Aging Parent* (New York, N.Y.: Pantheon Books, 1976),p. 29.

44. Ibid., p. 34.

45. Ibid., p. 35.

46. B. Isaacs, "Don't Bother—She Won't Notice," *Nursing Mirror* 149, no. 37 (November 1, 1979):24–25.

47. Mary Wolanin and L. Phillips, "Who's Confused Here?" *Geriatric Nursing* 1, no.3 (1980): 122–6.

48. Erving Goffman, "On Face-Work," *Psychiatry* 18, no. 3 (1955):218–9.

49. Erving Goffman, "The Nature of Deference and Demeanor," *American Anthropologist* 58, no. 3 (1956):483–8.

50. Ibid., p. 483.

51. Ibid., pp. 488–9.

52. Ibid., p. 490.

53. Ibid., p. 487.

54. Erving Goffman, *Behavior in Public Places* (New York, N.Y.: Free Press, 1963), p. 497.

55. Ibid., p. 87.

56. Dwight Frankfather, *The Aged in the Community* (New York, N.Y.: Praeger Publications, 1977), p. 78.

57. Rodney Coe, "Self-Conception and Institutionalization," in A.M. Rose and W.A. Peterson, eds., *Older People and Their Social World* (Philadelphia, Pa.: F.A. Davis, 1965), pp. 226–41.

Chapter 10

Coping and Decision Making

Chiyoko Furukawa

Coping and decision making are processes that older persons have experienced and practiced during their lifetimes. However, some individuals claim more success than others in dealing with life events that require adjustments and decisions to resolve problems. Furthermore, those individuals who were successful in earlier years tend to retain their ability to manage difficulties and changes related to the aging process. Some factors that contribute to the success are intelligence, life experiences, health, energy, and education. Individuals use these and other attributes to develop patterns of adaptation and problem solving that are beneficial for survival and congruent with their life styles. Thus, numerous patterns of aging may evolve, and there is no one design for successful aging. It might be hypothesized that elderly persons, who continue to cope and make decisions, manage to do so despite lessened resources and increased demands for adjustments by the aging process.

In successful aging, coping behavior gives a person protection from psychological, physical, and other insults. The protective function of coping behavior may be performed by eliminating or modifying conditions that lead to problems, by perceptually controlling the meaning of experience in order to neutralize problems, and by keeping psychological consequences from problems manageable.[1] Apparently, most elderly manage their problems using these or other processes. However, when demands of the aging process become life-threatening and require drastic, permanent changes, the coping mechanism for some older people may become exhausted. The decrease in energy, support, and resources, which is inherent in aging, contributes to reduced ability to adjust to changes. In particular, the loss of close interpersonal relationships with family members and friends is sorely felt in finding appropriate coping styles.

Decision making, as with coping, requires a concerted effort on the part of some elders, while others take it in their stride. Generally, the patterns established in youth continue to be used, and the process remains un-changed with age providing that the cognitive functions stay intact and unaffected by the adversities of becoming old. It is believed that aging in itself has little influence on the ability to make decisions. However, older people are more cautious about decisions and tend to choose a course of action that has a high probability of success.[2]

Guttman outlines four stages involved in an elder's decision making as it relates to life events.[3] These are particularly useful since dealing with changes in life events is the major concern of elderly persons. The stages as identified by Guttman are: first, the individual must be aware of the problem, need, stress, or crisis. Recognition and acknowledgment are nec-essary as a problem does not exist unless a person views it as such. Second, the problem must be analyzed to seek alternative information from self and others to determine costs, utilities, or values. This process allows the person to explore choices that might be available. Third, the best alter-native is selected, and this may include the decision to delay action. No action may also be viewed as a decision. When action is taken by using one of the selected alternatives, the fourth stage, which consists of eval-uating outcomes, follows. Specifically, this stage determines whether the action taken was or was not successful and satisfactory. The consequences of no action may also be evaluated, and other alternatives could be selected.

Guttman found that elders who took action clearly demonstrated a more intensive use of the decision-making process than those who were non-active.[4] He also contends that, contrary to what is reported in the literature, not all life events are seen as stressful by elders. Most older people living in a community are diverse and unique in their perception of life events and have a strong will to live and enjoy life.[5] However, society's views may differ as suggested by Harris' report that less than 41 percent of the people he surveyed considered the elderly to be active.[6] This implies that society has a misconception about the older population's ability to be self-sufficient, cope with their problems, and make decisions relative to their lives. The public must be educated about aging and shown that most older people live independently in the community, and few require confinement to institutional settings.

To understand the elder's coping and decision making requires the ex-ploration of the aged's dealing with losses, changes in life style, and psy-chological responses as a consequence of growing old.

DEALING WITH LOSSES

Major losses of work, income, physical and mental abilities, peers, and spouse can occur gradually over the years or in a relatively short period of time. However, when losses happen in succession, stress increases and the ability to establish coping behaviors may diminish because a complete resolution of previous losses may not have occurred. On the other hand, as individuals experience losses, coping behaviors may become strengthened as new information about adjustment capabilities is gained. However, professionals, family, and friends must provide assistance appropriate to each loss to the person who suffers multiple losses, and they must continue the support until a coping behavior is established.

Some strategies to assist the aged in coping with losses can be derived from Morgan's characteristics of older people who have been successful in coping.[7] These individuals seem to have an awareness of the aging process and are able to accept the limitations that accompany it. They do not attempt to continue activities that require abilities that are no longer available to them. There is a reevaluation of life goals, based on previous experiences, to establish modified, but realistic, pursuits for the remaining years. In these instances, individuals may forego goals of earlier years and identify new ones that are more appropriate to achieve. These goals usually serve as alternative sources for identity and self-esteem, and help maintain feelings of personal importance and self-worth. This activity is especially crucial for those people who relied heavily on their employment for their identity. Finally, the ability to reinterpret the meaning of self, when previous roles that sustained their position are no longer available, is important. This particularly applies to the earlier status of a parent and worker that has become inapplicable. Thus, new positions to replace former roles are necessary through self-evaluation and reassessment of life meaning in later years.

Similar individual characteristics of coping with losses inherent in aging are well illustrated by Fontana in her study of elderly participants of a senior center.[8] She identified the following four types of people: relaxers, do-gooders, joiners, and waiters. Each group demonstrated reactions to losses and the aging phenomena.

The relaxers showed no anger or signs of despair, and had a peaceful attitude toward aging. They selected and participated in activities that were of interest to them. They were content to meet their own needs by relaxing and doing what they wanted to do, and were not pressured by any social expectations. These people accepted aging and made adjustments to maintain their integrity.

The do-gooders viewed themselves as well adjusted and satisfied in retirement. However, they continued the work role by participating as volunteers for the benefit of other older people. They received fulfillment in helping others and found the role meaningful.

The joiners were people who spent most of their time and energy seeking fun through group activities arranged by others. Their new goal in life was to have fun, enjoy themselves, and stay away from activities that resembled work. This group had substituted work with recreation and found a role to satisfy their needs.

The waiters were mostly people who had experienced crisis in their lives, for example, work role loss, debilitating illness, or the loss of a loved one. The waiters had difficulty with life change adjustments and exhibited characteristic behaviors of reduced social contacts, such as inability to control some aspects of their lives, neglected personal appearance, grumpy disposition, and little concern for the welfare of others. The waiters' coping styles presented minimal redirection of their lives to find positive responses to alleviate the pain of losses.

A period of grieving usually follows a loss. Several experts provide descriptions of behaviors that usually occur. Table 10-1 illustrates the similarities of the stages and phases presented by Kubler-Ross, Lindemann, and Kavanaugh.[9,10,11] Although each theorist uses different terminology to describe the processes for coping with loss, the behaviors described are quite similar. All suggest behaviors to observe when assisting the older person to reach a resolution of loss by progressing through the mourning process. The grieving stages require care to avoid compartmentalization of human behavior and forced experience of each stage in the process of resolving losses. Some stages may be omitted, or a person may remain in a stage as a way of coping with losses.

LIFE STYLE CHANGES

Every older person has an established life style that contributed to the survival to old age. This is not to say that some may have survived despite themselves. However healthy or unhealthy a person's life style may have been, the important fact is that the individual was comfortable with it and

Table 10-1 Comparison of Grieving Stages

Kubler-Ross	Lindemann	Kavanaugh
Denial	Shock and disbelief	Shock
Anger	Developing awareness	Disorganization
Bargaining	Resolving the loss	Volatile emotions
Depression		Guilt
Acceptance		Loss and loneliness
		Relief
		Reestablishment

used the chosen style for a long time. This life style is unique to that individual. Therefore, it is natural for the older person to wish to preserve the chosen life style with full knowledge of the positive and negative features that affect the living pattern. These long-established living modes are particularly difficult to alter to accommodate different life events or to find appropriate coping behaviors.

Life style changes may be viewed as mandatory due to losses associated with the aging process. Generally, the losses become greater as an individual grows older and necessitate a more drastic alteration of the living pattern. It is ironic that the occasions requiring changes and adjustments are more frequent as a person loses adaptive abilities. The losses, which demand permanent supportive measures, are the most devastating changes for the elders. If appropriately planned, however, the major deviations in life pattern may be a positive experience. For example, retirement can offer freedom, which was not available during the working years, to engage in new activities or extend old ones. This change could be an enjoyable experience, as well as a satisfying alternative to the work role.

Researchers in gerontology agree on some of the factors that contribute to an individual's life satisfaction; however, the determination of the most influential elements appears uncertain. Factors such as age, physical and mental status, adequate income, participation in leisure, and self-esteem are mentioned as important determinants leading to selected life styles and life satisfaction in later years.

Life satisfaction research indicates that social and health factors are important. George studied the impact of personality and social status upon levels of activity and social well-being, and concluded that psychological well-being is associated with higher socioeconomic status; good health and being married also influenced activity levels and well-being.[12] Similarly, Markides and Martin found that health and activities are strong predictors of life satisfaction, with income an indirect influence that allowed participation in activities, for example, travel and hobbies.[13] Educational level played the least significant role. Palmore et al. investigated stress and adaptation in aging and indicated that psychological and social resources assisted in maintaining all the measures of life satisfaction.[14] Retirement was found to have the most negative social-psychological effect and some effect on physical adaptation. Furthermore, they reported that most of the potential stressors, that is, retirement, spouse's retirement, widowhood, departure of the last child from the home, and major medical events (illness requiring hospitalization) have less long-term outcome than the crisis occurrence might suggest.

In another study, Palmore researched the predictors of successful aging (defined as survival to age 75 with good health and happiness) and con-

cluded that the ability to participate in group and physical activities contributed to successful aging.[15] Group activities involved the physical,
psychological, and social aspects of the individual and provided for the
maintenance of physical health, mental stimulation, interactive skills, reality orientation, general mental health, sense of belonging, morale, purpose,
and social gratification. In support of Markides and Martin's model, Palmore found that education and intelligence by themselves contributed little
toward successful aging; the more important factor was how an individual
used intelligence or education.

The theories of aging offer some insight into the expectations of the
elderly person and the characteristics of successful aging or life satisfaction.
Currently there is no agreement on any one theory of aging; however, the
continuity theory provides an optimistic view on aging as well as taking
individual uniqueness into account. The main assumption of the continuity
theory is that a person wishes to maintain familiar and habitual patterns
of living and may be flexible about modification of patterns in response to
psychological, biological, and social factors that occur in growing old.[16]
Although a person may continue with earlier activities, changes in the
degree and method of participation indicate adaptation of past methods.
Frequently, an individual may or may not choose to replace lost or relinquished roles. However, high morale depends on successful adaptation to
new life situations.

The most distinguishing assumption in the continuity theory is that adaptation in any direction is possible, but research to test all the variables
adequately remains a difficult task because varied and complex experiences
among the aged are considered. The continuity theory remains unre-
searched, but its strength is the portrayal of the elders as having the ability
to adapt and cope with changes imposed by the aging process.

There is concern about life style changes for the elderly person who
becomes socially isolated. Isolation behavior of older people is complex
and must be seen within the context of life circumstances and personal
preferences, and in terms of voluntary, involuntary, lifelong, or recent
occurrences. This is suggested by Bennett's investigation of isolation patterns in which four types of older people were identified: (1) those who
maintain social contacts over a lifetime; (2) early isolates who were isolated
as adults, but are relatively active in later life; (3) the involuntary or recent
isolates who were active in earlier life, but as elders became isolated; and
(4) the lifetime or voluntary isolates who chose the isolated life style.[17]
The last behavior was illustrated in a recent study which revealed that
elderly residents of single occupancy hotels can be characterized as lifelong
loners who were unable to engage in effective relationships.[18] However,
the survey also indicated that these elderly residents did have a viable

personal network that provided both material and emotional support in time of need. This finding is contrary to the concept of isolation, which focuses upon deprivation of social contacts.[19]

The most common causes of isolation for the elderly person, which may also result in feelings of loneliness, are the death of a spouse, children who move away, chronic illness, and physical discomforts.[20] Loneliness is considered to be different from isolation in that it is a psychological state. Kivett discovered the feelings of loneliness in rural elders were quite complex and were confounded by many physical and environmental variables.[21] She suggests that integrating social activities, relationships, transportation, communication, and health may alleviate the situation. Decreased sensory input, such as visual and auditory loss, are also known to contribute to isolation and loneliness, unless proper interventions are instituted to prevent emotional stress. In addition, the inability to adjust to these stresses and the environmental changes required for coping may become the basis for bizarre behavior and self-imposed loneliness as a defense mechanism against further trauma.[22]

In selected instances, isolation behavior may be interpreted as an expression of independence by the elderly. Some older people value independence and will attempt to continue to adhere to this style as long as possible. Lopata found widows tended to live with loneliness and were unwilling to be economically and socially dependent on their children. They did not want to interrupt or interfere with their children's marriages and family life styles.[23]

Societal values also add to the confusion involved in an older person's independent status and often place the elders in a no-win situation. For example, one aspect of independence is removed when the individual must retire because of age. This can lead to financial strain, and in some instances the elders become dependent on supplemental income from governmental or family resources for life support. Another support system provided by marriage and a family becomes less effective following the death of a spouse or when grown children move away. The remaining parent is expected to function independently, but some degree of isolation or loneliness will invariably result.

Isolation and independence can be interrelated in a variety of ways. Older persons may fear isolation and use dependency to ensure that someone will continue to relate to them. This behavior is a coping mechanism to avoid social isolation and to remain in control. Lowenthal and Robinson express concerns about the aged who no longer can control their patterns of living and are forced to be with others when they prefer solitude or vice versa.[24]

Another issue that must be addressed is the notion that increased dependency with aging is bad, and independence is desirable. Most people, regardless of age, depend on others for some support to sustain their life styles. For example, no one questions the dependency of infants and children on the mother-father for meal preparation, clean environment, and nurturing in time of illness. It is time for society to acknowledge the reduced capabilities and resources of most elders and accept the responsibilities to assist them in maintaining their chosen life styles without any stigma.

Most would agree that role changes are inevitable in the aging process, and an individual's coping and decision making determines the relinquishing of old roles or accepting of new ones. The results of these actions influence behaviors of independence, dependence, and satisfaction with later life. Problems associated with aging might be minimized if an older person is able to replace lost roles with new roles. People often become victims of role loss upon retirement, and replacement of this role is crucial for positive adjustments; however, society has not provided adequate assistance in this direction.

Rosow contends that society has unspecified roles for the aged and does not allow a smooth transition to role changes and losses in contrast to earlier stages of life.[25] Individuals are prepared to progress from infancy through childhood to adulthood, but preparation for aging beyond adulthood is not apparent. Furthermore, Rosow views the systematic losses of status and the decline in competence, responsibility, and authority as major problems to the elderly group.[26] Because society has not clearly outlined norms for the aged to restructure their lives or to guide them in the establishment of new life goals, older individuals must use their own motivational abilities, creativity, self-development, and self-expression to identify new meanings of life while discarding previously used roles and norms as workers, parents, and spouses.

PSYCHOLOGICAL RESPONSES

Anomie, depression, and suicide are psychological responses to aging that are antithetical to life satisfaction. These adverse behaviors have no simple explanation and are believed to be associated with coping mechanisms and decision making that deviate from the usual behaviors of most older persons.

The concept of anomie, originally formulated by Emile Durkheim, has been widely discussed, critiqued, and used in the social sciences. Since some differences of opinion exist on whether anomie is experienced by the aged, an exploration of some of the interpretations of anomie may be helpful to decide if this behavior is seen in the elders.

Boor notes that anomie is a state of normlessness caused by rapid social change that leads to loss of social control and uncertain expectations from society.[27] A slightly different interpretation by Peretti and Wilson describes anomie as a feeling that life has broken down because norms and values have become meaningless and the world lacks the cohesiveness and solidarity associated with an integrated society.[28] Gliddens sees anomie, first, as a state of being demoralized. Second, he states that because society is the source of moral regulation, individuals who are inadequately integrated socially are in anomie. Third, aspirations cannot be reached because society creates potentialities that are incapable of actualization within the existing social framework.[29]

An opponent to the application of anomie, that is, normlessness, views the concept from the social structural position and maintains that the aged continue to have norms acquired throughout their lifetimes.[30] The normlessness position for the aged evolves from the younger cohorts rather than from the older people. Because society sets norms that can change with time, the aged's norms, established by past societal values, are in conflict with the prevailing newer and different norms. Anomie may exist in elders, but not with the majority of older people.

A proponent of anomie in aging claims that during periods of rapid societal changes, anomie becomes more of a problem because confusion occurs about appropriate and proper conduct.[31] Older people, who are particularly vulnerable, require clear-cut guidelines to feel good; unclear rules of conduct make them confused and disorganized. Deikman contends that anomie stems from the absence of a deeply felt purpose, and, as the body ages, the mind tends to grow restless to seek solutions to death.[32] For the aged, former goals become less or no longer significant, and life begins to appear as a random cycle of unimportant events and terminates in despair or dull resignation. Thus, older people become tired of keeping up with the times by changing customs, and they choose to depart from the scene of living.

Associated with the feeling of inability to keep pace and cope, there is evidence to suggest that people over 60 years of age have mild nondisabling feelings of depression that are rarely brought up for medical attention.[33] Some researchers have the opinion that the elder's inability to cope with multiple losses, feelings of helplessness, and reduced self-esteem is the basis for depression.[34] Gauer posits that a multitude of factors make elders, more than the younger population group, prone to depression.[35] Furthermore, depression is more prevalent in older men than women, while in the younger group, the reverse is true. The factors that most likely contribute to the depressive moods and stresses experienced by the elders are somatic illness, chronic physical and psychological disabilities, sensory deficits, general decline, economic and social disadvantages, frequent grieving, isolation, and self-overmedication with prescription or over-the-counter drugs.

It is estimated that nearly 20 percent of all elderly adults suffer from significant symptoms of depression.[36] The results of a psychiatric survey indicate only about 5 percent of the population over 65 have a well-defined depressive illness, but when the symptom check method was used in the population sample, the prevalence of depression increased to 11 percent.[37] This lack of agreement on the number of depressed elders is a concern that Jarvik explores.[38] He believes there is little understanding of the processes underlying depression despite the amount of evidence presented. The unexplored area regarding the age when the initial onset of depressive episodes occurs raises some unanswered questions, for example, "Why aren't all elders depressed?" Jarvik speculates that the answers to depression may be found in the interaction of the environment, life stresses, and the internal adaptive abilities of the aged person.

The difficulties in recognizing depression in elders are addressed by Hirschfield and Klerman, and Salzman and Shader.[39,40] It is estimated that only 25 percent of the people with depression receive treatment. One problem in diagnosing depression in the aged is attributed to the presence of a defensive ego mechanism or somatic symptoms, which disguise signs of depression. Another difficulty is that depression is often preceded by or associated with a variety of medical problems common to the older individual.[41] Therefore, depression can easily be overlooked, and the importance of examining cluster symptoms becomes evident for identifying depression in elders. To illustrate, Table 10-2 shows that clinical depression

Table 10-2 Comparison of Severe Depression and Senile Dementia Characteristics

	Depressed	Senile		Depressed	Senile
Depression	+ + + +	+ +	Confusion	+ +	+ + + +
Sleep and appetite disturbance	+ + +	+ +	Disorientation	+	+ + + +
Suicidal thoughts	+ +	±	Impaired recent memory	+	+ + + +
Emotional liability	+	+ + +	Decreased mental alertness	+ +	+ + + +
Anxiety	+ + +	+ +	Unsociability	+ +	+ + + +
Hostility-Irritability	+ +	+ + +	Uncooperativeness	+ +	+ + + +

Source: Reprinted with permission from C. Salzman and R. Shader, "Depression in the Elderly I. Relationship Between Depression, Psychologic Defense Mechanisms, and Physical Illness," *Journal of American Geriatric Society* 26, no. 6 (June 1978), p. 257

and senile dementia have similar characteristics; however, a given characteristic can be more prominent, as indicated by the greater number of plus signs in one characteristic as compared to another.

The signs of depression in elders may vary from facial expressions of sadness, apathy, disinterest, helplessness, and despair to withdrawal and refusal of food or drink. A person may remain in bed in severe depression and become nonparticipating in personal care or hygiene. Table 10-3 sum-

Table 10-3 Signs and Symptoms of Depression in the Elderly

Common signs or symptoms of depression	Differential diagnosis
Insomnia (early morning awakening)	Normal, particularly if there is daytime napping; dyspnea secondary to congestive heart failure; pain; many medical illnesses
Constipation	Normal, secondary to decreased autonomic innervation of (gatrointestinal) GI tract; dehydration; secondary to anticholinergic effects of drugs
Anorexia	Many medical diseases such as "failure to thrive;" chronic infection; malignancy; diabetes
Hopelessness, despair, gloom, sadness, apathy, withdrawal of interest	Many physical diseases such as cancer of pancreas, pernicious anemia, hypo- and hyperendocrine function; reaction to severe or chronic physical disease; secondary to sedating drugs; secondary to antihypertensive drugs or L-dopa
Memory loss	Mild forgetfulness normal; pseudodementia; true early dementia; secondary to medical drugs, for example, cardiac glycosides
Multiple somatic complaints and pains	Many medical diseases such as hyperparathyroidism; Addison's disease; rheumatoid arthritis
Withdrawal, mutism, retardation of affect and movement	Idiopathic parkinsonism; drugs, for example, akinesia secondary to phenothiazines; apathetic thyrotoxicosis; antihypertension agents; early congestive heart failure
Irritability	Secondary to benzodiazepine drugs, alcohol, and other disinhibitors; secondary to amphetamines; hyperadrenal function or cortisol drugs; drug withdrawal states (barbiturates, benzodiazepines, antipsychotics, antidepressants); many medical diseases; reaction to chronic illness
Decreased libido	Some decrease normal; secondary to physical illness; secondary to drugs, for example, phenothiazines, antihypertensive agents
Weight loss, pallor, increasing frailty	Chronic infection; diabetes; advanced metastatic cancer

Source: Reprinted with permission from C. Salzman and R. Shader, "Depression in the Elderly II. Possible Drug Etiologies: Differential Diagnostic Criteria," *Journal of American Geriatric Society* 26, no. 7 (July 1978), p. 307

marizes the signs and symptoms of depression that can be exhibited by elderly individuals. These manifestations provide clues for professionals working to evaluate the early detection of depression among older persons. In addition, the list of differential diagnoses in Table 10-3 is extremely helpful in determining normal functions from abnormal ones, and can be used in the health promotion and maintenance of the aging group.

Medications used for the treatment of chronic illnesses are known to predispose elders to depression. The drugs commonly used by the elderly group to treat a variety of conditions are listed in Table 10-4. Since the drugs can be used over an extended period of time, they might be considered, during reviews of drug therapy, as potential causes of depressive symptoms in older individuals. Adjustments of the medications as necessary may be the difference between continued depression and alleviation of the symptoms. When the focus of care is health promotion and maintenance care, this professional activity is an imperative intervention.

Depression in older people can lead to suicide. Suicide characteristics among elders are different from those in the younger age group in that

Table 10-4 Drugs Associated with Depression

Class and Generic Name	Trade Name
Antihypertensives	
Reserpine	Serpasil, Ser-Ap-Es, Sandril
Methyldopa	Aldomet
Propranolol hydrochloride	Inderal
Guanethidine sulfate	Ismelin sulfate
Hydralazine hydrochloride	Apresoline hydrochloride
Clonidine hydrochloride	Catapres
Antiparkinsonian agents	
Levodopa	Dopar, Larodopa
Levodopa and carbidopa	Sinemet
Amantadine hydrochloride	Symmetrel
Hormones	
Estrogen	Evex, Menrium, Femest
Progesterone	Lipo-Lutin, Progestasert, Proluton
Corticosteroids	
Cortisone acetate	Cortone acetate
Antituberculosis	
Cycloserine	Seromycin
Anticancer	
Vincristine sulfate	Oncovin
Vinblastine sulfate	Velban

Source: Reprinted with permission from *GERIATRICS* © 1979 Harcourt Brace Jovanovich, Inc. R. Hirschfield and G. Klerman, "Treatment of Depression in the Elderly," *Geriatrics* 34, no. 10 (October 1979), p. 54

older people make fewer attempts, communicate intentions of suicide less frequently, use more lethal methods, and are more successful than the young.[42] In addition, older people do not use suicide activity as a means to manipulate others and are less ambivalent; therefore, prevention is not possible in many instances.

Accurate statistics on suicide rates are not available because of underreporting, avoidance of stigma to the family, and, possibly, insurance implications. Nevertheless, the suicide rates for different groups and ages presented in Table 10-5 show that some consistent trends do exist in suicide activities. First, suicide rates are higher among males than females, regardless of race or age. Also, the suicide rate for both male and female groups is greater for the white population than for nonwhite people. Finally, Table 10-5 shows a significant and continued increase in suicide rate with age among white males, while for the rest of the population, the suicide rates attain a maximum at some mid-age and then decrease with age. The overall suicide rate in the U.S. has remained between 9 and 13 per 100,000 since World War II, but the rate for older white males has ranged from 40 to 75 per 100,000.[43]

The problem of geriatric suicides is a concern expressed by many experts. There apparently is no one factor that leads to suicide behavior, but rather a series of events and situations with which an elder must cope. Miller states, "The crucial factor seems to be how well developed and efficacious are the person's coping abilities."[44] He further explains it is the reaction of the person to a predicament rather than the trauma itself. Some older people are able to experience severe losses without ending their lives, while others decide on suicide as an answer to pain and suffering. Available evidence suggests that suicide is related to failure to cope with vital losses of income, spouse, or severe physical and emotional capacities.

Older people, for a variety of reasons, tend not to seek assistance for suicidal thoughts, although many are under a physician's care for other complaints. The reasons for not seeking assistance may be that most aged are unaware of mental health facilities and their services; transportation problems prohibit access to care; and suicidal behavior in older people is not perceived by mental health professionals. Some interventions to prevent suicide among older people include continued care to provide emotional support after major losses, delaying relocation decisions following the death of a spouse, parttime work after retirement, participation in religious or fraternal organizations and in senior centers, and other activities that encourage life values. Most important, immediate intervention is necessary when depressive behavior is identified or expressed, because the individual may be a potential suicide candidate.

Table 10-5 U.S. Suicide Rates by Sex, Race, and Age Groups: 1970 to 1976 (Rates per 100,000 population, 1977)

	Male								Female							
	White				Black and Other				White				Black and Other			
Age	1970	1974	1975	1976	1970	1974	1975	1976	1970	1974	1975	1976	1970	1974	1975	1976
All ages	18.0	19.2	20.1	19.8	8.5	10.2	10.6	11.0	7.1	7.1	7.4	7.2	2.9	3.0	3.3	3.2
5–14 yr.	.5	.8	.8	.7	.2	.4	.1	.3	.1	.2	.2	.2	.2	.2	.2	.4
15–24 yr.	13.9	17.8	19.6	19.2	11.3	12.9	14.4	14.7	4.2	4.8	4.9	4.9	4.1	3.9	3.9	4.0
25–34 yr.	19.9	23.3	24.4	23.7	19.8	22.9	24.6	22.8	9.0	8.7	8.9	8.6	5.8	6.3	6.5	6.5
35–44 yr.	23.3	23.8	24.5	23.6	12.6	15.6	16.0	16.8	13.0	12.1	12.6	11.0	4.3	4.5	4.9	4.7
45–54 yr.	29.5	28.3	29.7	27.7	14.1	11.9	12.8	13.5	13.5	14.1	13.8	13.8	4.5	4.0	4.5	4.3
55–64 yr.	35.0	32.1	32.1	31.6	10.5	12.5	11.5	12.3	12.3	11.0	11.7	12.1	2.2	3.4	4.1	2.8
65 and over	41.1	38.9	39.4	39.7	10.8	15.3	11.8	14.5	8.5	7.7	8.5	8.3	3.6	2.3	3.0	3.2

Source: George E. Delury, ed. *The World Almanac & Book of Facts* (New York, N.Y.: Newspaper Enterprise Association, Inc., 1980), p. 148

Note: World Almanac Source is National Center for Health Statistics, U.S. Dept. of Health, Education, and Welfare.

NOTES

1. L. I. Pearlin and C. Schooler, "The Structure of Coping," *Journal of Health and Social Behavior* 19, no. 1 (January 1978): 2.

2. Jack Botwinick, *Aging and Behavior* (New York, N.Y.: Springer Publishing Company, Inc., 1973), pp. 117–8.

3. David Guttman, "Life Events and Decision-making by Older Adults," *The Gerontologist* 18, no. 5 (October 1978): 462.

4. Ibid.

5. Ibid., p. 465.

6. Louis Harris, *The Myth and Reality of Aging in America* (Washington, D.C., National Council on Aging, 1975), p. 47.

7. John C. Morgan, *Becoming Old* (New York, N.Y.: Springer Publishing Co., 1979), p. 17.

8. Andrea Fontana, *The Last Frontier—The Social Meaning of Growing Old* (Beverly Hills, Cal.: Sage Publications, 1977), pp. 61–111.

9. Elizabeth Kubler-Ross, *On Death and Dying* (New York, N.Y.: Macmillan Co., 1969), pp. 39–137.

10. Erich Lindemann, "Symptomatology and Management of Acute Grief," *American Journal of Psychiatry* 101, no. 9 (September 1944): 141–8.

11. Robert Kavanaugh, *Facing Death* (Baltimore, Md.: Penguin Books, 1974), p. 107.

12. Linda K. George, "The Impact of Personality and Social Status Factors Upon Levels of Activity and Social Well-Being," *Journal of Gerontology* 33, no. 6 (June 1979): 840–7.

13. Kyriakos S. Markides and Harry W. Martin, "A Causal Model of Life Satisfaction Among the Elderly," *Journal of Gerontology* 34, no. 1 (January 1979): 86–93.

14. Erdman Palmore et al., "Stress and Adaptation in Later Life," *Journal of Gerontology* 34, no. 6 (November 1979): 841–51.

15. Erdman Palmore, "Predictors of Successful Aging," *The Gerontologist* 19, no. 5 (October 1979): 427–31.

16. Forrest Berghorn et al., *The Urban Elderly: A Study of Life Satisfaction* (New York, N.Y.: Universe Books, 1978), p. 17.

17. Ruth Bennett, *Aging, Isolation and Resocialization* (New York, N.Y.: Van Nostrand Rheinhold Co., 1980), p. 20.

18. Carl I. Cohen and Jay Sokolvsky, "Social Engagement Versus Isolation: The Case of the Aged in SRO Hotels," *The Gerontologist* 20, no. 1 (February 1980): 36–44.

19. Jack Botwinick, *Aging and Behavior,* p. 62.

20. Ibid.

21. Vera R. Kivett, "Discrimination of Loneliness Among the Rural Elderly: Implications for Interventions," *The Gerontologist* 19, no. 1 (February 1979): 108–15.

22. Edward Gfeller, "Pinpointing the Cause of Disturbed Behavior in the Elderly," *Geriatrics* 33, no. 12 (December 1978): 26–30.

23. Helena Z. Lopata, "The Social Involvement of American Widows," in Ethel Shanas, ed., *Aging in Contemporary Society* (Beverly Hills, Cal.: Sage Publications, 1970), p. 48.

24. Marjorie F. Lowenthal and Betsy Robinson, "Social Networks and Isolation," in Robert H. Binstock and Ethel Shanas, eds., *Handbook of Aging and the Social Sciences* (New York, N.Y.: Van Nostrand Rheinhold Co., 1976), pp. 432–56.

25. Irving Rosow, "Status and Role Changes Through the Life Span," in Robert H. Binstock and Ethel Shanas, eds., *Handbook of Aging and the Social Sciences* (New York, N.Y.: Van Nostrand Rheinhold, 1976), pp. 466–7.

26. Ibid., p. 471.

27. Myron Boor, "Anomie and U.S. Suicide Rates, 1973–1976," *Journal of Clinical Psychology* 35, no. 4 (October 1979): 703–6.

28. Peter Peretti and Cedric Wilson, "Contemplated Suicide Among Voluntary and Nonvoluntary Retirees," *Omega: Journal of Death and Dying* 9, no. 2 (1978–1979): 193–201.

29. Anthony Gliddens, *Emile Durkheim* (Kingsport, Tenn.: Kingsport Press, Inc., 1978), pp. 37, 52, 113.

30. James Birren, Notes from Gerontology Lecture, October 5, 1979, Albuquerque, N.M.

31. H. P. Resnik and Joel M. Cantor, "Suicide and Aging," in Mollie Brown, ed., *Readings in Gerontology,* Second Edition (St. Louis, Mo.: The C. V. Mosby Co., 1978), p. 122.

32. Arthur J. Deikman, "Sufism and Psychiatry," *Journal of Nervous and Mental Diseases* 15, no. 5 (November 1977): 318–29.

33. Stanley Goldstein, "Depression in the Elderly," *Journal of American Geriatric Society* 27, no. 1 (January 1979): 38–42.

34. Ibid., p. 38.

35. H. Gauer, "Depression in the Aged: Theoretical Concepts," *Journal of American Geriatric Society* 25, no. 10 (October 1977): 447–9.

36. R. Hirschfield and G. Klerman, "Treatment of Depression in the Elderly," *Geriatrics* 34, no. 10 (October 1979): 52.

37. H. Gauer, "Depression in the Aged: Theoretical Concepts," p. 447.

38. L. F. Jarvik, "Aging and Depression: Some Unanswered Questions," *Journal of Gerontology* 31, no. 3 (May 1976): 325.

39. R. Hirschfield and G. Klerman, "Treatment of Depression in the Elderly," pp. 51–57.

40. Carl Salzman and Richard I. Shader, "Depression in the Elderly I. Relationship Between Depression, Psychologic Defense Mechanisms, and Physical Illness," *Journal of the American Geriatric Society* 26, no. 6 (June 1978): 253–60.

41. Ibid., p. 257.

42. Marvin Miller, *Suicide After Sixty: The Final Alternative* (New York, N.Y.: Springer Publishing Co., 1979), p. 1.

43. Ibid., p. 3.

44. Ibid., p. 7.

Chapter 11

Alternatives to Institutionalization

Chiyoko Furukawa

The first option of the aged and their family when health care needs emerge is to choose noninstitutionalized care. Most literature indicates that only about five to seven percent of the elderly population are living in supervised facilities. The remainder are managing fairly well in the community and perceive themselves to be in reasonable health.[1]

Chronic illness is a major health problem of older persons, and many live with resultant effects of physical and mental decline. Although accurate statistics are unavailable for the number of disabled elders in the community, one report indicates that 45.0 percent of the older adults have limited activity and 38.3 percent have major activity limitations.[2] Heart conditions, arthritis, visual impairments, hypertension, and mental and nervous conditions are the primary causes of the disabilities.[3] These states of health require long-term support to maintain persons' optimal levels of functioning and to enable them to remain at home. However, as chronic conditions worsen and physical reserves to combat illnesses or diseases lessen with time, many become homebound and bedfast. Brody reports that eight percent of the noninstitutionalized older population are in this situation.[4]

MAXIMIZING COMMUNITY AND FAMILY RESOURCES

The availability of community services influences decisions about alternatives to institutionalization. Some communities are more attuned to the needs of the aging and have developed an array of services to assist with the health maintenance of the older population. Each community creates the types of services that are believed to be essential in meeting the needs of its elderly citizens.[5] The services in most communities include senior centers, transportation, shopping assistance, home delivered or congregate

193

meals, home maintenance, friendly visitors, mobile library, information and referral, home health, and homemaker services.

The expansion of existing services is desperately needed to optimize assistance not only to maintain the aged, but to support the family and primary care givers. For example, additional day care centers that provide effective and comprehensive services could benefit the aged and the family. The elder's mental status would be improved through contacts with other older persons, and the change of environment from the home to other settings may provide additional stimulation. Day care centers that offer a variety of services such as medication review; diet counseling; dental programs; and referrals to obtain hearing aids, glasses, and other assisting devices are especially beneficial to the elders and their families. These centers also allow family members to continue their occupations during normal working hours by assuming responsibilities for the older member who requires some supervision. Unfortunately, the utilization of day care centers in most communities is minimal and needs to be increased through more active promotions and advertisements. Burnside believes further development of options to institutionalization is needed for the older peoples' safety and socialization; for continual assessments to delay or prevent physical or mental deterioration; for the convenience of the family; and to lower costs below institutional care for everyone concerned with the aged.[6]

Home health services are another community service that may be expanded to offer assistance during the evening hours or the weekends. The extension of this service to longer hours can relieve family caretakers on a periodic and short-term basis, and can be seen as maximizing home care support as an alternative to institutionalization. Rossman asserts that home care may be preferable even when patients are acutely ill; after care and day care are frequently the best long-term plans for the older person.[7]

Several communities have demonstrated the ability to maintain older people who needed assistance with activities of daily living by using available local resources.[8,9,10] As an example, institutionalized persons in La Crosse, Wisconsin, returned to their homes as a result of improved working relationships between the nursing homes and community services.[11] The Domiciliary Care Program in Pennsylvania placed dependent adults in certified homes where room; board; companionship; and daily help with personal care, dressing, and medications were provided.[12] This particular program also demonstrated the cost effectiveness of deriving maximal use of community services in that custodial home care reduced care costs from $25 to $35 per day in the nursing home to approximately $9 per day.[13]

In many cases, an older person requiring institutional care at a later time is a high probability. Thus, care providers who are involved in planning for long-term care must consider the total spectrum of community services including institutional settings. This approach offers an opportunity to prepare the older individual and family members to plan and seek extended services for the existing health conditions of the elder. Furthermore, the method enhances and assists in sustaining the independence of the community's aged adults for as long as possible.

To prepare for the expected growth of the older population, communities must plan additional services in advance in order to maximize their resources. In the past, there has been a notable lag in the development of community services to assist families in keeping their older relatives out of institutions.[14] Increasing services to meet the needs of the aging population requires more funds to initiate new programs. However, when a large portion of public resources is directed toward elderly care, there is a possibility for a backlash from the younger group. Some may view the services for the elders as expensive and needlessly prolonging the life of persons who are no longer paying their way in society. This type of thinking does not recognize older persons' past contributions and is a simplistic way to resolve problems associated with scarce resources.

Family Assistance

Family studies have shown that kinship associations continue despite spatial separation resulting from contemporary life style and that the degree of association is influenced by residential propinquity.[15] Moreover, parents are visited more frequently by offspring in the working class, as compared to middle class; families and the offspring of still lower class families visited most often.[16] Also, when parents become extremely elderly, infirmed, or financially deprived, the family members who have resources assist more than others.[17]

These studies have demonstrated that most families take the responsibility to care for their aged parents or relatives, and institutionalization is the last alternative. Brody states that "families are not 'dumping' older people into institutions," and 80 percent of the health care to older people is provided by their families.[18]

Seelback and Neugarten believe that elderly parents generally rely upon filial responsibility for support and care when the need occurs.[19,20] Female relatives, for example, daughters, daughters-in-law, nieces, or granddaughters, become the primary helpers with the necessities of life, such as shopping, cooking, cleaning, personal care, and transportation for health care. In many instances, these activities continue on a long-term basis because many reject institutionalization as a stigma on the family. Family philosophy and negative public opinion about institutions tend to nurture this viewpoint. These opinions are also supported by reports of the U.S. Senate investigations revealing that some nursing homes provide less than adequate care and by publications that vividly describe exploitations of the institutionalized elders.[21,22,23,24,25] There are institutions that provide humane and quality care, but these establishments receive relatively little publicity.

Family members attempt to avoid admission of older relatives to nursing homes at any cost. A particular concern is the care givers who are also elders but continue to be responsible for the care of the dependent aged. In order to maintain the physical and mental health of the elderly care giver, it is essential to provide assistance, support, and relief on a systematic basis. The type of assistance needed will depend on the individual situation and may be limited to giving verbal support or to taking over the total responsibility of care for a few days or a week. These supportive activities by family members often reinforce relationships or create new bonds that strengthen the support for each other further.

Families are often faced with dilemmas that occur when the needs of an elderly relative are too much for the primary care giver. Silverstone and Hyman provide insights into the dynamics of family harmony or discord, sibling rivalry, money matters that create conflicts, persons who play the martyr role, and difficulty with the caretaker's own family relationships.[26] They also state that the first step for the family is to gain new insights during trying times, and the second is to develop new approaches to problems that concern family members. Continued efforts by the family are necessary to find successful solutions. Families are rewarded with resolutions of problems that otherwise would not have resulted if members had not worked in concert with each other.

Cost Effectiveness and Quality of Life Preference

The cost of institutional care is quite expensive, and the higher the level of care, the greater the cost.[27] The levels of care meeting the requirements for Medicare and Medicaid payments can be categorized as: (1) extended care (ECF) requiring professional nursing care covered by Medicare insurance; (2) Medicaid coverage for skilled nursing facilities used by eligible individuals for long-term or terminal care; and (3) intermediate care for those requiring custodial care with little professional assistance. (Medicare coverage is not available for this third level of care, but in some instances Medicaid support may be available.)[28] The cost of these levels of care ranges from $320 per month for the rest-home facility to more than $900 per month for skilled nursing or ECF care.[29] In many instances, care cost only includes room and board, and services such as medical care, drugs, laboratory fees, and other special needs become additional costs. Currently, the lack of funding resources to assist the aged in facilities for long-term chronic problems is an unresolved issue. Older people and their families are known to have exhausted lifetime savings before becoming eligible for welfare support and Medicaid benefits. The limited supply of Medicaid facilities poses another problem, although 40 percent of the federal Medicaid allocation is expended for the services to the elders.[30]

Despite these problems with financing institutional care, some elders must be admitted to inpatient facilities because other alternatives are no longer adequate. Kastenbaum and Candy contend that once an individual reaches the age of 65, there is a one-in-four chance of an older person entering a nursing home some day.[31] Although this may not be the choice for a family, institutional care from a cost standpoint may be comparable to home care if all aspects of the latter are considered. Unfortunately, consensus among experts regarding the costs to help elders within the community is unavailable to make precise comparisons. However, Rossman, in his argument to support noninstitutional care for the older population, estimates that home care cost at Montefiore averages $12 to $14 per day compared to $45 per day for a skilled nursing facility in New York City.[32] Day care costs may average $23 or $25 per day, which is approximately the cost of an intermediate care facility. Both day and home care are not 24-hour care and have added costs to families and the aged that are not taken into account, such as housing and meals. The difficulty of comparing the cost of institutional care versus community care is supported by Kane and Kane, who state:

> There is currently a great enthusiasm for the development of alternative models for institutionalization of the elderly. There is less evidence, however, that any type of technology is being transferred to buttress this enthusiasm on a foundation of meaningful information. Until the issues noted above are more widely discussed and some level of reconciliation achieved, it is unlikely that a great deal of progress will be made.[33]

Skellie and Coan report some progress toward identifying information regarding the effectiveness of alternative care.[34] They investigated the relationship between the use of comprehensive community care services and mortality for a sample of elderly individuals who were eligible for nursing home care. When compared to a randomly assigned control group, death rates among those referred to community care services were lower within the first six months after enrollment and were maintained throughout the first year. The difference in death rates was attributed to specific long-term services that were recommended and received to support the functional health status of the patients. Moreover, the preliminary mean direct cost of community care in 1978 was $169 per month, which compared with Medicaid's estimated monthly cost of $500 for nursing home care at the same time period.

When inpatient and outpatient care are compared, the elders' preference for quality life must be considered. Older people prefer their own homes to institutional settings. This fact is often overlooked, and the tendency is to transfer people to other institutions from acute-care settings. Rossman notes: "One reason may be that physicians and other professionals mistakenly regard the home environment too primitive for delivery of adequate care."[35] Furthermore, he maintains that the home setting may be the therapeutic locale with the least risk for some persons. Often professionals are unaware or underestimate the difficulty that arises for many elderly from admission to a nursing home. Institutionalization frequently connotes abandonment or impending death to the aged.[36] It is not uncommon for a marginally independent older person or couple who have temporary health problems to lose their independence permanently during this episode.[37] These people may be able to continue living in the community with intensive temporary assistance until functional abilities return. Otherwise, persons' preferences to live a few more years in their homes will have been usurped. Elderly individuals must, with appropriate support, be given the right to choose their preferred life style even in time of crisis. Experts who have studied the long-term care problems of elders conclude that public policy has failed to produce either satisfactory institutional care or alternatives for chronically ill older individuals.[38]

Mental Health Resources

The mental health status of older persons may depend on the degree to which a person is satisfied and has a positive outlook on life.[39] Sometimes the observed mental health problems are not necessarily as serious as they seem. Forgetfulness and poor judgment in older people are quickly interpreted as mental deterioration, while these same observations in younger people are accepted as an "off day" occurrence. Consequently, families and care providers, in their efforts to be helpful, tend to institute and foster dependency behavior on the part of the elderly, and the aged person becomes maladjusted.

The extent of mental disorders in old age is considerable.[40] However, many older persons in need of mental health services do not receive adequate assistance because of problems associated with mental health programs.[41] Estimates show that only three percent of the aged with mental problems are under care by any type of institution, and only one percent are in mental hospitals.[42] A 1971 American Psychiatric Association estimate revealed that at least 3 million, or 15 percent, of elders need mental health services.[43] This finding is believed to be a conservative one, and the real need for mental health services is not documented, particularly since many older people who have chronic illness also have concomitant emotional reactions that need attention. Additionally, a number of elderly individuals live in the lower social stratum, and the resultant loss of self-esteem can influence the maintenance of mental health.

Eisdorfer presents the problems related to the mental health services for the aged.[44] First, there is the dilemma of professional and social views on the tolerance of deviant behavior and early intervention, and the right of the individual to accept or reject treatment. Second, geographical orientation often influences mental problems. For example, the aged, who is adapted at home, may exhibit a behavior that indicates the need for custodial care when admitted to an acute care setting. A related concern is the hidden population of older adults who are frail, poor, nonambulatory, and unknown to community services.

Eisdorfer suggests the following ways to improve mental health services to the aged in order to alleviate these types of problems:

- Develop psychological tools that will accurately measure the aged's mental status. The tools available for the younger population are not suited as clinical guides and norms for the aged.

- Eliminate professional biases about the aged's inability to learn, their poor therapeutic risk, and misconceptions about incurable brain damage. Focus upon the individual's adaptive capacity rather than pathology.

- Consider that no single professional can provide the complex care needed by the older person. Many professionals who see problems differently can contribute to the mental health care.

- Overcome societal views that older people are superfluous because their life expectancy has been shortened; are not suitable for therapeutic sessions; and are brain damaged, impotent, and incomplete.

- Increase professionals' knowledge about the aged, and decrease the political ploy of playing one group against another in determining service needs between the young and old.

Mental health professionals are not totally at fault; older people have also contributed to the underutilization of mental health services. Their reluctance to accept care when symptoms indicate the need for professional assistance is well known. The longstanding social climate, in which the stigma attached to mental illness has been the accepted norm for many older people, is difficult to reverse. In addition, the elder's primary care physicians tend to view mental health problems as a part of being old rather than as an abnormal condition that warrants referral to mental health specialists. Thus, early consultation and differential diagnosis of mental illness precipitated by physical conditions are frequently delayed or over-looked. Butler and Lewis claim older people are not seen, in proportion to their emotional and psychiatric needs, as outpatients in psychiatric clin-ics, in community mental health centers, and in the offices of private psychiatrists or other mental health experts.[45] They estimate that two per-cent of the persons seen in psychiatric clinics are over 60 years old and about four to five percent of the clients in community mental health centers are over 65 years old, but only about two percent of private psychiatrists' time is directed to older people. In all of these settings, elderly adults are seen for routine diagnostic purposes and rapid disposition rather than for treatment. These findings not only indicate the underutilization of mental health care by the aged, but also the tragic deprivation of health services to promote and maintain the well-being of older people. This situation is particularly applicable to those individuals who develop reversible mental illness, such as depression and paranoid tendencies, late in life.[46]

There are older mentally ill persons who have been institutionalized all their lives because their illness occurred before the discovery of modern therapy. The continued care for these elders becomes precarious with each determination of budgetary priorities. In recent years, communities, ill-prepared and with inadequate resources, have been forced to provide care and support to the long-term institutionalized elders whose type of care is different than more recently diagnosed persons. The institutionalized groups are more dependent and will require continued support, as they have little or no independent life experiences that could assist their maintenance in the community. The mental health resources are essential for comprehen-sive community services and vital to the older people's quality of life and promotion of health.

MAXIMIZING INDIVIDUAL RESPONSIBILITIES FOR INDEPENDENCE

The first preference of elders is to have privacy and independence in their own homes, followed by desires, in descending order, to live with another person of the same sex, to live near or with the family, and to live in an institution.[47] Palmore's 20-year study of 207 normal aged persons found that although their chances of needing institutional care before death were approximately one in four, increase in age was not a strong determinant because a person's aging was offset by the decrease of years before death.[48] Other factors cited (living alone, having never married, being separated, having no or few children, and being female) increased the chance for institutionalization, while adequate finances, education, and being white increased access to institutions. A common fear shared by a number of older persons is that of becoming so dependent for personal care that institutional living is the only choice left for them. Palmore recommends further study of the admission and discharge rates for various groups to understand the factors that affect institutionalization. He sees a requirement for finding the best mechanism to assist those in need with access to institutions and to decrease unnecessary admissions to long-term facilities.[49]

There is no single right answer to the question of when institutionalization should become the choice because each aged person is unique, and circumstances, resources, finances, and other factors must be considered to maintain independence. The most important activity is the involvement of the elderly individual in the decision-making process on whether to enter a facility or select alternatives to institutional care. The right to make choices is paramount, regardless of concern for the health of the person.[50]

Elderly individuals are considered to be adults who are responsible for their own decisions.[51] Butler and Lewis support this contention and state that "human beings have a fundamental right to make their own decisions, enter into contracts, vote, make a will, and refuse medical or psychiatric treatments."[52] They see each of these decision-making activities as representative of persons controlling their own lives with the knowledge that the results could be favorable or unfavorable. Family members and professionals are in a position to assist the aged to make satisfactory decisions by supplying relevant information and indicating the consequences of the different options. Despite the presence of confusion or appearance of difficulty with comprehension, efforts must be made to give elders an opportunity to participate in the decision-making process. The only occasion when the right to make a decision becomes inapplicable is whenever illness invalidates an individual's capacity to make choices or when there is a potential of danger to self and/or others. However, family members tend to make the decision for institutional care and influence the elder's choice under the guise of their overprotective behavior.[53] When this occurs, the family is attempting to show concern and care, but it is possible for the aged to interpret such events differently, particularly if they perceive an institution as a place for dying.

Often conflict arises among the family, professionals, and older persons about an elder's desire to remain at home, especially when there is difficulty with self-care. In this instance, the amount of risk taken by elders may be more important for their mental health than most people realize. Elderly individuals have the option to take the risk, and it is essential to listen to their views and interpretations of the situation. The best approach to assisting in decision making is to be honest and objective with the aged person, but it is difficult for some families to follow this course because they wish to avoid confrontation.

Another essential activity is the assessment of the older individual's ability to function independently in the community. The assessment should be done in the home setting rather than in an acute care facility, and should be applied to both the activities of daily living (ADL) and mental abilities. A home setting is chosen because inpatient settings frequently disrupt continuity and lack the familiarity of the home. When elders are in customary surroundings, there is less probability for them to become disoriented or confused. Kleh suggests that the fundamental considerations for ability assessment should include observations in the home, street, store, and other environments where the elderly person lives.[54] In addition, the family relationship and the type and amount of available support must be assessed to ensure adequate maintenance.

The evaluation of an elder as an invalid is an example of the decision-making process that operates without order and careful consideration of all facets of the aged's life circumstances. Brody is critical about employing the crisis approach for determining the need for institutional care.[55] This approach is often preceded by long periods of strain for the family and the elderly individual. In the early discussion stage, the lack of community services and professional assistance to provide the rationale for decision making adds to the frustrations. Brody notes: "few old people receive careful preparation for discharge to a new living situation or even are afforded the opportunity to participate in the decision-making process, though participation is known to be a critical predictor of their subsequent adjustment and well-being."[56]

Murray et al. concur with Brody's viewpoint and discuss the beneficial effects resulting from an elderly individual's participation in the selection of a nursing home or other alternative settings.[57] An important outcome is that the person remains in control by acquiring advance knowledge about the new place of residence. Thus, any need to fantasize or guess about the change in environment is eliminated. Also a degree of independence, which the individual can still manage, remains intact and provides for continued self-esteem and positive self-concept. On the other hand, when an elder's choice is to remain in familiar surroundings within the community, lifelong habits can be retained to the extent of the individual's capabilities. This status sustains the identity and independence as long as possible by eliminating environmental hazards; providing additional supports, such as assistance with meal preparation, personal care, and transportation; and contributing to increased interactions with family members.

Barney describes the coping process of the elderly individual to maintain independence as:

> Older persons (and those close to them) may typically fail to perceive the decline or may mask it by adjusting their life style to change in capacities, resources, and interests. It has been seen that older people living together often develop support systems, informal and fragile, yet highly effective in prolonging autonomous living. For all these aging persons trying to maintain their independence, the question is more and more pressing: How is it possible to secure more help without accepting more control?[58]

According to Butler and Lewis, "we know very little about the survival traits, but tend to think of survival in terms of capacity for independence."[59] People who lived independently frequently adjust poorly to a highly structured environment that expects dependent behavior and damages the individual's self-reliance.[60] However, if a person has been more dependent in the earlier part of life, there is better adjustment to the institutional life. It appears that neither the highly independent nor the highly dependent person has the resiliency to make changes late in life. The resistance to changes in later years is believed to be related to past and lifelong personality traits rather than to old age.[61]

A literature review on the impact of relocation clearly showed that studies of home-to-institution moves identified different results between voluntary and involuntary relocation.[62] Those subjects who moved voluntarily consistently fared better than those who were moved involuntarily. Locker and Rubin found that family participation assisted the aged to understand the meaning of a relocation.[63] Also, some decision making on the part of the elderly residents, no matter how minor, was an important activity to counteract feelings of helplessness. Even moves within an institution were found to require careful preparation and long-term support to ensure adjustment to a new location.[64] Adjustment behaviors to change, such as straightening of clothes and other personal belongings as a compensatory activity, were observed even in apparently smooth relocations.[65] Adaptation to a different location is a process that requires new and old coping styles for adjustment to occur.

There is evidence that confused, disoriented, and physically disabled elderly individuals lack adaptation capabilities to relocation. Furthermore, the resultant disorganization during and immediately after a move increases mortality.[66] A technique to assist the confused person has not yet been fully developed, and the available methods to convey information about an impending move are insufficient to reduce the consequences of a relocation. It is believed that the mentally impaired individual is unable to prepare for change because personal resources necessary for coping are unavailable. Thus, the lack of cognitive function in persons with mental shortcomings causes them to be extremely vulnerable to the negative effects of residential change.

NOTES

1. Robert L. Kane and Rosalie A. Kane, "Alternatives to Institutional Care of the Elderly: Beyond the Dichotomy (United States)," *The Gerontologist* 20, no. 3 (June 1980): 249.

2. U.S. Department of Commerce, Bureau of Census, *Statistical Abstract of the United States* (Washington, D.C.: U.S. Government Printing Office, 1980), Table 202, p. 127.

3. Cary S. Kart, Eileen S. Metress, and James F. Metress, *Aging and Health—Biological and Social Perspectives* (Menlo Park, Cal.: Addison-Wesley Publishing Co., 1978), p. 10.

4. Stanley J. Brody, "Resources for Long-Term Care in the Community," in Elaine M. Brody, ed., *Long-Term Care of Older People* (New York, N.Y.: Human Sciences Press, 1977), p. 62.

5. Ruth, Murray, M. Marilyn Huelskoetter, and Dorothy O'Driscoll, *The Nursing Process in Later Years* (Englewood Cliffs, N.J.: Prentice-Hall, Inc., 1980), p. 161.

6. Irene Mortenson Burnside, *Psychosocial Nursing Care of the Aged* (New York, N.Y.: McGraw-Hill Book Co., 1980), p. 157.

7. Isadore Rossman, "Options for Care of Aged Sick," *Hospital Practice* 12, no. 3 (February 1977): 107.

8. "Supermarket of Services Allows Dependent Adults to Avoid Institutions," *Forum* 2, no. 4 (1978): 17–21.

9. "Dependent Adult Helped to Live in Community," *Forum* 2, no. 2 (1978): 22–27.

10. Ruth Shepherd, "Nursing Home Costs Halved by Home Maintenance Program," *Forum* 2, no. 2 (1978): 32–35.

11. "Supermarket of Services Allows Dependent Adults to Avoid Institutions," p. 19.

12. "Dependent Adult Helped to Live in Community," p. 22.

13. Ibid.

14. Elaine M. Brody, *Long-Term Care of Older People* (New York, N.Y.: Human Sciences Press, 1977), p. 308.

15. Vern Bengtson, Edward Olander, and Anees Haddad, "The Generation Gap & Aging Family Members: Toward a Conceptual Model," in Jaber F. Gubrium, ed., *Time, Roles & Self in Old Age* (New York, N.Y.: Behavioral Publications, Inc., 1976), p. 250.

16. Ibid., p. 251.

17. Ibid., p. 254.

18. E. M. Brody, *Long-Term Care of Older People*, p. 308.

19. Wayne Seelback, "Gender Differences in Expectations for Filial Responsibility," *The Gerontologist* 17, no. 5 (October 1977): 421–5.

20. Bernice Neugarten, "Old and Young in Modern Societies," in Ethel Shanas, ed., *Aging in Contemporary Society* (Beverly Hills, Cal.: Sage Publications, Inc., 1970), p. 20.

21. Frank Moss and Val Halamendaris, *Too Old, Too Sick, Too Bad* (Germantown, Md.: Aspen Systems Corporation, 1977), p. 14.

22. Jon Hendricks and C. Davis Hendricks, *Aging in Mass Society* (Cambridge, Mass.: Winthrop Publications, 1977), pp. 282–83.

23. Carobeth Laird, *Limbo* (Novato, Cal.: Chandler & Sharp Publishers, Inc., 1979), pp. 1–2.

24. Cary S. Kart, Eileen S. Metress, and James F. Metress, *Aging and Health: Biological and Social Perspectives* (Menlo Park, Cal.: Addison-Wesley Publishing Co., 1978), pp. 206–08.

25. M. A. Mendelson, *Tender Loving Greed* (New York, N.Y.: Vintage Books, 1974), pp. 3–33, 177–94.

26. Barbara Silverstone and Helen K. Hyman, *You and Your Aging Parent* (New York, N.Y.: Pantheon, 1976), pp. 40–63.

27. Ellen Brubeck and Robert Walton, "When an Elderly Needs Extended Care," *Geriatrics* 34, no. 2 (February 1979): 93–100.

28. C. S. Kart, E. S. Metress, and J. F. Metress, *Aging and Health—Biological and Social Perspectives,* pp. 199–200.

29. E. Brubeck and R. Walton, "When an Elderly Needs Extended Care," p. 99.

30. R. L. Kane and R. A. Kane, "Alternatives to Institutional Care of the Elderly: Beyond Dichotomy (United States)," p. 249.

31. R. Kastenbaum and S. Candy, "The 4% Fallacy: A Methodological and Empirical Critique of Extended Care Facility Population Statistics," *Aging and Human Development* 4, no. 1 (1973): 15–21.

32. I. Rossman, "Options for Care of the Aged Sick," p. 116.

33. R. L. Kane and R. A. Kane, "Alternatives to Institutional Care of the Elderly: Beyond Dichotomy (United States)," p. 257.

34. F. Albert Skellie and Ruth E. Coan, "Community-Based Long-Term Care and Mortality: Preliminary Findings of Georgia's Alternative Health Service Projects," *The Gerontologist* 20, no. 3 (June 1980): 372–9.

35. I. Rossman, "Options for Care of the Aged Sick," p. 107.

36. Ibid.

37. Ibid., p. 116.

38. E. Percil Stanford, "The Politics of Providing Health and Mental Health Care for the Aged," in Adina M. Reinhardt and Mildren D. Quinn, eds., *Current Practice in Gerontological Nursing* (St. Louis, Mo.: The C. V. Mosby Co., 1979), p. 27.

39. Ibid., pp. 29–30.

40. Robert N. Butler and Myrna I. Lewis, *Aging & Mental Health,* Second Edition (St. Louis, Mo.: The C. V. Mosby Co., 1977), p. 52.

41. Carl Eisdorfer, "Mental Health Problems in the Aged," in A. N. Exton-Smith and J. Grimley Evans, eds., *Care of the Elderly: Meeting the Challenge of Dependency* (London, England: Academic Press, 1977), p. 62.

42. E. P. Stanford, "The Politics of Providing Health and Mental Health Care for the Aged," p. 27.

43. R. N. Butler and M. I. Lewis, *Aging & Mental Health,* p. 52.

44. C. Eisdorfer, "Mental Health Problems in the Aged," p. 63.

45. R. N. Butler and M. I. Lewis, *Aging & Mental Health,* p. 53.

46. Ibid.

47. R. M. Coe, A. F. Rosen, and H. M. Rosen, "The Geriatric Patient in the Community," in E. V. Cowdry and F. U. Steinberg, eds., *The Care of the Geriatric Patient,* Fourth Edition (St. Louis, Mo.: The C. V. Mosby Co., 1971), p. 287.

48. Erdman Palmore, "Total Chance of Institutionalization Among the Aged," *The Gerontologist* 16, no. 6 (June 1976): 504.

49. Ibid., p. 507.

50. R. N. Butler and M. I. Lewis, *Aging & Mental Health,* p. 69.

51. Cynthia A. Anderson, "Home or Nursing Home? Let the Elderly Patient Decide," *American Journal of Nursing* 79, no. 8 (August 1979): 1448–9.

52. R. N. Butler and M. I. Lewis, *Aging & Mental Health,* p. 207.

53. C. A. Anderson, "Home or Nursing Home? Let the Elderly Patient Decide," p. 1448.

54. Jack Kleh, "When to Institutionalize the Elderly," *Hospital Practice* 12, no. 2 (February 1977): 124.

55. E. M. Brody, *Long-Term Care of Older People,* p. 46.

56. Ibid.

57. R. Murray et al., *The Nursing Process in Later Years,* p. 177.

58. Jane Barney, "The Prerogative of Choice in Long-Term Care," *The Gerontologist* 17, no. 4 (August 1977): 309–14.

59. R. N. Butler and M. I. Lewis, *Aging & Mental Health,* p. 120.

60. Robert N. Butler, "Looking Forward to What?" in Ethel Shanas, ed., *Aging in Contemporary Society* (Beverly Hills, Cal.: Sage Publications, Inc., 1970), p. 120.

61. R. N. Butler and M. I. Lewis, *Aging & Mental Health,* p. 26.

62. Richard Schulz and Gail Brenner, "Relocation of the Aged: A Review and Theoretical Analysis," *Journal of Gerontology* 32, no. 3 (May 1977): 322–33.

63. R. Locker and A. Rubin, "Clinical Aspects of Facilitating Relocation," *The Gerontologist* 14, no. 4 (August 1974): 295–9.

64. Elaine M. Brody, Morton H. Kleban, and Miriam Moss, "Measuring the Impact of Change," *The Gerontologist* 14, no. 4 (August 1974): 299–305.

65. Beverly Patnaik et al., "Behavioral Adaptation to Change in Institutional Residence," *The Gerontologist* 14, no. 4 (August 1974): 307.

66. E. M. Brody, *Long-Term Care of Older People,* p. 133.

Chapter 12

Beyond Ethnicity

Dianna Shomaker

ETHNICITY

The elderly, just like the young and middle-aged, come in all shapes, sizes, and colors, and from a wide variety of national backgrounds. In an effort to provide holistic health care and avoid stereotyping, ubiquitous attention has been given to developing awareness of people's ethnicity.

Nursing programs, especially in the western half of the United States, prodded by the Western Interstate Counsel of Higher Education in Nursing (WICHEN), have made concerted efforts to incorporate concepts of ethnicity into their curriculums. Branch and Paxton spearheaded a drive to continue growth in sensitivity to the needs of "ethnic people of color."[1] Their book became a text for many colleges of nursing. Bullough and Bullough expressed a similar goal.[2] Community health texts followed the trend. Anthropologists and sociologists also explored what everyone was calling "ethnicity."

In all of these attempts, differences between ethnic groups were listed and compared. The result of many of these efforts was the very thing the endeavors were designed to avoid. Stereotypes were either reinforced, or new ones were developed. The goal had been to recognize individuality, but the unconscious limitation that arose was an emphasis upon individuality among groups, not between individuals. Moreover, there seemed to be no complete agreement as to the definition of ethnicity or its value. Those who were stereotyped were justifiably angry; those who preferred their own culture were embarrassed; and those who tried to help often made the mistake of prejudicing the cause.

The elderly have all too often been stereotyped, but even more complicated is the plight of those older persons who claim membership in an "ethnic group;" they are doubly stereotyped. It is important to recognize differences and similarities in those for whom a person is providing care

207

and to be aware of cultural proclivities. Care givers should do more than just acquaint themselves with information about each general group, though. They should have an understanding of basic universal principles and concepts of race, individuality, ethnocentrism, prejudice, stereotyping, and ethnicity in order to provide successful support and interaction.

Concept of Race

In the latter part of the nineteenth century, scholars were divided on the issue of race, but the influence of evolutionary ideology provided not only a ground for agreement, but the basis upon which to perpetuate the notion of racism, white supremacy, and social stratification. Both groups of debaters believed in the cultural and biological inferiority of the non-Caucasian, but whether or not it was reversible was an irreconcilable chasm; race determined a person's association with culture and subsequent behavior.[3]

There have been many attempts to classify people into groups based on similarities. During the 1930s and 1940s, education about the world consisted of learning about four races: Negroes, Indians, Orientals, and Caucasians. People were defined and classified according to race. A race, according to Hooten, was: "A great division of [hu]mankind, the members of which though individually varying, are characterized as a group by a certain combination of morphological and metric features, principally non-adaptive, which have been derived from their common descent."[4]

Categorizations were directly related to the color of the skin, but the colors of the hair and eyes were implied. This was part of a centuries-old belief. Negroids were associated with curly or woolly hair and long legs; Caucasians with finer, straighter, and lighter hair; and Orientals and Indians with straight black hair shafts. Anthropometric measurements were categorized, as were the size and shape of the nose, lips, and eyelids. Even toes and fingers and length of members were categorized by race. It was often arbitrary and inaccurate, and all factors led to deceptive categorization at best. Little regard was given to genetic similarity or dilution. Skin was often colored by dirt, grease, makeup, sun, wind, and mutation.

Stereotypes of appearance and behavior were accepted with little or no attempt to isolate those attributed to individual personality differences. Each race became associated with certain food preferences and behavior characteristics that were isolated and unique to them, and usually not shared with the other three races. Sometimes the characteristics were limited to a subgroup within a race; other times they were insensitively attributed to the entire race. "Negroes are said to be libidinous; whites intelligent; Germans industrious; Japanese imitative; or Yankees mechanically ingenious."[5]

Governments classified people politically as one race or another based on little logic. For example, in the United States people are classified Indian if they have as little as one-fourth Indian blood, regardless of supposed racial makeup of the other three-fourths. However, if a child is born of other mixed heritage, race becomes a personal choice. Thus census accounts by race become a subjective tally and reflect personal preference, not race per se.

Race is an inapplicable concept today in its original sense. Because of such arbitrary factors, race as an indissoluble nomenclature of people and cultures has received severe criticism. Montagu objected to it because it implied all issues of changing people and culture had been resolved.[6] Races were hypothetical postulates and arbitrary classifications that did not reflect reality, and categorization into such groups implied a preconceived notion of finality. He prefers the term "ethnic group," while others have chosen to attempt redefining racial groups by tracing gene frequencies.

Hooten's definition eventually fell from favor and was replaced by blood grouping data and gene frequency. "The concept of race seemed to him to be of no use in describing or explaining human genetic variability."[7] Today, in an attempt at greater clarity and precision in determining the racial association of an individual, biological differentation is the criterion rather than superficial color, language, or social similarities. It is based on blood factors, principally the ABO blood type system, the M-N series, and the Rh factor, as well as various hemoglobins, enzymes, and amino acid excretions. Particular combinations occur in some groups and not in others, making information contained in the blood chemistry the major dependable means of determining membership in a race and the racial sources of an individual's forbears.

This is particularly useful in tracing the origin and mixture of groups. For example, the Rh-negative gene is commonly found among Europeans, especially Basques, and R_o in Africa. These can assist in demonstrating "white" and "black" admixture. In ABO blood groups, B is absent among American Indians and Australian Aborigines, but common in Africa, India, and Asia. If using the M-N series among inhabitants in the Pacific, heredity can be traced; M is common among Japanese and Europeans, but rare among Australian Aborigines. N is absent among American Indians. So once again, admixture between various areas can be more objectively traced by analyzing blood factors, and the technique can serve as a basis for identification of original "racial" groupings.[8]

Medical problems are attributed in part to particular genetic propensities that persist in biologically similar people, who also share a common environment of longstanding. In areas where breeding is isolated either by law, population density, or geographic location, there is greater genetic similarity, but where migration and emigration have occurred, genetic purity has been replaced by heterogeneity. Those who remain in an area may, over many generations, gain adaptation to a disease. A commonly discussed example is the person who carries the gene for the sickle-cell trait and has protection against malaria as a result of sickle cell. That person's red blood cells are unsuitable for reproduction of the malaria parasite.[9]

Due to evolution, races are constantly changing. What were originally thought to be four discrete and unique races are now seen as complex blends. Based on past standards, these races have become dilute, compromised, contaminated, unclear, and diffuse; based on today's knowledge it is evident, if a person insists on the term "race" as a category, that there are more than four. Moreover, some races have become extinct, and others have emerged, influenced by environment, history, geography, mobility, religion, technology, urbanization, industrialization, and political alliances.

Racism, Stereotyping, Prejudice, and Discrimination

Racism is an international, centuries-old phenomenon.[10] Just as there has been conflict in rationale for determining race and racial characteristics, so has there been conflict between various groups throughout history. Even though the concept of "race" has improved and progressed, the virulence of racism among populations persists, perpetuated by myths and stereotypes. Basically racism is the dislike of a person or group of persons to which people have attributed characteristics that are a threat to their own status. For example, people see others doing things in a different way and often speaking in a different language. The threat arises when people see this as different from their own behavior and consider it inferior. Because people need to see their own behavior displayed in others to validate their characteristics as good, different behavior is evaluated as having the potential of replacing their own behavior.

Racism is a form of social stratification composed of many complex variables. Archer and Fleshman identify racism on two levels: individual and institutional.[11] Individual racism governs personal behavior toward others, whereas institutional racism is the overarching umbrella of policy and politics that condones discriminant behavior by dominant society members in relationship to those with less power and status. The two are complementary forces. One cannot exist without the other.

Kitano analyzes racism as being stratified on three levels: (1) fear of difference due to color dissimilarity; (2) discrimination as a byproduct of economic, social, political, and psychological factors; and (3) a product of rapid social change due to improved technology, increased urbanization, and industrialization.[12] Racism increases in depth and complexity as a person is influenced by a greater proportion of these variables. Each individual's perspective toward another is shaped by past experience, emotions, and needs. There is more than one valid means of viewing a situation. As many interpretations and perspectives as possible should be weighed if attenuation of discrimination is to be achieved.

Prejudice, dislike of another's ways, or evaluation of another's inferiority may come about for two reasons. In the United States a primary reason is the historical need for low-cost labor, exemplified by blacks brought from Africa as slaves and bearing a stamp of social inferiority placed on them by their owners and the government. There were also laborers who emigrated from Italy, Ireland, Japan, and China. They came, willing to work for less, speaking another language, and often looking different, with unfamiliar food preferences and the influence of foreign educational systems. They were paid less to work hard for others. They had limited living standards, education, and personal freedom, by both tacit social patterns and the immigration laws. From the outset they were labeled inferior, and there was no expectation that their status would change.

Nonetheless the fear that they might change threatened the status of those who preceded them. The reverse happened with Native Americans. They were here first and were overpowered by immigrants with the single-minded purpose of establishing a new country. Each new wave of persons bearing some degree of similarity in language, location, physical traits, or food preferences was lumped together by others and identified by commonalities different from the observers. Whether or not the commonalities persisted, the characterizations remained in the form of stereotypes.

Stereotypes are merely sweeping, overgeneralized statements predicated on applying one value system upon another behavior. But they are far more complex in reality. Both stereotypes and their validity are hard to discern.[13] These extreme statements and beliefs not only cripple society, but they halt growth of interpersonal relationships in the future because they blind people to the recognition of diversity in others.[14]

> The myth of the extremes flourish[es] everywhere, sometimes in the head of the same person, even though they seem to contradict each other and cancel each other out . . . the truth about . . . all people lies in the whole range of diversities between the two extremes. The stereotypic extremes of views often result in destructive—even bizarre—treatment.[15]

Application of stereotypes is not reserved for a particular group. Harris claims that "condensed psychological portraiture slipping imperceptibly into stereotypes has always been a vice of learned as well as vulgar observers of cultural phenomena."[16] Epstein concurs stating: "We have, historically, forced certain groups of people into unproductive behaviors, and then we have attributed those behaviors to some innate determinism."[17]

The other origin of prejudice is blind overzealousness in ethnocentrism, that is, preferring one's own culture to the point of obliterating any ability to see another's advantages. Ethnocentrism in itself is not prejudice. It is, rather, preference for one's own ways. It is normal, and emotionally and socially a healthy attitude. All people should prefer their own cultural values above those of others; they were raised in the cultural milieu and taught a profound worth for certain habits, customs, religion, traits, food, and problem-solving devices. Those items that served the needs of a group persist over time and are in turn taught to their children. Pride in one's own culture is important. The problem arises when a person is not able to allow others, who are different in background, appearance, or values to have an equal pride and opportunity to display it. At that point, those who foster prejudice say, "I don't like them because they're not like me." "A better way is the way I do it . . . they're dumb, stupid, inferior, for practicing such a behavior; when they become like me, I'll like them." Obviously this implies an inferiority status bestowed on the "different" one, and a degree of personal preference so strong it negates any possibility of understanding another. Persistence in this attitude will prohibit growth of sensitivity, awareness, or appreciation for any others than those cast from an individual's own mold. Any motivation to accept those who are dissimilar is clouded. Those rare few who escape such a blind person's cultural cage will be allowed because they are exceptions. The exceptions become the subjects of superficial contradictions used to show that the person is not prejudiced: "I'm not prejudiced, I've even got a white (or black, or red, or yellow) friend." Although prejudice has often been attributed to those who are members of the dominant society, prejudice and stereotyping can be reciprocal behavior among all persons of various differences, equally virulent in ability to limit positive reception of other's individuality and differences. The dislike can flow both ways.

Another perspective of this issue is the myth that persons of a particular type, group, race, and so on, stick together. In fact, there are many Germans who can't stand each other; many Japanese who don't willingly seek the companionship of one another; and many Chicanos who have no desire to understand another Chicano. These are differences often mistakenly represented as cultural but in fact have greater credibility as personality and psychological uniqueness. The conflict, which transcends cultural or racial boundaries and is influenced by other factors, is not solely limited to a person's ethnic identity.[18]

Hall maintains that cultures collide because people ignore each other's nonverbal communication, not because they lack a deep knowledge of another. In order to gain sensitivity to another, there must be an openness to weigh observations objectively, rather than according to an individual's own value system.[19] It is peoples' own cultures that make them subjective. To know others, people must know themselves first. That is a challenge people often avoid.

> Much of our culture operates outside our awareness, frequently we don't even know that we know. . . . We unconsciously learn what to notice and what not to notice, how to divide time and space, how to walk and talk and use our bodies, how to behave as men and women, how to relate to other people . . . this applies to all people.[20]

Brownlee states that people create or perpetuate stereotyping and generalizations when they make decisions or reach conclusions after partially exploring data; when they generalize from one instance or person to an entire group; or when blindness and urgency obliterate awareness of variation and change in individuals and cultural behavior.[20a]

Concept of Ethnicity

In popular thinking, the concept of race is still very much alive, but the number of "races" has increased considerably beyond four, and the complexity of definition has expanded to incorporate blood types and other biological factors. In an effort to avoid the negative connotation attached to "race," people have turned to the word "ethnicity." It is ubiquitous. The groups are more discrete and the categories more numerous. The goal of clear boundaries of particular groups remains just as elusive, and even with "ethnic groups" discrimination is just as probable. As many have observed, it is just as easy to be ethnically prejudiced as it is to be racially prejudiced. However, Montagu defends the switch from "race" to "ethnic group."[21] He asserts that not only does it remove some of the erroneous stigma of race, but "ethnic group" carries with it a degree of purposeful vagueness that stimulates questions and reflection and makes the questions to be solved more evident. Cohen observes that ethnicity is a term with vague definition that implies cultural roots, national identity, and socially linked behavior, but that it also carries the implication of marginal status in politics and class.[22] It calls to mind subcultural differences and identity in such things as "foreign" names, accents, food habits, and links with another country. Also, according to Cohen, it obscures ethnicity of those in whom no immediate difference can be ascertained. Cohen further asserts that ethnicity is behavior and identity rather than diverse national background, that even white, Anglo-Saxon Protestants (WASPs) are ethnic, although it is seldom that a WASP is referred to as a member of an ethnic group. Ethnicity is a means of focusing on organizational functions of symbolic patterns of behavior. It is more than a conceptual tool; it is an ideological quest for a just and equitable society.[23]

Ethnicity is used to generate support of issues and political candidates. It is used in competition for scarce resources and to validate meaning in a group or a movement. People may be related to a group by ascription, wherein they identify themselves as members of the group; or a person may be related to a group via genetics. In both ways a sense of sharing is preferred because it counteracts alienation. But merely being identified as a member of a group does not identify the degree of acceptance by members of one another. Membership can be and often is fluid. But the result of uniting in a group is one of the more successful means of identifying inequities. "Organized ethnic groups can fight for equal rights, or persons within them can leave and try to become members of more privileged groups; but many inequities remain group-determined."[24]

Everyone uses the term "ethnicity." It often replaces terms like race, tribe, culture, and minority. Not only does it refer to ascriptions that people place on themselves, it is also a fluid concept that expands and contracts in relation to specific needs, and becomes a way of asserting one's rights. According to some it is based on inequality of power and access to resources; others describe it as a concept of social stratification and conflict, and the conflict can be due to geography, economics, ethnic identification, or religion. The label "ethnicity" only indicates differences between groups, not similarities; but it implies boundaries that define a group, mutual interests, and common values, as well as real or presumed standardized behavior. Unending discussion surrounds attempts to clarify the definition of ethnicity, ethnic group, ethnic identity, ethnic categories, and criteria for inclusion and exclusion of membership.[25]

One of the major contradictions regarding ethnic groups lies in the means of becoming a member. Barth, who developed most of the initial major components of the concept of ethnic groups and their boundaries, maintains that even though groups are largely biological in origin, perpetuation of membership can also be by ascription and self-identification.[26] Members share cultural values and forms that become a field of communication for each other. Groups have requirements for membership, and these are both inclusive and exclusive. "They are defined by their non-membership as well as by the rules of membership."[27] They are neither exclusive in use of territory nor developed in isolation to other ethnic groups.

Feldman and Thielbar suggest that members of an ethnic group see themselves alike owing to real or imagined common ancestry.[28] They claim however, that: "The only way to gain membership in an ethnic group is to be born into it. It does not matter how devout a convert one is, or how well one has mastered the group's life style, full membership in an ethnic group can occur only through the process of ascription."[29] Both Feldman and Barth agree that ethnic life is more often than not genetically as well as culturally influenced. Both must be considered. According to Knutsson, "Any concept of ethnic group defined on the basis of 'cultural content' will not suffice as a tool for the analysis of ethnicity in its various interactional contexts."[30]

In the final analysis it is the interpersonal relationships within and between groups that generate the most evident traits by which a person may characterize a group without stereotyping and listing traits of behavior. "Ethnicity becomes not one single universally applicable term, but rather a wide range of interrelations in which the dominant reference is to an ethnic status. . . ."[31]

BEYOND ETHNICITY

What are health care providers to do when given a heterogeneous group of persons, a vague and arbitrary set of definitions of race and ethnicity, and personal value systems that may be in conflict with that of the client? Better care is given when the individual, rather than the group, is considered, but the process by which a person integrates into a group and establishes continuity and solidarity with it should not be neglected.

Within the United States, persons react to stimulus both as individuals and as members of groups. Under identical stimuli, a person's response as an isolated individual is predictably dissimilar to that of a person who is reacting as a member of a group. Provision of a health maintenance system is generally initiated on an individual basis with secondary group influence in the form of family and institutional concern. Individual care is complicated by personality, and social and cultural systems of both the provider and the client. In the present emphasis on individualism apart from cultural group, an individual must wrestle with the relationship of all factors as an integrative process. In trying to avoid stereotyping and inappropriate care, the concept of individualism as defined by Talcott Parsons may be valuable:

Individualism: the belief that an individual possesses some fundamental rights that arise from his [or her] inherent worth and are not derived from his [or her] membership in kinship or other social groups. This belief is supported by a form of social organization in which individuals participate as individuals rather than as representatives of groups.[32]

In the case of the elderly, the care giver confronts the peak of several decades of experience, grooming of personal values, and relationships. An elder cannot survive without dependencies and interdependencies, even as an individual who values independence.[33]

If the momentum of childhood is to increase, the sense of "getting somewhere," of unending achievement, is to be sustained in adulthood and on into maturity, it must involve an accumulation of more than physical growth: skill or knowledge, power, honor and the right to property. It must involve loyalties to kin and friendship. All such accumulations are culturally defined as extensions of one's self.[34]

Although there is a sound argument made for individuals as members of groups, contact will be with an individual and should be founded on sensitivity, which will be satisfactory in dealing with both personality and cultural or ethnic uniqueness. This contact removes the mask often erected by assessment of group interaction. Care givers are striving for depth of encounters with individuals in a cultural frame of ideology, where individuals play out different histories.[35] This is important because the members of social chains are continuously moving and changing. Many ties are broken through death, altercation, mobility, and inertia.[36] In the end individuals will arrive at personal decisions and behavior useful for their own specific needs.

There are several means by which to begin growth in awareness. Murphy offers sage advice in directing the individual to attain greater understanding by looking at what things are *not* as well as attempting to analyze what they are.[37] In modern society a person often discovers greater meaning in behavior and its motivation if it is viewed beyond the superficial and obvious, to the reversal of the obvious. To look at what these are as well as what they are not is referred to as dialectic reasoning, a means of understanding opposite perspectives of the same issue. For example, dialetic reasoning suggests that differentiating and separateness are means by which a person may relate and associate. By separating from some people, a focus is created whereby others are singled out for association. "Closeness to some requires distance from others and the active assertion of difference and opposition are ways of relating."[38] In attributing meaning to relationships with clients, then, individuals must become aware of how meaning is conveyed in their life experiences. Everyone has unspoken and hidden assumptions about values and philosophy. Not everything said and done is the sum total of those values. Just as often, the use of something depends on its lack of meaning as much as possession of meaning.[39]

Dealing with individuals with such a potential spectrum of diversity is awesome and frequently frustrating. There must be some guidelines for the health care provider that transcend ethnic boundaries. It is a new concept to go beyond such boundaries, given the amount of attention they have received in the past. However, to observe dogmatically only the obvious and common behavior within the limits of a group does not allow recognition and worth of the group heterogeneity.

To come to grips with individuality within another's ethnic group does not require lists of traits specific to the group's behaviors. In fact this is counterproductive. Those traits change over time as do nuances surrounding them. The list would become archaic faster in some areas than in others; moreover, some members of the group may never have embraced such traits, or at least not as fully as others. Further, the last person to recognize changes, subtle or overt, would be the outsider, who lives in a rhythm out of phase with the group. If that outsider is the care provider, care and response to cultural or ethnic needs would be in jeopardy of being out of harmony with reality. In addition, outside individuals may find commonalities from one culture to another and unconsciously transfer expectations crossculturally.

To return to the original question, how does a care provider assess aging crossculturally without slipping into stereotyping and inadequate assessment of a person's needs?

Maxwell and Maxwell studied 95 random sample cases from 185 distinct areas worldwide.[40] The position of the older persons in families was analyzed specifically to determine "negative deference," or contempt, toward elderly persons. The following eight predictors for such attitudes were found:

1. physical deterioration—sickness, loss of strength
2. mental deterioration—senility, offensive behavior
3. deterioration of appearance—wrinkles, gray hair, ugliness
4. assumption of negative traits—witchcraft, sorcery
5. lack or loss of skills
6. lack or loss of children/family support
7. loss of wealth
8. hoarding wealth

The last two were dropped from the final analysis because of minimal occurrence. Lack or loss of children was the strongest predictor of a contemptuous attitude toward a person on the part of others, and of course the converse also holds: a person's family support system becomes the first line of defense against contempt toward the elderly. Deterioration of appearance was the next greatest predictor, and physical deterioration the third most common predictor. The authors hypothesize that similar patterns would be demonstrated among other cultures than the 95 studied.

Moving beyond differences in ethnically related behavior in search of crosscultural universals related to older people, there seem to be two opposing views. One is that the world view of each culture harbors important variations. The other is more absolute in insisting that there is a consistency between cultures.[41] In both arguments it is clear that aging is part of an entire life span that must be considered within that context, not in isolation.[42] Meyerhoff and Simic see aging as a dynamic, growing process, during which a person accumulates relationships, accomplishments, knowledge, honor, intimacy, and other assets in the process of living.[43] Within this context they attempt to identify common themes of life and threads of experiences that transcend superficial and situational differences. These are valuable not only to see older people in a different light, but to serve as a basis for understanding individual elderly on a different level than used before.

Some universal truths identified crossculturally included:

- The aged are a minority.

- Older women outnumber their male peers.

- Widows form a high proportion of the older population.

- Every society classifies some people as old and prescribes appropriate behavior toward them on the part of others.

- With old age, there is a shift from participation in economic production to sedentary, advisory, or supervisory roles.

- Some older people continue to assume positions of leadership.

- Adult children and older people share a relationship characterized by mores and some form of mutual responsibility.

- Each culture clearly defines appropriate behavior, influence, and responsibility for men and women.

- Dichotomy of roles, divided according to sex, punctuates entire life cycles.

- Male and female life cycles have separate developmental history.

- Roles of males and females are usually complementary, with power peaks for each sex in different areas at different times in a given culture.

- Rewards depend a lot on individual ability, resourcefulness, good judgment, and luck at every point in the life cycle.

- Old age is no more homogeneous than any other phase of life.[44]

Each culture and ethnic group has unique processes by which these universals are manifested. According to Meyerhoff and Simic, if a person makes trait lists, the differing processes by which these universals are achieved are lost or distorted through inaccurate interpretation of the degree of completeness and credibility of behaviors.[45] "Aging in its sociocultural aspects subsumes a multiplicity of attitudes, values and modes of behavior."[46] It is best to weigh the impact of each on individuals as single entities. Aging is not an immediate, dramatic shift from youth, but is a serial process of growth upon past phases of life. Meyerhoff admonishes readers not to focus on what has survived the test of time, for the observer will miss the process whereby events are generated, transformed, and integrated into personal reality. The process is relevant to the experience of all phases of life, carrying with it a dynamic reciprocity between values and events. The process is not always logical or harmonious, primarily because humans, regardless of age, are not passive objects or receptacles, but active, unpredictable beings who channel, negotiate, and manipulate the forces of the sociocultural milieu.[47] "Norms are fluid, and maximum opportunities exist for individual innovation, exploitation, and experimentation. Resourcefulness of individuals may be maximally exercised and often becomes very influential in accounting for differential success in aging as a career."[48]

Meyerhoff and Simic posit that analysis of individual continuities and discontinuities is an effective means of understanding the cultural process and is readily applicable to the older individual in a society or ethnic group. "Cultural continuity implies contact with, and access to, a coherent and relatively stable body of ideas, values and symbols."[49]

There is a degree of reciprocity that assists in creating solidarity of human connections and involvement through establishment of confidence, trust, and promise of future mutual support.[50] It is present, but not always evident. It is to be found in functions assumed in later life, in the degree of cultural gap in generational ties, and in the quality of effort exerted to establish a place for older persons in a society. It is a process and degree of linking and integrating events and ideas.[51] In some cultures, success in old age relates to physical viability in order to maintain social relationships.

In others, old age is not judged by physical agility, but by the competence displayed in building "reciprocal relations over the years with their decendants and collateral kin."[52]

Continuity demands varying forms depending on the specific cultures. It is this crucial factor that the care provider must hone to a fine degree of awareness and sensitivity in assessing and analyzing the reciprocal impact of culture and individual older persons.

> Though each culture places somewhat different demands on its members as they grow older, and adorns the concept of success with various visible signs, nevertheless, the aged seek universally a sense of participation, self-esteem, external recognition, and verification of their accomplishments. Unfortunately, in no society do all persons meet with equally good fortune in this quest, nor are all social settings similarly amenable to granting this bounty to their aged.[53]

Discontinuity is the disruption of the continuous process of relationships, connections, and events. Older people tend to incur greater degrees of discontinuity than other age groups because of mobility of younger family members and greater frequency of death in their immediate sociocultural environment. Evidence of concerted attempts to reestablish continuities may be found. This may be to alleviate the instability, uncertainty, and lack of trust precipitated by the interference in social mechanisms that accompanies discontinuity.[54] The older person is now in the position of reinterpreting conflicting norms, values, and relationships in order to survive. Care providers must look at ways individuals express concern for continuity when it is absent or disrupted.[55]

Establishment of patterns of continuity and discontinuity is most readily evident when the full life history of the elderly individual is considered. Careful attention should be given to whether or not a behavior is due to the inevitability of the physiological phenomena of aging, whether it is a unique psychological trait of the individual, or whether it is a cultural manifestation. "Certainly, the mere enumeration and contrasting of formal statuses occupied by the aged and of ritual signs of respect paid them, are not sufficiently adequate measure and may in fact be utterly misleading."[56] Continuity of customs and social forms may appear to the unaware care provider as stagnation or a return to the past.[57] Moreover, some discontinuity is the product of cultural and social change, as well as physical change that accompanies aging. The form taken by continuity and discontinuity differs in content, significance, and style in each society. For example, depending on demographic and structural organization, the sequence of generations may be a significant factor in altering the social milieu, as it often is in stable traditional villages.[58] In others, time or space may be the basis upon which social continuity is predicated, as it is in a time-oriented scheduled existence in some sectors of United States society.[59] Where clock time is not a factor, seasonal time may be.

Space as a measure of communicating continuity or discontinuity is often expressed in terms such as "close" or "distant" friend, or "aloof" or "stand-offish" friend. The degree of emotional involvement can be indicated by the physical distance maintained between self and another.[60]

Individuals' idealization of their roles can conflict with reality. The test of a continuous and shared role with others often comes about with aging. In Kenya, to be old tests the ability and willingness of children to care for elders. Uncertainty and insecurity cause delay of such testing as long as possible, while continuity is nurtured. The threat to continuity arises because of rapid social change across the country.[61]

Continuity and solidarity can often be rekindled when people discover an historic tie preceding or external to the group in which they are active. A tie may be a common language, social organization, or family pattern. Once this shared set of meanings exists, the individuals become part of a unit with its own communication and solidarity.[62] The value of the tie must be decided by the person actively involved with it.

A break with past ties can be initiated by migration. Jews who have emigrated from Europe[63] and Mexicans who have settled around Los Angeles[64] suffer discontinuity as a result of this movement from their land of origin. Because they are as heterogeneous within their ethnic groups as they are in relation to society-at-large, establishing a new pattern of continuity in their own lives now must be a purposeful effort. Simic sees "people making and negotiating meaning in constantly changing circumstances, and using cultural materials as the fabric from which to spin new 'webs.' "[65] These webs are significant because they provide continuity and mend discontinuity and disruption.

In conclusion, older people are not a homogeneous group, nor is each so-called ethnic group. Yet programs are designed as though old people, and more specifically the old of particular ethnic groups, are homogeneous. They are doubly handicapped by prejudice and society's view of old age. Racial prejudice and democratic ideals are in conflict, as are continuity and discontinuity, ethnicity and individuality.[66] Health care providers must acquire skills to assess and assist the elderly by observing their individual ethnicity in greater depth. Effectiveness of such efforts is distorted and diluted if the care provider relies heavily upon trait lists and the concepts of race and ethnicity. By moving beyond this into the processes that create change and integration, a person can more greatly appreciate the value of individual diversity regardless of culture.

NOTES

1. Marie Branch and Phyllis Paxton, *Providing Safe Nursing Care For Ethnic People of Color* (New York, N.Y.: Appleton-Century-Crofts, 1976).

2. Bonnie Bullough and Vern Bullough, *Poverty, Ethnic Identity and Health Care* (New York, N.Y.: Appleton-Century Crofts, 1972).

3. Michael Crawford, "The Use of Genetic Markers of the Blood in the Study of the Evolution of Human Populations," in M. H. Crawford and P. L. Workman, eds., *Methods and Theories of Anthropological Genetics* (Albuquerque, N.M.: UNM Press, 1973), p. 29.

4. Marvin Harris, *Rise of Anthropological Theory* (New York, N.Y.: Thomas Y. Crowell Co., 1968), pp. 82–100.

5. Ibid., p. 82.

6. Ashley Montagu, "The Concept of Race," *American Anthropologist* 64, no. 5, part 1 (1962): 919–29.

7. Crawford, p. 30.

8. S. M. Garn, *Human Races,* Third Edition (Springfield, Ill.,: Charles C. Thomas, 1971), pp. 55–58.

9. H. C. Bickley, *Practical Concepts in Human Disease* (Baltimore, Md.: Williams & Wilkins Co., 1974), p. 167.

10. Charles Marden and Gladys Meyer, *Minorities in America,* Fifth Edition (New York, N.Y.: D. Van Nostrand Co., 1978), p. 97.

11. Sarah Archer and Ruth Fleshman, *Community Health Nursing* (North Scituate, Mass.: Duxbury Press, 1979), pp. 533–5.

12. H. L. Kitano, *Race Relations* (Englewood Cliffs, N.J.: Prentice-Hall, 1974), pp. 3–6.

13. Barbara Devine, "Old Age Stereotyping," *Journal of Gerontological Nursing* 6, no. 1 (January 1980): 25–32.

14. Ann T. Brownlee, *Community Culture and Care* (St. Louis, Mo.: C. V. Mosby, 1978), p. 23.

15. Charlotte Epstein, *Learning to Care for the Aged* (Reston, Va.: Reston Publishing Co., 1977), pp. 66–67.

16. Harris, p. 399.

17. Epstein, p. 46.

18. Beverly Bonaparte, "Ego Defensiveness, Open-Closed Mindness and The Nurses Attitude Toward Culturally Different Patients," *Nursing Research* 28, no. 3 (May–June 1979): 167–71.

19. Edward T. Hall, "How Cultures Collide," *Psychology Today* 10, no. 2 (July 1976): pp. 66–74.

20. Ibid., p. 69.

20a. Brownlee, p. 23.

21. Montagu, pp. 926–7.

22. Abner Cohen, "Ethnicity in the Politics of Stratification," in Irwin Press and M. Estellie Smith, eds., *Urban Places and Process* (New York, N.Y.: Macmillan Pub. Co., 1980), pp. 397–401.

23. R. Cohen, "Ethnicity: Problem and Focus in Anthropology," *Annual Review of Anthropology* 7 (1978): 402.

24. Ibid., p. 402.

25. Ibid., pp. 379–95.

26. Fredrik Barth, *Ethnic Groups and Boundaries* (Boston: Little, Brown and Co., 1969), pp. 10–27.

27. Robert Murphy, *The Dialectics of Social Life* (New York, N.Y.: Columbia Univ. Press, 1971), p. 137.

28. Saul Feldman and Gerald W. Thielbar, *Life Styles in Diversity in American Society* (Boston, Mass.: Little, Brown and Co., 1972), pp. 272–273.

29. Ibid., p. 273.

30. Karl Eric Knutsson, "Dichotomization Integration," in F. Barth, ed., *Ethnic Groups and Boundaries* (Boston, Mass.: Little, Brown and Co., 1969), p. 99.

31. Ibid.

32. Talcott Parsons, *Evolution of Societies* (Englewood Cliffs, N.J.: Prentice-Hall, 1977), p. 250.

33. Sally Falk Moore, "Old Age in a Life-Term Social Arena," in B. Meyerhoff and A. Simic, eds., *Life's Career-Aging* (Beverly Hills, Calif.: Sage Publications, 1978), pp. 67–9.

34. Ibid., pp. 66–67.

35. Ibid., p. 71.

36. Ibid., p. 73.

37. Murphy, pp. 118–37.

38. Ibid., p. 135.

39. M. Kearney, "World View Theory and Study," *Annual Review of Anthropology* 4 (1975): 261–2.

40. Eleanor K. Maxwell and Robert J. Maxwell, "Contempt for the Elderly: A Cross-Cultural Analysis," *Current Anthropology* 21, no. 4 (August 1980): 569–70.

41. Kearney, p. 260.

42. Barbara Meyerhoff and Andrei Simic in B. Meyerhoff and A. Simic, eds., *Life's Career-Aging* (Beverly Hills, Cal.: Sage Publications, 1978), p. 240.

43. Ibid.

44. Ibid., pp. 14, 240–5.

45. Ibid., p. 233.

46. A. Simic, "Aging and the Aged in Cultural Perspective," in B. Meyerhoff and A. Simic, eds., *Life's Career-Aging* (Beverly Hills, Calif.: Sage Publications, 1978), p. 18.

47. Ibid., p. 19.

48. Ibid., p. 21.

49. Meyerhoff and Simic, p. 232.

50. David Jacobson, "Mobility, Continuity and Urban Social Organization," in J. Friedl, ed., *City Ways* (New York: Thomas Y. Crowell Co., 1975), pp. 358–59.

51. Meyerhoff and Simic, p. 236.

52. Ibid., p. 241.

53. Ibid., p. 242.

54. Jacobson, p. 360.

55. Meyerhoff and Simic, pp. 234–41.

56. Simic, p. 18.

57. A. Cohen, p. 401.

58. Moore, pp. 24–25.

59. Hall, pp. 71–73.

60. Hall, p. 72.

61. Frances M. Cox and Ndung'u Mberia, *Aging in a Changing Village Society: A Kenyan Experience* (Washington, D.C.: Int'l Federation of Aging, 1977), p. 8.

62. R. Cohen, pp. 397–8.

63. Barbara Meyerhoff, "A Symbol Perfected in Death: Continuity and Ritual in the Life & Death of an Elderly Jew," in B. Meyerhoff and A. Simic, eds., *Life Career-Aging* (Beverly Hills, Calif.: Sage Publications, 1978), pp. 163–205.

64. Jose Cuellar, "El Senior Citizen's Club," in B. Meyerhoff and A. Simic, eds., *Life's Career-Aging* (Beverly Hills, Calif.: Sage Publications, 1978), pp. 207–30.

65. Simic, p. 21.

66. Brownlee, pp. 61–63.

Chapter 13

Working with Groups of Elderly

Dianna Shomaker and Chiyoko Furukawa

PRINCIPLES OF GROUP WORK WITH THE ELDERLY

For centuries people have attempted to work out conflicts and arrive at resolutions; their methods and reasoning have come from every extreme. Some have been more successful than others. In the early 1900s, Pratt decided that problems could be resolved in groups rather than individually, but the technique was stimulated by a need to rehabilitate soldiers as quickly as possible after World War II. Therapy in groups was expedient and economically more feasible than individual therapy. The emphasis was on treatment of the entire person and not a particular disease, as had been the focus in the past. The goal was to increase the individual's interpersonal competencies by building on strengths rather than weaknesses. The assumption was that people will do whatever is necessary for survival, whether that action is efficient or effective. Moreover, they tend to draw upon past problem-solving techniques for present resolutions.

Regardless of age, everyone must deal with feelings and complex problems that arise as new goals and needs evolve. In order for therapy to become more effective, maladaptive habits and fears must be overcome and this frequently requires assistance oriented toward modification of adaptive techniques and methods. Everyone has the basic capacity to seek growth and adapt new ways of functioning.[1] In a group setting, individuals can gain understanding of their behaviors and their methods, at which point growth can begin.

Today there are many types of interaction groups designed to give assistance to their members, and many have been adapted to the needs of the elderly. They include such approaches as life review, reminiscence, remotivation, music and art therapy, and life cycle groups. Some serve the needs of the elderly, others the needs of their families. Groups form to resolve problems of common interest or dimension. Once the purpose for the group has been achieved, it will dissolve or form a new purpose. It is crucial to keep the goal of the group in mind as it functions, and, as the needs of the group change, to discuss with its membership the need to reassess the goals and direction. If it is feasible, goals, purpose, and direction can be changed to meet new needs and interests. It is detrimental to pursue those ends that no longer meet the needs of the clientele. Generally the goal is to decrease suffering, improve behavior, decrease interpersonal friction, increase capacity for making and keeping friendships, and motivate persons to increase productivity and creativity in order to gain a sense of purpose and identity.[2]

No single definition of a therapy group has ever been agreed upon, but there are some areas where agreement does exist. The group is a microcosm of the present in which to work out conflict.[3] It is drawn together to solve individual or common problems in a group effort. It can be organized for many reasons, and need not be only for mentally disturbed hospital patients. People are in the group because of a disruption in some facet of coping.

Modification can occur effectively in group work.[4] The mechanism is thought to be involuntary adaption as a release of emotions, encouraged by the specialized setting and process, occurs. "Repressed and painful material is subject to verbal review and catharsis, in a sense taking the sting out of the past by recapturing it and altering one's perception."[5] Participants gain greater objectivity regarding their interpersonal relationships and how they have evolved.[6]

Freedman outlines group therapy as an interaction in a group setting that applauds the growth of self-awareness and knowledge of interaction mechanisms.[7] A group forms to provide support for its members while exploring past and present feelings, and consequences of action; encouraging objective need for change; and evaluating shifts in relationships.

Ebersole elucidates the group's supporting role in assisting the participants to gain greater self-esteem where declining physical capacity has eroded it; to cope with grief from losses; to retain a sense of identity; and to reevaluate past events in light of current needs, fears, and interests.[8] Smolensky and Haar caution the advocate of group therapy not to expect all persons who enter a group to find resolution; each individual will change differently and in a different degree from the other members.[9] Those who experience change must have a strong sense of belonging to the group, and of course information, plans, and consequences of change must be relevant to the individual's needs if group therapy is to be useful. Most important, the impact of change must be recognized as a disruption of the status quo that will produce strain in other areas and may require additional related adjustments.

The desired end product of group therapy, then, is a fuller understanding of interpersonal relations, better coping and adaptation to the environment, and correction of past distortions of assessments. The group serves as a means of clarifying and decreasing distortion in each member's ability to assess. This ultimately increases self-esteem, autonomy, and efficacy.[10]

FORMATION OF GROUPS

Membership

Spontaneous groups of individuals sometimes have aspects similar to therapy groups and may indeed act as such under some circumstances. However, where groups are formed for problem resolution or therapy, members must be selected carefully in order to avoid attrition and disruption. This mandates that leaders interview all potential members beforehand. Behavior and needs of the members and the goals of the group activity must be compatible. The leader must determine if the group will actually benefit each person considered, and whether each person will make a valuable contribution to the group goals.[11] Burnside advocates a balance of personality types, while others emphasize a need to omit disruptive, disturbed, wandering, incontinent, psychotic, hypochondriacal, or abusive persons because of the strain and intimidation they bring to the meetings.[12] However, when possible, requests to join the group should be honored. Group therapy may not be appropriate for some problems, however, especially persons with mental illness who can better profit from hospital or private therapy. Also, it is important not to mix complexities of problems. For example, if the group is to deal with adjustment to the death of a spouse, would it be prudent to include a recent widow who is noticeably depressed?

As rapport develops among members and communication barriers become less formidable, members will demonstrate greater relaxation and confidence in relation to other members. Sensitivity to each personality will become more spontaneous, and self-consciousness will diminish. Ideally, all will grow in their abilities to be forthright and open with each other, confronting as need be, supporting spontaneously, inquiring for clarification, and finally responding nondefensively and granting each other nonjudgmental acceptance. Factionalism will occur in the group as people or subgroups of friends. This is inevitable and does not particularly signal a problem. These are emotionally supportive relationships that often strengthen group functioning.[13]

One means of establishing a basic plan for the group and minimizing issues that could become disruptive to the group process is to establish a contract, either verbal or written, between each member of the group and the group leader. This is to provide everyone with clear guidelines for the group's meeting schedule and the obligations of the members individually and collectively. Moreover, it will delineate the function of the leader and the purpose of the group. This is necessary in any well-run group, regardless of whether the arrangement is called a contract or takes the form of basic announcements at the beginning of the first session. The additional function of a contract, however, is to establish agreement on each point with all members individually as a condition of becoming members of the group. Burnside also advocates the contract in that it will encourage interaction between the prospective member and the leader for assessment.[14]

The contract should include the expected number of members, whether attendance is mandatory, the purpose of the group, and how meetings and socialization will be structured. Any scheduled activities and deviation from schedules should be anticipated and explained at the time of the organization and presentation of the contract. The final, and an important, item is a guarantee of confidentiality among group members and the leader; all information must be kept strictly within the confines of the group. This clarification of the roles of members and leader serves to reduce anxiety among members, and support or negate expectations and assumptions at the onset of the group formation. With less energy dissipated in anxiety and uncertainty, there is more available for the development of the human component so essential in group dynamics. The group can begin earlier and with less confusion to develop a culture of its own, with its own norms, introspection, and self-understanding.[15]

Group Leadership

The function of the leader in group work is primarily to maintain stability and offer suggestions for development of the group's norms.[16] It is assumed that the role will be played by a nonmember. Yalom, in his classic book on group therapy, points out that groups do not develop structure and cohesion automatically or inevitably.[17] The role of the leader in attaining these begins well in advance of the first group meeting. Burnside sees the leader as the glue for group cohesiveness, setting the tone and climate of the group through personal qualifications and careful selection of its membership.[18] At the point of convening, the leader does not direct the group, but oversees the total development of its movements through time, assisting in creating norms early in the life of its existence.[19,20]

The leader is a role model, a facilitator of movement and growth, an expert who observes and interacts objectively, a resource person, an exemplar of more objective thinking that should develop into patterns of communication that will enhance forward progress.[21,22,23] Leaders do not supply the answers; they encourage group members to think and talk through their problems, intervening only when there is danger to the group because a member is too aggressive or is violating the terms of the contract or its implied equivalent, or when the group has reached an impasse or plateau in its interaction.[24] The leader monitors group effect, gives social reinforcement, and keeps the group moving calmly toward its goal, but conversation is neither directed by nor channeled through the leader.[25] Interaction should be direct from one participant to the others.

Group interaction is also a learning process, and effective leadership can extend and enrich that learning among the members.[26] This can be accomplished in part as the leader from time to time interprets for the members and assists them in integrating knowledge.[27] Rephrasing and asking for clarification are two roles shared by the group and the leader. This process keeps information more objective and helps individuals avoid forming opinions and conclusions based on inaccurate assumptions. Once feelings are verbalized to the group, and recast and clarified by the leader and members, awarenesses are formed that might not have been possible for an individual acting alone in attempting to assess a situation and its consequences. It is this new awareness that the leader helps the members integrate into their banks of prior knowledge.

A group does not usually convene as an ideally matched set of members, and the members are not always ideally qualified for group discussion. This is one of the growth processes that results from group work. Initially it is often necessary to ask each person's opinion on an issue in order to stimulate conversation. Some find it valuable to use exercises that will open the group to better discussion patterns.[28] For example, group members may be given two minutes to learn as much as they can about the person next to them and then to introduce the person to the group; or members in the group may be asked to give thumbnail sketches of themselves to the group.

People are more secure when a meeting is conducted in a warm atmosphere. A small circle is not only a good configuration in which to foster such a feeling, but it also allows better visual and auditory contact among members. For some, security is enhanced by having the circle around a table rather than open to the group. Name tags are valuable in the beginning; they facilitate acquaintance and use of names among members. The use of names when addressing one another, "hello" and "good-bye" and other polite conventions, and the use of touch and smiles all create a warmer atmosphere for growth and sharing. In addition, recognition of each other's positive traits, and sincere praise and compliments are not only vital to each member's self-esteem and self-image, but also to effective group process.

The size of the group depends on the capabilities of the members and the leader. In general, smaller groups produce less anxiety. There needs to be a realistic appraisal of how well one leader can successfully guide a group that is undertaking multiple, overlapping, long-range problems of all dimensions of several members at once. A person does not enter a group problem-solving process with a single, isolated conflict or dislocation to be resolved; the nominal problem to be dealt with is always complex and interwoven with all other aspects of a person's being.

It takes skill to retain sensitivity while providing direction, role modeling, and feedback, yet not dominate the group.[29,30] The ability to be an attentive listener, to exercise patience, and to be sensitive to a change in group tone are vital to effective leadership. In order to develop a sensitivity to each member's needs, it is necessary to know the medical, social, and familial history of each person in moderate depth before the first meeting convenes. Individual rapport is developed in this way, but must continue to be nurtured and reinforced often during the group contacts. In addition, the participants need to know the leader and his or her feelings, ideas, goals, and background. Sharing information increases the strength of any bond between them and allows for more honest, open, and direct communication.[31]

Burnside has found it valuable to differentiate between agitation and anxiety in group members, that is, the difference between hostility and fear, and what they do to the group stability.[32] Initial anxiety is common in new groups, but can be resolved through group discussion. Long-term anxiety, or anxiety that appears later in the group history, is often symptomatic of new triggers that are not always related to the group process. These should be explored in the same manner.

Anxiety often reflects fear of a threat to a person or something perceived as a threat by that individual. It is demonstrated by nervous mannerisms or avoidance patterns. Common symptoms include hand and body movements that are carried to extremes, such as pulling at hair, wringing hands, tapping fingers or feet, fiddling with objects, putting hands to the face or over the mouth while talking, and restless movements. Talking too fast, interrupting others, chain smoking, monopolizing the conversation, and excessive or inappropriate laughter and joking may also be symptoms. Avoidance may occur in any degree on a continuum. A person may visually avoid others by lack of eye contact or by staring off into space, or physically avoid others by turning partly away or sitting away from the group or by not coming to the meeting at all. If members are absent, the leader should contact them immediately; the cause of absence may be, but should not be assumed to be, anxiety. There may be another cause. A member may forget, have an emergency, be ill, or have no transportation. On the other hand, the group may be a threat to that person. Given the age of the membership of a group composed of elderly persons, worry of a person's own or another's death may be a source of anxiety. If anxiety occurs in the group, the members should be encouraged to ventilate, to recognize their feelings, and to mourn if need be. To stay away from the group is counterproductive to the stability of the membership and the process.[33]

Agitation is disruptive to the group in another manner. It often is demonstrated by verbal or physical abuse to self or others, and by vacillation with depression or apathy that often mask anger. Causes may be found from all dimensions of an individual's existence, from medication to social injustice. Agitation should be dealt with directly and immediately. The first step is discussing it within the group. If it is too destructive to group cohesion, the affected participant should be guided toward other resources for resolution, that is, individual counseling, medical evaluation, treatment, and so on.

It is not easy to be a group leader. A leader never stops growing in sensitivity and organizational skills, many of which are gleaned from the participants of each new group experience. A leader also grows in appreciation for a need to not only be consistent, punctual, patient, gentle, and flexible, but tenacious and compassionate as well. The ability to handle all manner of emotions and communication styles is honed by constant, changing interaction with the dependent and the independent, the aggressive and the meek, the angry and the loving, and the healthy and the ill older persons. Knowledge of group process and of normal and pathological aging are only the beginning qualifications. Time and experience will create and test many of the remaining skills.

GROUPS FOR THE ELDERLY POPULATION

As with any age cohort, there will be diversity in the rate of acceptance and participation in group activities designed for therapeutic purposes. Older people tend to be more reluctant to join groups because their past experiences in this process may be limited. Many are also cautious about associating with groups that may involve divulging personal information. It has been found that group activities are utilized at a relatively low rate by senior citizens and probably attract the more gregarious older people.[34]

To assist older people to participate in functions that may meet their specific health and social needs, it is helpful to note their behavioral characteristics with regard to group activities. The elderly group members are more likely to focus their discussions on physical complaints, conflicts, past or impending losses, and reminiscences about their lives. Listening to these concerns conveys the caring attitude; but during these discussions, older people are more tolerant with individuals who monopolize conversations.

The use of touch is also important in working with older people and should be done in a spontaneous manner combined with a sincere effort to compensate for the emotional, social, and sensory deprivation many must endure.[35] Elders are quick to project warmth to a group leader, and test and assess the leader's personal security; ability to cope; and feelings about life, death, and themselves.[36] However, the aged will develop trust slower and look for an honest approach.

There are a number of therapeutic groups, with varying degrees of success, planned and organized for older people. Most groups aim to provide an opportunity for sharing experiences, feelings, problems, support, and ultimately for personal growth. Professionals must assess the particular needs of the client in assisting individuals and family to select a suitable group whose purposes can resolve specific problems.

Generally, the types of groups available for therapeutic purposes may be categorized by situational and developmental issues, that is, aging, debilitating conditions, or crises confronting older persons. Life review, life cycle, or reminiscent groups may be appropriate for persons dealing with adjusting or coping with the aging process. Remotivation and reality orientation activities are more congruent to those elderly individuals who might be debilitated with severe losses and confined to institutional settings. In crisis situations, family and individual therapy may be in order to assist in the resolution of critical problems.

THERAPEUTIC USE OF GROUPS

The activities and processes used for the life review and reminiscent groups are quite similar. Each group attempts to allow elderly individuals to verbalize and share their experiences. Initially, when the tendency for older people to direct their thoughts to the past and to self-reflect was observed, it was believed to be an indication of loss of recent memory.[37] However, a therapeutic quality emerged as the consequences of the life review process were scrutinized. Butler postulated that reminiscence was a normal part of life review evolving from the elder's realization of approaching dissolution and death.[38] The process is characterized by a conscious effort to recall past experiences, and, in particular, unresolved conflicts are reexamined and reintegrated. The ability to reintegrate and find resolution to conflicts gives new significance and meaning to a person's life and eventual preparation for death by mitigating fear and anxiety.[39]

Life review activities may include obtaining older persons' extensive biographies from them and other family members. Some instruments useful in the life review process are family albums, scrapbooks, memorabilia, genealogies, and other remembrances that may expedite reawakening of key memories and responses.[40] The recalling activity is conducive to assisting the older family member summarize life's work and frequently, the process allows for shared feelings about parenting with their offspring. Hence, the goals and effects of life review are "expiation of guilt, resolution of intrapsychic conflicts, reconciliation of family relationship, transmission of knowledge and values to those who follow and renewal of ideas of citizenship and the responsibility for creating a meaningful life."[41] In many respects, the life review process has a psychotherapeutic quality beneficial to the participants.

The reminiscing process is viewed as a developmental milestone that allows a person to gain an understanding about life. A reminiscing group is useful to older people because it offers an opportunity to share experiences with each other, to gain an insight of self and others, and to review historical events of the time.[42] The sharing of memories often promotes a bonding among the participants, assists to reaffirm individual identity and personal worth, and reduces loneliness and isolation.

Reminiscing groups may be long- or short-term, formal or informal, and structured or spontaneous.[43] Short-term groups have a limited number of participants, and topics are selected to meet the special needs of the participants. Generally, sessions for this group are held to less than ten weeks.[44] Long-term reminiscing groups have a more formal structure, require a periodic assessment and review of their goals, and admit new members only upon individual group member's approval.[45] A weekly meeting is also conducive to establishing a reminiscing group and provides an event that older people may anticipate on a regular basis. Spontaneous reminiscing groups are usually informal and often serve as entertainment with nostalgic qualities stimulated by special occasions.[46] A democratic and open climate is necessary for sharing memories and is essential for all types of reminiscing groups.

Ebersole recommends that reminiscing groups have an equal number of males and females to show the importance of sexuality as experienced throughout life in interactions.[47] This composition of the group allows for a variety of experiences from both the male and female viewpoints.

The reasons for developing reminiscing groups for older people are to:

- form cohort affiliation
- enhance socialization
- exchange ideas

- augment interaction
- promote intergenerational understanding
- facilitate recreation
- expedite reality orientation and remotivation
- encourage therapeutic life review
- work toward self-actualization and creativity
- serve as a springboard for starting other types of groups.[48]

The need for psychotherapeutic groups may result from crisis events, such as severe physical and mental illnesses, losses from death or divorce, radical changes in personal relationships, and the loss of employment. Often older persons who have lifelong anxiety or are unhappy react with panic to unexpected tragedies, and need the support and friendship of other people or a therapy group to adjust to the crisis. If this fails, special therapy sessions are required to assist in gaining insights into their problems and to provide support until emotional equilibrium can be achieved. A psychotherapeutic approach, which includes discussion and personal interchange, is required to allow expression of severe anger, hurt, astonishment, and so on. In many instances, this may be the first opportunity the elderly persons have had to participate in self-examination with skilled help, or this may be the first time that events have compelled them to seek assistance.

Group therapy with elders should focus on reality with frequent, brief sessions rather than hour-long sessions.[49] The reality issues should address age-related life situations and problems, and should capitalize on the strengths of the participants while keeping the limitations of the group in mind. The group must be structured to give clients positive reinforcement for effective coping and nonreinforcement for ineffective coping. Supportive encouragement is particularly important for the latter manifestations.

Some form of remotivation is also appropriate for group therapy with older people. This approach has been found to be superior to the conventional methods used with younger age groups. If motivation can be tied in with life review and reality, the process provides an opportunity for demonstrating past coping successes and gives insight into present resources that can be used to resolve the immediate problems.

MAINTENANCE USE OF GROUPS

Groups that help provide health and well-being to older people are required on a continuous basis or, at least, when individuals seek them.

Much of the thrust of maintenance groups is directed to meet a person's holistic needs and support. The life review and reminiscing groups that were discussed earlier can be used for meeting those needs if they can be structured on a long-term basis.

Senior citizens' activities are also excellent as additional types of maintenance groups. Most senior centers have planned functions such as card games, bingo games, sewing, shuffleboard, book reviews, and other pursuits that can evolve into structured or unstructured groups. Over a period of time, these events attract the same persons to participate in the activities, which leads to a cohesive group. In many instances, the groups evolve through the dynamics of group development with its trials and tribulations of jockeying for leadership, accepting or deleting members, and resolving differing opinions.

An important technique to mention here is the life cycle crisis approach to group therapy. This approach is neither strictly psychoanalytical nor an encounter process. The goals are to ameliorate suffering, overcome disability, provide an opportunity for new experience of self-fulfillment and intimacy, and verbalize emotions. The group therapy, as conceived by Butler and Lewis, has experimented with age integration on the basis that rich exchanges of feelings are possible between generations.[50] They describe life crisis as "the near-normal to pathological reactions to adolescence, education, married or single life, divorce, parenthood, work and retirement, widowhood, illness, and impending death."[51] Therefore, the life cycle group is concerned not only with psychiatric problems, but also with the preventive and remedial treatment of people as they experience life events.

FAMILY AS A GROUP

Family therapy is a complex and involved process because of the different generations of participating individuals. This situation may bring together many viewpoints, individual problems, relationship difficulties, and interaction skills. Issues in family therapy may center on decision making regarding an older person's welfare, feelings of guilt and abandonment, longstanding family conflicts, the necessity to provide continuing care, and involvement with the older family member.[52] Some families of the aged are faced with formidable problems that require professional assistance to find amicable solutions for all persons concerned. However, in most instances, family situations provide for support that old people can expect and receive despite the mobility and instability of the modern family.

In family counseling, it is essential to remember that external support does not provide lasting effects, and the ultimate goal is to mobilize the family unit to move toward a solution.[53] The role of the therapist is primarily one of a facilitator, as family problems are often longstanding. For example, a neurotic old person is likely to have a neurotic family with prolonged experiences of interplay with personality problems and long-existing symptomatology.[54] Often these people have developed negative behaviors that exacerbate one another. In this instance, the therapist would do well to achieve some semblance of an agreeable solution. It may be too much to ask for a caring and supportive attitude for the aging parent.

On a more positive side, most families are quite capable of discussing their feelings about one another with some guidance. Vocal tension in families is believed to be a more favorable prognosis than exaggerated tolerance and concern.[55] All members, even those who are not living together, must participate in family discussions as all human relations are characterized by ambivalence when illness of older members occurs. This event conjures up feelings of hostility, concern, guilt, or affection. Because some tension and ambivalence are normal between generations, skill and empathy on the part of the therapist are required to determine when family therapy should be directed to overcome normal disagreements and when to suggest radical solutions for the resolution of problems.

An important outcome of group therapy is the reduction of family problems to manageable size and new strategies that can be used for future concerns. Ideally, this is accomplished in an atmosphere where all the participants are free to ventilate. Every individual problem should be addressed in this environment, as both the young and old can benefit from this interchange. Moreover, this process gives the therapist an opportunity to identify relatives with serious emotional problems that may have been overlooked in individual therapy sessions.

GROUP PROCESS IN LONG-TERM FACILITIES

Group activities in institutional settings have been in existence for some time. Initially, groups were formed for recreation and entertainment. More recently, health care legislation has required that long-term facilities employ an activity director to develop therapeutic programs that offer interaction opportunities for clients. Also, resident councils and committees are established in many facilities to provide a mechanism for residents to participate and give input to the administration of the institution.

The number and types of groups that can be formed in long-term care settings are almost endless, and there may be considerable overlapping. The Philadelphia Geriatric Center is an example of the kind of group that can be organized to meet the needs of residents, potential residents, and their families. The center has developed useful principles for group work involving older people.[56]

There are two specially designed group techniques—remotivation and reality orientation—for the frail aged living in long-term care facilities. These techniques may be used jointly or singly depending on the needs of the older person to improve his or her quality of life.

Remotivation therapy was established in the late 1950s to remotivate mentally disturbed patients.[57] It is a simple form of group work that can be used in many settings where elderly people live. The purpose of re-motivation therapy is to stimulate and revitalize individuals who have lost interest and are uninvolved in the present or the future.[58] The therapy is structured and uses objective materials to which the persons are encouraged to respond. To stimulate thinking, the person is required to focus upon simple and common objects of daily life.[59] The experience is reality-based and offers the older person a bridge between the individual's self-percep-tion and the perception of others. Remotivation strengthens individuals with encouragement to describe themselves concretely as people who have roles and specific social functions, and to speak factually about past and present experiences.[60]

It is recommended that remotivation therapy be held once or twice a week for 12 sessions. Topics should be varied for each session to stimulate client motivation, and discussion should last from 30 minutes to one hour depending on the response of the group. Ideally, there should be 15 par-ticipants who are able to interact with others and not be totally regressed. The following five steps are recommended for each motivation session:

1. "Create a climate for acceptance" by using about five minutes to acknowledge the participants by name, express pleasure for attend-ance, and make other remarks of encouragement.
2. "Create a bridge to the world" by using about 15 minutes to talk about general interest topics selected by the group during a previous meeting. Each participant is given an opportunity to respond.
3. "Share the world we live in" by using about 15 minutes to further develop the topic under discussion with the use of visual aids.
4. "Appreciate the work of the world" by using about 15 minutes to deliberate on jobs that relate to the topic being discussed, how ma-terial objects are produced, and types of related jobs done by the participants.
5. "Create a climate of appreciation" by using about five to ten minutes to convey pleasure about attendance and contributions. Make plans for the next meeting that allow for continuity and give participants something to anticipate.[61]

Reality orientation is an intervention strategy based on repetition and relearning to reorient moderately confused geriatric patients. The goal is to increase the person's sense of reality by providing consistent and accurate information about himself or herself and the environment. Some advantages to reality orientation as a therapeutic and meaningful activity are that it is a simple technique that can be easily learned, can be implemented jointly with nursing activities and training sessions, and can be modified to fit several different settings, for example, home, day care centers, senior centers, and others.[62]

The number of participants for a reality orientation session should be between three to five persons. All participants should possess some verbal skills, but may have varying degrees of interactional abilities. Sessions should be held on a daily basis with each meeting lasting about 30 minutes. Strict adherence to time and selected meeting place must be exercised. The environment should be conducive for the sessions and accommodate the participants comfortably. Materials required for reality orientation are clocks, calendars, bulletin boards, and other articles useful for stimulating the mind. Family members should also be included in the overall plan of treatment to promote continuity and consistency of the therapy. It is imperative that family members give accurate information at all times. Staff techniques for handling difficulties should be shared with the family so the members may use the same strategies when needed to achieve the goals of reality orientation.

Music and art therapy groups are relatively new techniques used in long-term care settings. These activities provide for another dimension of pleasure and creativity for institutionalized elderly persons. The sound of music is believed to be therapeutic and has the potential to arouse the regressed or withdrawn persons who are unresponsive to verbal stimuli. Art therapy allows elders to express feelings and to create drawings, collages, sketches, and paintings that ultimately enhance self-esteem and confidence.

Leadership in art and music therapy, unlike reality orientation or remotivation groups, requires a person with subject expertise in addition to the qualities that are essential to successful direct group activities.

SUMMARY

Group therapy techniques were originally devised for younger age groups, but with the growing number of elderly demonstrating the need for emotional support and problem resolution, the principles of various types of group therapy have been adapted to the needs of the elderly. It has proven to be successful in community settings, where in the past these needs were often overlooked or masked by the philosophy of bearing the normal burden of aging.

Those techniques most commonly developed for the older persons are reality orientation, remotivation, and reminiscing. One of the more recent and progressive techniques is the life cycle crisis approach developed by Butler and Lewis. This approach requires intergenerational integration of families and individuals, and is based on life span events, not in isolation, but as life experiences.

Group therapy techniques are such that both professionals and non-professionals can implement them successfully, and this has been one of the more positive aspects of groups for the resolution of problems. These group therapies have improved the quality of emotional support systems for elderly individuals, affecting their physical, social, and attitudinal aspects of daily living; opening avenues to coping and adapting better; and enhancing self-esteem and self-image.

NOTES

1. J. R. Ellis and E. A. Nowlis, *Nursing: A Human Needs Approach* (Boston, Mass.: Houghton Mifflin Co., 1977), pp. 85–86.

2. Alfred Freedman and Harold Kaplan, *Comprehensive Textbook of Psychiatry* (Baltimore, Md.: Williams and Wilkins Co., 1967), pp. 1237, 1578–9.

3. Irvin Yalom, *The Theory and Practice of Group Psychotherapy* (New York, N.Y.: Basic Books, 1970), pp. 30–31.

4. Irene M. Burnside, *Working With the Elderly* (Belmont, Cal.: Wadsworth Publishing Co., 1978), pp. 101–5.

5. Priscilla P. Ebersole, "A Theoretical Approach to the Use of Reminiscence," in Irene M. Burnside, ed., *Working With the Elderly* (Belmont, Cal.: Wadsworth Publishing Co., 1978), p. 144.

6. Yalom, pp. 32–33.

7. Freedman, pp. 1237–9.

8. Ebersole, p. 147.

9. J. Smolensky and F. Haar, *Principles of Community Health* (Philadelphia, Pa.: W. B. Saunders, 1972), pp. 62–63.

10. Yalom, pp. 30–31.

11. Burnside, p. 63.

12. Ibid., pp. 55–62.

13. Ibid., p. 119.

14. Ibid., p. 199.

15. Yalom, pp. 89–90.

16. Burnside, p. 118.

17. Yalom, p. 83.

18. Burnside, p. 72.

19. Freedman, p. 1240.

20. Burnside, pp. 118–120.

21. Ibid.
22. Yalom, pp. 92–95.
23. Freedman, p. 1240.
24. Ibid., pp. 1240–2.
25. Yalom, p. 83.
26. Burnside, pp. 118–9.
27. Yalom, p. 83.
28. Ibid.
29. Ibid.
30. Burnside, pp. 63–72.
31. Ibid., pp. 81–84.
32. Ibid., pp. 63–64.
33. Ibid., pp. 118–9.
34. Robert N. Butler and Myrna I. Lewis, *Aging and Mental Health* (St. Louis, Mo.: The C. V. Mosby Co., 1977), p. 270.
35. Ruth Murray, M. Marilyn Huelskoetter, and Dorothy O'Driscoll, *The Nursing Process in Later Maturity* (Englewood Cliffs, N.J.: Prentice-Hall, Inc., 1980), p. 113.
36. Ibid., p. 113.
37. R. Butler and M. Lewis, *Aging and Mental Health*, p. 269.
38. Ibid., p. 49.
39. Ibid.
40. Ibid., p. 269.
41. Ibid.
42. Priscilla P. Ebersole, "Establishing Reminiscing Groups," in Irene M. Burnside, ed., *Working with the Elderly* (North Scituate, Mass.: Duxbury Press, 1978), p. 241.
43. R. Murray, *The Nursing Process in Later Maturity*, p. 111.
44. Ibid., p. 244.
45. Ibid.
46. Priscilla P. Ebersole, "Establishing Reminiscing Groups," p. 243.
47. Ibid., p. 247.
48. Ibid., p. 251.
49. T. L. Brink, *Geriatric Psychotherapy* (New York, N.Y.: Human Services Press, 1979), p. 214.
50. R. Butler and M. Lewis, *Aging and Mental Health*, pp. 271–2.
51. Ibid., p. 271.
52. Ibid., p. 273.
53. John H. Herr and John H. Weakland, "The Family as a Group," in Irene M. Burnside, ed., *Working With The Elderly Group Process and Techniques* (North Scituate, Mass.: Duxbury Press, 1978), p. 335.
54. T. L. Brink, *Geriatric Psychotherapy*, p. 71.
55. Ibid., p. 72.
56. Elaine M. Brody, *Long-Term Care of Older People* (New York, N.Y.: Human Services Press, 1977), pp. 199–207.

57. Marcella B. Weiner, Albert J. Brok, and Alvin M. Snodowsky, *Working with the Aged* (Englewood Cliffs, N.J.: Prentice-Hall, Inc., 1978), p. 113.

58. Helen Dennis, "Remotivation Therapy Groups," in Irene M. Burnside, ed., *Working With The Elderly Group Process and Techniques* (North Scituate, Mass.: Duxbury Press, 1978), p. 219.

59. Ibid.

60. Ibid., p. 220.

61. R. Murray, *The Nursing Process in Later Maturity*, p. 106.

62. Lucille R. Taulbee, "Reality Orientation: A Therapeutic Group Activity for Elderly Persons," in Irene M. Burnside, ed., *Working with the Elderly Group Process and Techniques* (North Scituate, Mass.: Duxbury Press, 1978), p. 207.

Part III

Delivery of Health Promotion and Maintenance Service

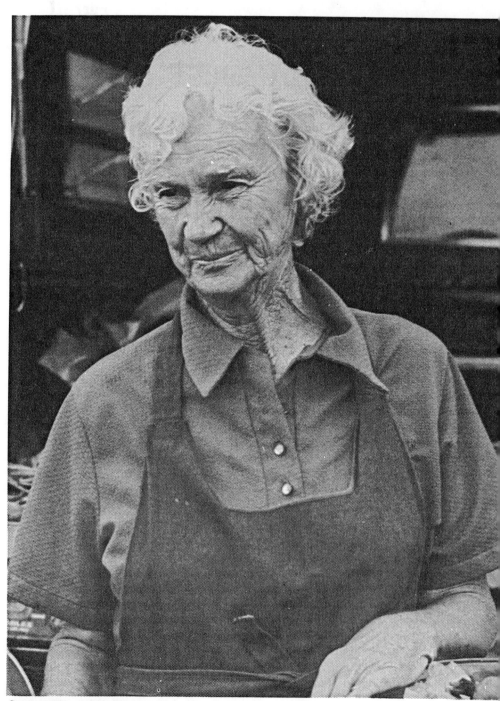

Courtesy Albuquerque News

Chapter 14

An Application of Health Promotion and Maintenance Model

Chiyoko Furukawa

Critics have stated that chronic and long-term health problems of the aging are insufficiently addressed by the Medicare program.[1,2,3] Considering that approximately 80 percent of all older Americans have one or more chronic conditions, the apparent inadequacy of Medicare benefits to provide for long-term care led to the development of several alternative health programs especially designed to provide services to support the elderly who have or are prone to chronic conditions.[4,5,6,7,8] Although these programs vary from an informal two-nurse system to a multidisciplinary model, a common theme is the promotion and maintenance of health with emphasis on long-term care.

The Adult Health Conference (AHC), a community-oriented health promotion and maintenance program, has been developed and implemented by the Boulder County Health Department in Colorado. The reasons for using this program as a model are two-fold: (1) As supervisor of the Home Care Program for the county, the author initiated the program and is therefore intimately familiar with all aspects of the services; and (2) The program is well suited to serve as a comprehensive model to illustrate the application of the philosophy and conceptual framework described in Chapter 1.

OVERVIEW OF THE ADULT HEALTH CONFERENCE

The AHC is a nursing service initiated in 1972 as a counterpart to the agency's Well-Child Conference, a service that is generally traditional with municipal and county health departments. The designation of "Adult Health Conference" was selected over the more prevalent term "Well-Oldster Clinic" to deemphasize the clinic atmosphere with its implication that a person must be acutely ill to participate. It also appeared at the time that the elderly were exceptionally sensitive to being labeled as "old people;" thus, the word "adult" was selected as a recognition of their preference. This feeling of being aged has ebbed with time as familiarity with the program and its services by both the elderly and the community has increased.

The program is now in its ninth year and provides a monthly or bimonthly service at fourteen locations within Boulder County. The frequency of services at a particular location is determined by the number of participants attending the conference; bimonthly services are provided only when attendance exceeds the staff's capabilities to provide proper services at a single meeting. A conference site is usually staffed with two nurses who give care to approximately 30 clients within a half-day schedule. Each site is assigned a specific date for its conference, such as the third Tuesday or the first Thursday of a month; this provides a meeting on a regular basis and minimizes any confusion that might result from a schedule on a more random interval.

The initiative for the AHC evolved from the agency's experience in providing home health care. In particular, the Medicare regulations prohibited continued care to avoid supporting independent living after an elderly's health problems stabilized. The agency perceived this as a serious lack of concern because subtle exacerbation of chronic illness among the elderly is difficult to detect and could readily progress to acute illness. Professional observation and judgment to evaluate the signs and symptoms of regression from health to illness were found to be important in preventing health complications, alleviating individual apprehensions and insecurities, maintaining independence, and providing support. It was clearly evident that some health services were necessary, particularly to assist in those instances where the nature of the problem strained or extended the capabilities of an elderly's financial and social resources.[9]

The agency believed that the elderly were entitled to care that encompassed every aspect of the aging process and ensured an optimal level of functioning. The philosophy underlying the AHC used the concepts of holism, prevention, and high-level wellness in the following way:

- Health care is a basic individual right.
- Elderly persons are unique individuals with feelings and reactions to social changes and the aging process.
- Protection of the client's rights is imperative.
- Health care practices require mutual goal setting.
- An holistic approach is necessary for the care of the individual, family, and community.

The 1972 program objectives, which supported the agency's philosophy, were to provide health promotion and maintenance care to 1,200 persons in the 65-years-and-over group within Boulder County by the application of the following six nursing interventions:

1. Detect early signs of unrecognized problems through the use of interviews, examinations, observations, and selected screening methods.
2. Monitor individuals with chronic conditions to ensure that continued medical care regimens were followed and to assist in maintaining the level of health status selected by each individual.
3. Offer health education on nutrition, exercise, safety, medical care, physical examination, and self-care. (Health topics for the classes were to be decided by the elderly group.)
4. Utilize community resources for services of other professionals when mutually identified as a need for high-level wellness.
5. Furnish follow-up nursing care to aid individuals with health problems and to facilitate actions of community agencies to abate difficulties influencing any individual's wellness.
6. Encourage consumer referral of individuals in need of any community health services.

These program objectives were designed for implementation by the agency's nursing staff because the funding situation limited the use of professionals whose expertise and contributions were needed to deliver comprehensive health care. This required the nurses to be responsible for seeking and coordinating the services of other health professionals as the need arose.

The Adult Health Conference is heavily oriented to the nurse's role in health promotion and maintenance care, but is based on availability; assistance from allied professionals in the community was eagerly sought. The services of professionals such as clinical psychologists, occupational therapists, and podiatrists were not used so are not included in this discussion. However, if these services were needed, these professionals would also have been approached for their assistance.

THE ROLE OF HEALTH PROFESSIONALS

Role of the Nurse

The AHC services were offered with the community's elderly group activities at a variety of settings including senior citizens' meal sites, recreational facilities, and subsidized housing units. These different sites offered an interesting challenge for initiating nursing care in a nonclinical setting. Although an attempt was made to explain the role of the nurses in a presentation outlining specific health and other services, the first elderly group participating in the program was puzzled by the nurses' presence. Many individuals were familiar with the nurses' role in institutions, for example, in hospitals, clinics, and physicians' offices, but they had little or no previous experience with community health nurses. The elders' initial behavior indicated both a reluctance to approach the nurses and a nonverbal cue of "I don't know why you should be here." These apparent feelings were further enhanced by the emphasis on health promotion and maintenance care, an uncommon concept for many who were more familiar with illness care. Moreover, the notion that nurses were offering these services rather than physicians, who were their normal primary health care person, was confusing.

In this situation, the elderly perceived the nurse's role as unclear, without sanction, and substantially different from the normative role, that is, a "hospital nurse" under the supervision of an institution or a physician. Stryker's view on role expectation offers some explanation to the behavior of the elderly group.[10] He states, "Role theory 'locates' role expectations in the culture of the larger society within which interactions occur. Roles are taken as the 'givens' of interactions as existing in institutionalized form prior to interactions." The AHC setting and the nurse's role in health maintenance within the community structure of the health care system were new experiences for the elderly. The nurse working independently within the AHC program failed to conform to the nurse's role expected by the elderly.

A strategy that allowed ample time for both the elderly and the nurse to become acquainted was employed to clarify the nurse's role. A low-key informal approach was used to increase opportunities for communication and interaction, and getting to know each other was basic to establishing a relationship as well as understanding the roles of both parties involved. During this phase of interaction, the protection of a client's rights and self-choice to request for nursing was put into operation.

The nurses accepted the role of participant-observer to enhance the interactive process. They participated in the recreational functions, had lunch at the meal sites, and interacted socially with the elderly. Every opportunity to facilitate an understanding about the nurses' function was sought. The nurses also used their observational skills during this time to assess unobtrusively the nutritional habits, general health status, attitudes toward nursing care, and the group's social interaction characteristics to obtain a holistic view of the elderly. Most of the elderly enjoyed the social contact with their peers, nurses, and recreational and meal-site workers.

Some knowledge about the importance of "balanced" meals was evident among the clients; however, many appeared overweight. The general health statuses were functional with few ambulatory difficulties, ventilation problems, or other overt signs of health problems.

This initial phase of becoming acquainted benefitted both the elderly and the nurses. Getting to know the nurse as a person first was important to develop trust, a precursor to imparting personal and family health problems for seeking professional advice. Some elderly established rapport with the nurses in a short time, while others preferred to wait and see. The nonparticipants viewed the participants as adventurous and kept a watchful eye on the latters' interaction with the nurses. They were especially curious about the care received by the participating members of their group.

On the other hand, the nurses listened attentively to the concerns expressed by the elderly, and special efforts were directed to assist those who indicated potentially serious health problems for themselves and/or their family member. A careful assessment of the problems and guidance to find specific solutions acceptable to each individual were a nursing priority. During this process, the nurses facilitated communication by emphasizing the confidential nature of the information given to them by the elderly. This time was also used to explain the differences between medical and nursing care and to clarify the nurse-physician relationship within the health care system. Individuals were also encouraged to continue their physician care and treatment.

As the program progressed, the AHC nursing role emulated the independent nurse practitioner functions described by Agree.[11] The nurses demonstrated a commitment to help those who sought assistance, and teaching and counseling were a major tool for this effort. More emphasis was directed to health rather than illness, and the thrust of the nursing practice focused on treating the whole person and the prevention of health problems rather than only on specific physical complaints.

The interdependent practice, another nursing approach similar to the Primex nurse, influenced the role of the AHC nursing staff.[12] The emphasis of care was on achieving a level of wellness appropriate to the elderly and their significant others. The plan of care was established with full participation and decision making by the elderly.

In summary, the nurses' role in the Adult Health Conference included the following functions:

- obtaining and evaluating a health history, and recording pertinent findings;
- performing a physical assessment using a variety of examination techniques to detect health deviations from the norm;

- providing surveillance and guidance in health care to individuals and families;

- instituting care to maintain and promote health while preventing recurrence of illness and disability;

- supervising rehabilitation measures for the elderly who required long-term follow up;

- coordinating and collaborating with other health professional services to provide appropriate care as required for the elderly;

- identifying and making referrals to community resources to achieve high-level wellness for the clients and their families.

Role of the Physician

The AHC program necessitated a more creative role for the physician who traditionally diagnosed and found cures for diseased conditions. "Medical education's Flexnerian emphasis is on physiochemical reduction and the experimental laboratory orientation. This approach stresses cures, not health, and is not at all conducive to the development of care plans for chronic diseases."[13] Since this was not consistent with the AHC program objectives, which were primarily concerned with health promotion and maintenance care, physicians were also required to assume a collaborative and consultative posture in addition to the usual diagnostic role.

Consultation requires communication with the physician to discuss progress or status of condition, while collaboration emphasizes input from all concerned, namely, the nurse, physician, and elderly, to determine continuation or change in the treatment plan. Medical expertise would be sought by the nurse and/or the elderly when signs or symptoms of abnormal deviation from health or chronic conditions manifested. The physician's diagnosis and treatment plan for acute exacerbation are essential for regaining health or maintaining chronic conditions in order to achieve optimal level of functioning.

The decision on the physician's role within the AHC program evolved from discussions among the agency's medical director, nursing director, nursing staff, and members of the Board of Health. There was agreement that medical care would be included and sought on an individual basis from the client's physician. However, one particular concern of the group was the possibility of the nurses' infringing upon medical practice, thus, potentially creating a nurse-physician problem. These concerns were resolved by defining the nursing roles and clearly communicating by means of printed brochures that the services of the AHC were a complement, rather than a replacement, to medical care.

Also debated was whether the agency should seek the local medical society's sanction and approval for the program. This action was deferred because the existing relationship of the medical community with the agency did not guarantee obtaining support for the new program. The alternative approach, which was implemented, was to initiate the program and to offer clarification to the physicians as the need arose. This method proved to be effective as indicated by the increasing client referrals from physicians to AHC for periodic surveillance and monitoring of elderly health maintenance needs.

The nurses were responsible for initiating active participation by the physicians in the activities of the health conferences. This was fairly easily accomplished as most nurses had a working relationship with the medical community through their involvement in the agency's home health care program. A major consultation activity was to obtain an annual physical examination from a physician to ascertain the elderly client's health status. This activity continued until the nursing staff was qualified to conduct clients' physical examinations independently. An initial comprehensive examination and evaluation are essential in health maintenance care, with subsequent periodic reexaminations depending on each person's medical history.[14]

In the area of preventive care, the physician's expertise was sought to verify treatments such as medication dosages, dietary and activity restrictions, and timely progress report or evaluation. This approach was designed to give consideration to the physicians' attitudes toward the prevention of disease.[15] The approach complemented the nurses' viewpoints supporting health maintenance care, and the two philosophies served to provide for the needs of the elderly clients.

Another significant contribution by several physicians was the donation of their time for group teaching activities, in which the topics for each class were selected by the elderly on the basis of their interests and concerns. The subjects ranged from minor ailments to more serious illnesses such as diabetes, arthritis, and heart disease. The presentations were enthusiastically received, and the elderly asked questions without feeling intimidated. This is in contrast to reports that elderly patients were reluctant to ask questions during their visits to the physician's office.

The physicians' role in providing health care to the aged as described in the literature parallels the experiences of the AHC and the agency's home health care program in that few physicians were found to be committed or interested in geriatric practice. Although accurate statistics are unavailable, there is a relatively small number of physicians in this country specializing in elderly care.[16] An increase in physicians for geriatric care remains uncertain as medical students continue to receive limited schooling and clinical experience on aging. Geriatric medical practice is also perceived to be less prestigious, less rewarding, a "waste of time," ineffective, or a burden to the community-at-large.[17] However, some consideration for expanded geriatric content and experience in medical curriculums is beginning to emerge. For example, Freeman suggests the following topics for a geriatric medical curriculum:

- epidemiology of aging;
- the nature of senescence or aging process;
- morphology of aging;
- physiologic mechanism of the aging body;
- pharmacologic therapy for the elderly;
- patterns of health and disease in elderly persons and the elderly organ system;
- psychology of aging;
- common and uncommon syndromes in major organ systems;
- surgical and anesthetic principles and the elderly;
- general characteristics of aging that necessitate special considerations at home or in the hospital, such as finances, family, and environment.[18]

In line with Freeman's suggestions, 75 percent of the physicians in a 1976 American Medical Association survey responded that there was a need for special training in geriatrics.[19] In addition, there is reason to be somewhat hopeful for the growth of geriatric medical practice since Congress and the public are joining forces to improve medical and health care of the aging. Until these plans become a reality, however, the main role of the physician in health promotion and maintenance care of the older population will be that of a consultant and collaborator for nurses and other health professionals.

Role of Other Health Professionals

The AHC implemented a team approach to health care by incorporating the services of several professional disciplines for scheduled periods. The aim of this team effort was coordinated care to assist the elderly in coping with specific health concerns and health deviations, or in maintaining optimal functioning. The health professionals participating in the AHC program were physical therapists, nutritionists, mental health workers, social service workers, and dental hygienists. Most services were nonchargeable and were made as an in-kind contribution by the professionals or by the service organizations they represented.

Consultation services for physical therapy came from therapists on contract to the agency for home health care. Whenever health problems requiring extensive individual followup were identified, the therapist made arrangements with the physician to establish a plan of care and received Medicare payment for services. There were few elderly attending the AHC who required extensive physical therapist services; most only needed some guidance to maintain their physical activity. A major contribution in this regard was made by the physical therapist who assisted the nursing staff in establishing guidelines for counseling the elderly about the safe limits of exercise and range of motion; for example, the "finger walking routine" on a wall surface was recommended to encourage and maintain range of motion for the fingers, hand, and upper extremities. These guidelines were developed to maintain the elderly's activities of daily living.

The services of nutritionists for the AHC were obtained from the following community resources: the Colorado Department of Health; the Boulder County Extension Agent; the Tri-County Health Department; and a Community Action Program. These nutritionists offered individual and group counseling for concerns such as weight reduction and diabetic and cardiac diets. They also made suggestions to the nurses for improving the method of nutritional assessment using dietary history, height and weight, dental health, physical signs of nutritional deficiency, and hemoglobin screening information, which were obtained from the health history and physical examination. Many factors must be considered when nutritional assessment is done since the identification of nutritional problems and the determination of treatment rarely have simple solutions. Particularly significant are individual differences in nutritional status that result from a lifetime of insults from diseases, variations in body structure and metabolism, and diversity in physical activity.[20] Also, whenever extreme alterations in nutritional habits occur, a referral for medical evaluation is necessary because the loss of taste, a common complaint among the aged, may be the result of lesions on the facial nerve, medulla, thalamus, and temporal lobe, or of atrophy of taste buds from the normal aging process.[21]

Closely aligned to nutritional status is dental health which was incorporated in recent years and has become an integral part of the AHC's health promotion and maintenance care. The dental hygienist's role focused upon the health of the oral cavity, recognizing its contribution to the individual's total wellness state. Because oral tissue also undergoes changes with aging, surveillance activity is vital for early detection of problems. Observation of changes affecting occlusion, teeth, oral soft tissues, saliva, perioral skin and muscles, and the entire stomatognathic system are essential.[22] For many elderly, observation and assessment by the hygienist may be the only dental appraisal available, as dental care is a low priority for them. Moreover, the exclusion of dental care from the current elderly health care benefits is a major threat to physical and mental wellness. The AHC attempts to remedy this dental care shortcoming, and whenever problems are identified by the hygienist, referrals are made to empathetic dentist members of the Boulder Dental Aid, Incorporated, a voluntary organization that enlists dentists to offer a 50 percent discount on dental services to the elderly.

Another team member, the social service worker, acted upon referrals from the nursing staff to determine eligibility for assistance with supplemental income, food stamps, homemaker services, and transportation needs. The elderly's reluctance to accept supplemental income and food stamps has been an unresolved problem. The homemaker and transportation services were accepted more readily because there were no apparent money transactions involved for these benefits. The elderly tended to view any social services as charity whenever a sum of money was directly a part of the benefit.

Since the elderly tended to reject social services assistance, the AHC staff was particularly careful to assess the elderly's mental health status. The inability to meet the psychosocial necessities of life adequately may lead to serious consequences that require the care of mental health professionals. Referrals of this nature, especially for those problems that were beyond the scope and practice of nursing, were made to the mental health agency. Severe reactions with adaptation to old or new life circumstances, namely, retirement, role changes of family members as a result of terminal or chronic illness, death of a spouse, loneliness, and depression were some of the reasons for mental health services referrals. Frequently the referrals included the family as well so that they would also receive support and assistance in coping with the client's mental health problem. This process was followed because treating the elderly can be a complicated problem requiring medical services in conjunction with psychosocial guidance for the elderly and family members.[23]

The mental health agencies established priorities to meet the demands for services according to age groups. In this situation, low priority is frequently placed upon the elderly caseload because of the service demands made by the younger population. This was the apparent reason for the lack of service to AHC clients. Also, in addition to the natural reluctance of the elderly to seek mental health services, this low priority contributed to the low completion rate for referrals to the mental health agency.

This inequitable distribution of mental health services is seen in many communities, and it is evident that a number of state or area planning efforts in aging, social services, or health resources give low priority to the problems of the mentally ill elderly.[24] Furthermore, outreach programs to identify persons with mental illness are often excluded from service models. The current less-than-desirable staffing for new programs undoubtedly results from the outmoded or stereotyped misconception that there is no hope for the mentally ill and the elderly.[25]

Other health professionals and agencies available to the elderly included audiologists from the University of Colorado Speech and Hearing Department for evaluation of hearing problems; occupational and speech therapists for rehabilitation needs; Family Planning Clinic Services for Pap smears; and the Alcohol Counseling Services for addiction problems. Legal aid was also considered a part of the AHC, and when required, the elderly were referred to the Legal Aid Society or the District Attorney's Consumer Affairs Department for assistance, particularly with matters concerning unfair or fraudulent practices. These resources were extremely important in providing the elderly with legal protection and services.

COLLABORATION WITH HEALTH PROFESSIONALS AND THE COMMUNITY

Collaboration in health care is a joint venture by two or more professionals and/or organizations in an attempt to overcome fragmentation of services and to improve the quality of care for clients. Collaboration links agencies as support groups to establish a new, or strengthen the existing, community health care system. Collaboration also requires cooperation by the involved parties, with each acknowledging clearly established roles and functions. Ideally, collaboration requires a commitment from all those involved to achieve the predetermined mutual goal successfully. Archer and Fleshman describe collaboration:

> . . . a collegial relationship with other nurses, health discipline members, and clients. Inherent in collaboration is the belief that each person has a unique contribution to make and should participate equally in decision-making. Collaboration thrives in settings where communication is open and participants hold a mutual respect for one another.[26]

Critics of existing elderly health care approaches point to the lack of collaboration among social and health agencies.[27,28,29] They contend the diverse needs of the community elderly, for example, medical, emotional, social, financial, and spiritual, seem especially amenable to professional and community collaboration for instituting coordinated services. These exigencies, which are inherent in the aging process, require an interdisciplinary team approach if assistance to the elderly and family are desired. Thus, the goals of holistic care and achievement of high-level wellness mandate communities to plan coordinated services. There are few, if any, community agencies that can boast of single-handedly providing the multitude of elderly services.

Collaboration with existing community agencies was expedited by the multidimension and holistic approach of the AHC program. The guiding theme of the program from its inception was the "piggyback" approach to the delivery of health services. This approach espouses joining of forces, personnel, facilities, and resources to link services to offer multiple benefits within a particular setting. Each service remains distinct from others, but becomes mutually supportive in a number of ways. The setting of AHC is an example of mutual support and fulfills the following purposes:

- delivery of health care to the target population through joint planning of services with existing groups to combine social and health services offerings in one location;

- demonstration of agency personnel's cooperative spirit by assisting each other in the variety of activities beneficial to the elderly;

- containment of service costs by sharing facilities and using in-kind contributions;

- identification of potential users of the services through the participants attending the functions;

- dissemination of health services information by the participants to nonparticipating community elderly;

- resolution of transportation problems by sharing the available established services.

Collaboration efforts by the nurses and the directors of the Senior Citizens' Center, retirement home, and recreation and meal programs ranged from arrangements for safe environment, privacy, interpreters for the minority elderly, and appointments for health assessments, to counseling and exploring with the elderly in identifying health topics for group teaching. In addition, pertinent articles about AHC services were written and distributed by the directors in the recreational and housing unit newsletters. Whenever special group activities were held, nurses were invited to speak about the services of the AHC. In collaboration with many agencies, every possible avenue was used to inform the community about the health service.

The collaboration was successful because each person and agency had an understanding of the responsibilities and tasks that would benefit the recipients of the services. Moe asserts that for collaboration to be effective, each agency must actively relate what it does to the work of the other agencies and organizations.[30] This was quite evident in the community where the AHC program was initiated.

The collaboration was facilitated by the Boulder Senior Citizens' Co-ordinating Council, which played a major role to nurture collaboration among all the member agencies concerned with the elderly's welfare. The council met monthly to update eligibility requirements for each member agency's services, discuss each agency's concerns, find solutions for mutual client problems, assess progress or status of specific referrals, and, most importantly, give continued support to each member agency's personnel and programs.

Moe gives insights into the level of cooperation and collaboration achieved by the Boulder agencies.[31] He explains that the high interest in relationships among organizations and agencies as units or parts of the community is influenced by two significant factors. The first deals with the nature of the problems people confront. The second concerns the nature of responses by organizations and agencies to problems, and whether the responses made are viewed or not viewed to be sufficiently comprehensive and specific to make a difference in resolving problems. Moe further suggests that the community is the smallest unit in which to view problems holistically and to find ways to resolve them.[32]

Since a community has problems that are unique to itself, problem resolutions must be matched to the resources available in the community. This process occurred with the Boulder Senior Citizens' Coordinating Council, which was able to identify mutual concerns about the status of the elderly, and then to cooperate and collaborate with agencies to improve the life style of the target population. The continued support for the AHC by the council contributed to many agencies and organizations working together to make an improved difference in the quality of life for the community's elderly. Another result of collaboration was the relatively low service cost for AHC. The cost to the program per client visit was $3.66 in 1973 (the initial year) and $5.40 in 1978.

PARTNERSHIP COMMITMENT WITH THE AGED

The philosophy of the AHC supports the partnership role of the elderly consumers with the nurse and other health professionals. Decision making by the elderly, an important component of this partnership, was encouraged by openly sharing findings and alternatives to assist the elderly with problems and concerns. Thus, the elderly were placed in an associate position, where they had the opportunity to weigh alternatives, and accept or reject possible solutions according to their own judgment. This partnership role was a new experience for many elderly as society tends to place them in a dependency role, particularly with respect to health needs. The youth-oriented outlook and work ethic value of society apparently take precedence and contribute to degradation of the elderly's confidence in their decision-making capabilities; therefore, the elderly tend to relinquish their rights to make decisions. One consequence of this action cited by Eisdorfer is that when sons and daughters intercede for their parents in giving health information, it may be distorted by the children's defensive attitude.[33] This suggests that misinformation about health problems may occur when family members are eager to help. Health professionals are in a key position to encourage full participation by the elderly and to assist the family in accepting their role as an important helper rather than as a decision maker for the elderly. Most elderly are capable of becoming partners in health care when support and practice are available to them.

The partnership commitment with the elderly was enhanced by the one-to-one relationship between the nurse and the elderly, which conveyed trust and encouraged free expression of thought. As closer relationships were established, the reluctant elderly began to participate more in the AHC services. This suggests that the nurses were influential in affecting the health care seeking behavior of the elderly. Moehrlin's study of the elderly health care use pattern found that the community health nurse not only positively influenced the choice of using health services, but elderly participants who enrolled in the health services were more knowledgeable about other services available to them than those who did not have contact with a nurse.[34]

The appropriate use of health services—another partnership commitment with the elderly—required educating the elderly about the importance of a physical examination. Although this was a new concept since most of them related examinations only to times of illness, many agreed with the benefits and sought physical examinations from their physicians once the rationale was given.

The development of partnerships with physicians was another matter. In particular, the elderly were reluctant to ask questions freely, as might be expected of a "partner" of a physician. After it was explained to them that the fee for office visits entitled them to pose questions, some of the elderly were encouraged to pursue answers on their next visit. Support and education are needed to encourage the development of the elderly's full partnership potential in health promotion and maintenance care.

CONTINUITY OF CARE

Continuity of care involves all health-related activities required to prevent disruption of care. It encompasses communication of relevant information from the record system, treatment and medication plans, client and family data pertinent for follow-up care, health teaching results, and other activities essential for the welfare of the clients. Continuity of care also facilitates the exchange of information with other health team members to maintain consistency in carrying out care procedures or routines, and to reduce feelings of uncertainty and neglect on the part of the client and family.[35] The continuity of care is supportive in nature and assists in achieving high-level wellness because essential care is provided as long as necessary to facilitate attainment of health.

The achievement of high-level wellness in health promotion and maintenance care requires followup or continued care as an integral part of the services and long-term contact with the client. One illustration clearly shows the benefit of the record system to expedite continuity of care. A client health record, with documentation of vital signs, health history, and screening results, assisted in the early identification of an elder's undetected severe cardiac problem. The symptoms of decreased pulse rate and difficulty with normal activity level were compared with the baseline health data, and differences were identified. An immediate referral was made for medical evaluation and resulted in the implantation of a pacemaker to alleviate a heart block. In this instance, the record system provided for continuity of care, and, without the baseline information as a reference, the health status deviation may not have been detected.

Baseline information in the records of the elderly with chronic conditions is important for maintenance of health because it allows early recognition of exacerbation of problems. For instance, the use of periodic urine and blood screening for several diabetic clients facilitated the physician's adjustment of treatments before the occurrence of serious health deviations. Furthermore, this activity involved the exchange of information between the physician and the nurse in order to maintain the elderly client's health. Similar continuity in the care plan was offered to AHC participants who had hypertension. The participants' periodic blood pressure results and the effects of medications were communicated to the physician for necessary adjustments of the treatment plan.

Home visits were another continuity of care activity for the AHC program and were made to clients with: (1) mobility problems to assess their daily living activities in the home environment; (2) complex health problems requiring urgent nursing evaluation; (3) emotional problems that could not be assessed at a conference site due to time and space constraints and the lack of privacy; and (4) confusion about the dosage, effects, and side effects of their medication. These home visit activities amplified the caring aspects of nursing, often strengthened the assessment process, and expedited the use of pertinent information, which the elderly and the nurse employed to make mutual decisions about health care needs.

HEALTH ASSESSMENT AND SCREENING ACTIVITIES

The development of the AHC's health assessment tool used the concepts of holism, prevention, and high-level wellness, and viewed the elderly's health status within the context of the physical, psychological, sociocultural, and environmental dimensions. The elderly's abilities for adaptation/coping, decision making, and acceptance of responsibility were appraised during the process of gathering data to determine the health status of each individual.

The collection of health status data began with an explanation to the elderly about the purposes of documenting the data and about the confidentiality of the information. Assurance was given that the health data were to be shared with others only with permission from each client and only on a need-to-know basis. Moreover, the purposes of the health assessment were conveyed as a need to: (1) determine the current health status; (2) identify potential health problems; (3) aid in promotion and maintenance of health; and (4) assist the elderly to achieve optimal health or high-level wellness.

The health assessment was conducted as an interactive process between the elderly and the nurse. This required the use of good communication skills and techniques to establish rapport, develop a sense of mutual trust, and ensure that the interactions did not turn into just a "question and answer" session. Each elder was viewed as a unique individual, and the nurse conveyed interest, concern, and care early in the health assessment process. The nurse also provided explanations and encouragement for mutual decision making and shared responsibility for health care.

Although the list is not in priority order, the assessment tool contained the following:

Physiological Dimension

- Past medical and health history, and review of body systems—illnesses, hospitalizations, surgeries, traumas, fractures, diagnostic tests, frequency of medical care, date and purpose(s) of last visit, vision and hearing examinations, immunizations, and allergies

- Medication patterns—prescriptions, over-the-counter drugs, herbs, ointments, suppositories, laxatives, dosages, length of time on medication, time of day medication is taken, and mode of medication intake

- Nutrition and fluid intake—number of meals per day, food preferences and dislikes, amount and type of beverage intake per day, description of appetite, food allergies, weight gain or loss, usual weight, preferred weight, height, and body type

- Sleep and rest patterns—number of hours per night, number of naps per day, interrupted sleep, and difficulty getting to sleep

- Elimination pattern—urinary pattern (day/night), bowel habits (regular/irregular), diarrhea, and constipation

- Reproductive—number of children, pregnancy complications, sexual activities, and satisfaction and dissatisfaction

- Family health history—medical problems (cancer, hypertension, diabetes, stroke, and heart) and other familial conditions (sickle cell anemia, hemophilia, and so on)

- Activity level—amount of exercise, ambulation problems, and recreational participation and preference (golf, swimming, tennis, cards, and so on)

Psychological Dimension

- Adaptation/coping—aging process, retirement, decreased income, loss of friends/family member, response to change and stress, self-control, anxiety, anger, depression, and loneliness

- Family relationship—marital, offspring, relatives, and residence of family members

- Support person(s)—relative, friend, health professional, neighbor, and so on (primary and secondary support persons)

- Mental status—orientation, attention span, memory, and recall

- Sexuality—opportunity for expression and preference, and so on

- Life and health goals—short- and long-term

Sociocultural Dimension

- Ethnicity—primary language, cultural values, and beliefs
- Educational background—future goals, and so on
- Place of birth
- Marital history
- Past work experience and income source(s)—income adequate/inadequate
- Religious preference—ability to attend church services
- Living arrangements—type of home (apartment, home, boardinghouse, and so on), own, rent, and others living in household
- Hobbies and interest(s)—new or lifelong and established
- Activities and outings from home—daily, weekly, monthly, and so on

Environmental Dimension

- Rural or urban—type of neighborhood and relationship with neighbors
- Accessibility—to medical care, recreational facilities, grocery store, relatives, friends, and other life essentials
- Pollution problems—water, air, garbage and trash, noise, and chemicals
- Transportation—private, public, and other
- Home safety—stairs, bathroom facilities, type of cooking facilities, ventilation, heating and cooling, and home and yard maintenance

Subjective and Objective Data

- Chief complaints or concerns expressed
- Vital signs—blood pressure, pulse, and respiration
- Physical examination findings

- Screening results—blood (hemoglobin, blood glucose) and urine (sugar, albumin, nitrite)

With respect to health screening, which yields important baseline health information, the AHC limited the activities to urine testing, hemoglobin values, blood pressure reading, and pulse and respiration rates. Urine screening for sugar and albumin was conducted using the reagent method, with normal and abnormal results determined by the manufacturer's guidelines. The nitrite test for bacteriuria was added to the screening activities in subsequent years to monitor for asymptomatic infections of the renal system, which are believed to be prevalent in the elderly.

The Sahli hemoglobinometer was employed for hemoglobin screening with normal values established as 14-18 gram percent for men and 12-16 gram percent for women. The clients were requested to share the results for comparison with the AHC findings whenever a hemoglobin check was ordered in the physician's office.

Appropriate health screening activities are selected after the completion of the health assessment or upon request for a specific screening procedure by the elderly. Blood pressure reading was the most frequently requested screening activity of the AHC program. Repeatedly, it was during the procedure of taking blood pressure that the elderly would begin to verbalize problems and concerns. This is an indication that the elderly may possibly have used blood pressure screening as an aid to express their concerns.

When the AHC program was initiated, the guideline for abnormal blood pressure was established to be: systolic reading—165 or over; diastolic— 95 or over. Since then, the AHC has adopted the following for blood pressure screening:

Normal:	under 140/90; over 90/60
Abnormal:	160/95; under 90/60 (65 years and over)
	150/90; under 90/60 (45–64 years)
Questionable:	140/90 to 160/95 (65 years and over)
	140/90 to 150/95 (45–64 years)

It should be noted that whenever individuals with abnormal findings are identified, follow-up care is provided using the established protocol for rechecks and referrals for medical evaluation and care.

TEACHING AND COUNSELING

The basic process for teaching and counseling activities requires active client participation and heavily depends on the client's abilities to accept responsibility and make decisions beneficial to their health status. Frequently, the teaching and counseling activities for the elderly were integrated and jointly accomplished. More often, it was necessary to start with counseling to identify specific teaching topics. Once the topic was identified and the learner's knowledge base was ascertained, the content for teaching was delineated with the elderly to include the most important information in the lesson plan. The teaching sessions were informal, involved demonstration and return demonstration when appropriate, and, in most instances, provided handouts of written information for the elderly. Efforts were made to clarify any misunderstanding, and terminology familiar to the elderly was used to ensure comprehension, to give explanations, and to expedite a change in behavior.

A change in behavior is necessary for learning to occur in teaching situations, but the change is most difficult for the learner because previous secure and familiar actions must be discarded.[36] This is especially applicable to the elderly who have more deeply ingrained lifelong habits to change in most learning situations.

However, the AHC experience found that the elderly who sought information were ready to attempt changes, particularly in regards to medications and diets. This is indicated in Figure 14-1, which summarizes the relative frequency of health-related topics selected by the elderly during the program's first year. Diet and medication (25 percent and 24 percent respectively) were the most frequently chosen topics of concern. One interpretation of this was that the elderly were interested to learn about diets as a part of health care, although it may have meant changes to their long-established eating habits. Similarly, learning about medication might have led to changes other than to accepting passively prescribed treatment. However, the elderly were interested in obtaining information on medication as a matter of health maintenance and prevention.

An important aspect of teaching is the evaluation of any changes in behavior on the part of the learner. The measure for such evaluation within the AHC was primarily based on elderlys' reports on how the teachings affected them and on objective data such as weight loss, decrease in blood pressure, and increased hemoglobin value, which may be related to dietary teaching for some individuals. These evaluations were made by the elderly and the nurse, and generally included discussions on the value or appropriateness of a given topic. After clear delineations of possible consequences were offered by the nurse, decisions were mutually made for terminating or continuing a particular subject that was previously selected to attain established teaching goals. Regardless of teaching outcomes, the nurses continued to support and to direct their efforts to give assistance to individuals on any topic chosen by the clients.

An informal approach, which was directed to the resolution of specific problems that often resulted from situational or interpersonal difficulties,

Figure 14-1 Frequency of Health Teaching and Counseling Topics

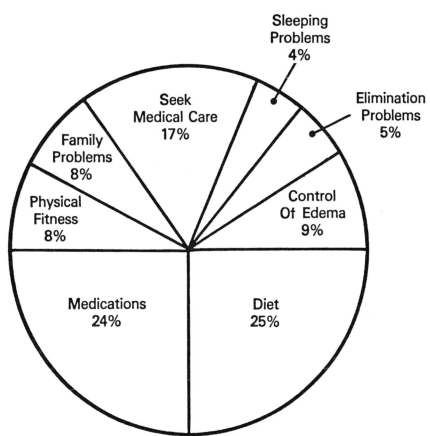

Source: C. Furukawa, "Adult Health Conference: Community-Oriented Health Maintenance Care of the Elderly," *Family & Community Health* 3, no. 4 (February 1981), p. 114.

was also used in counseling services. The nurses attempted to direct and assist the elderly in finding acceptable solutions in the resolution of difficulties. No attempts were made to conduct in-depth sessions to explore ways to change longstanding feelings and attitudes. The elderly were assisted in becoming aware of their own feelings, but the sessions were not a replacement for psychotherapeutic sessions. Problems that required psychiatric assistance were referred to the mental health agency for assistance from the experts in the field of mental health services.

SUMMARY

The development and implementation of the Adult Health Conference were closely aligned with the philosophy and conceptual framework described in Chapter 1. Health promotion and maintenance care were emphasized in achieving high-level wellness for elderly clients. The elderly were considered as partners to the nurses and other health professionals, and they participated in the decision making and took responsibility for meeting their own health needs. The adaptation/coping abilities of individual clients were incorporated into the mutual planning and decision for health teaching and counseling activities.

In recognition of the holistic needs of the aging, the AHC collaborated and coordinated with several community agencies to provide comprehensive health services. The collaboration efforts with the agencies and their personnel contributed to the effective sharing of the available community resources. Some of the resources shared included facilities, transportation services, personnel, interpreters, and publications.

NOTES

1. Sara K. Archer, "Health Maintenance Programs for Older Adults," *Nursing Clinics of North America* 3, no. 4 (December 1969): 730.

2. Jerome Hammerman, "Health Services: Their Success and Failures in Reaching Older Adults," *American Journal of Public Health* 64, no. 3 (March 1974): 255.

3. Cary S. Kart, Eileen S. Metress, and James F. Metress, *Aging and Health: Biological and Social Perspectives* (Menlo Park, Cal.: Addison-Wesley Publishing Co., 1978), p. 297.

4. Percil E. Stanford, "The Politics of Providing Health and Mental Health Care for the Aging," in Adina M. Reinhardt and Mildred D. Quinn, eds., *Current Practice in Gerontological Nursing* (St. Louis, Mo.: C. V. Mosby Co., 1979), p. 27.

5. R. R. Stortz, "The Role of a Professional Nurse in Health Maintenance Program," *Nursing Clinics of North America* 7, no. 2 (June 1972): 207–23.

6. E. Anderson and A. Andrews, "Senior Citizens Health Conferences," *Nursing Outlook* 21, no. 9 (September 1973): 580–2.

7. Floyd Garetz and Peter Reth, "An Outreach Program of Medical Care for Aged High-Rise Residents," *The Gerontologist* 14, no. 5 (May 1974): 404–7.

8. Archer, "Health Maintenance Programs for Older Adults," pp. 729–40.

9. Stanley J. Brody, "Evolving Health Delivery Systems and Older People," *American Journal of Public Health* 64, no. 3 (March 1974): 245–8.

10. Sheldon Stryker, "Fundamental Principles of Social Interaction," in Neil J. Smelser, ed., *Sociology: An Introduction* (New York, N.Y.: John Wiley & Sons, 1973), p. 538.

11. Betty C. Agree, "Beginning Independent Nursing Practice," *American Journal of Nursing* 4, no. 4 (April 1974): 636–42.

12. V. E. Stolar and Reva Rubenstein, "Developing the Science Component in a Primex Program," *Nursing Outlook* 21, no. 5 (May 1973): 325–7.

13. Kart, *Aging and Health,* p. 273.

14. H. J. Rosen, "Modern Care Delivery for the Aged: A Program in Total Health Maintenance," *Journal of the American Geriatric Society* 20, no. 10 (October 1972): 505–9.

15. Stanley J. Brody, "Comprehensive Health Care for the Elderly: An Analysis," *The Gerontologist* 13, no. 4 (April 1973): 412–8.

16. Kart, *Aging and Health,* p. 270.

17. Ibid.

18. T. J. Freeman, "Gerontology's Educational Profile," *Geriatrics* 31, no. 10 (October 1976): 115–6.

19. Kart, *Aging and Health,* p. 273.

20. D. Weir et al., "Recognition and Management of the Nutritional Problems of the Elderly," in Austin B. Chinn, ed., *Working With Older People,* Vol. IV (Rockville, Md.: U.S. Department of Health, Education and Welfare, 1971, reprinted 1974), p. 267.

21. Kart, *Aging and Health,* p. 76.

22. Arthur Elfenbaum, "Dentistry for the Elderly in Health and Illness," in Austin B. Chinn, ed., *Working With Older People,* Vol. IV (Rockville, Md.: U.S. Department of Health, Education and Welfare, 1971, reprinted 1974), p. 338.

23. Samuel Granick, "Psychological Study in the Management of the Geriatric Patient," in Austin B. Chinn, ed., *Working With Older People,* Vol. IV (Rockville, Md.: U.S. Department of Health, Education and Welfare, 1971, reprinted 1974), p. 323.

24. Stanford, "Politics of Providing Health and Mental Care," p. 35.

25. Ibid.

26. Sarah E. Archer and Ruth P. Fleshman, *Community Health Nursing Patterns and Practice* (North Scituate, Mass.: Duxbury Press, 1979), p. 11.

27. Brody, "Comprehensive Health Care," pp. 412–8.

28. Carl Eisdorfer, "Observations on Medical Care of the Aged," in C. R. Boyd and C. G. Oakes, eds., *Foundations of Practical Gerontology* (Columbia, S.C.: University of South Carolina Press, 1973), pp. 68–76.

29. Hammerman, "Health Services: Their Success and Failure," pp. 253–6.

30. Edward O. Moe, "Agency Collaboration in Planning and Service: The Emerging Network on Aging," in Adina M. Reinhardt and Mildred D. Quinn, eds., *Current Practice,* p. 175.

31. Ibid., p. 178.

32. Ibid.

33. Eisdorfer, "Observations on Medical Care," p. 75.

34. Barbara A. Moehrlin, "Utilization of Health Care Services by the Elderly," in Irene Mortenson Burnside, ed., *Psychosocial Nursing Care of the Aged* (New York, N.Y.: McGraw-Hill Book Co., 1980), p. 173.

35. Ruth B. Murray, M. Marilyn Huelskoetter, and Dorothy L. O'Driscoll, *The Nursing Process in Later Maturity* (Englewood Cliffs, N.J.: Prentice-Hall Inc., 1980), p. 353.

36. Barbara K. Redman, *The Process of Patient Teaching in Nursing,* 2nd Edition (St. Louis, Mo.: C. V. Mosby Co., 1972), p. 91.

Chapter 15

Health Promotion and Maintenance in the Institutional Community

Dianna Shomaker and Chiyoko Furukawa

If health care is to benefit individuals, all resources of potential use to those recipients must be designed with maximum concern for each person's unique needs and potential. Also, every health care program and facility must encompass a basic belief that users will continue to grow and develop to the maximum of their capabilities. There is little reasonable support for the erection of a facility or institution that no longer encourages or allows a user to continue growing and developing. Such a detrimental health care approach would be an inhuman paradox. If this is not correct, then all facilities could be built with the intent that the user enter with no reason, need, or desire to leave. This premise suggests that the individual's growth has reached its maximum capacity and ability so that the next step is to await death. If it were certain that life had been completed, there would be no need to stimulate social and psychological factors for health care recipients within the institution or society.

To date no populace has been shown to have been so healthy through life that individuals arrive at their first need for health care facilities in such a terminal state of perfection. However, many facilities exert no effort to foster growth, which implies that further continuance of the individual's horizons is either impossible or unnecessary.

Health care facilities admit people for the express purpose of curing them for discharge back into the community as functional citizens. The guide is a medical model. People who enter are sick, a role that is not generally preferred by the people entering or the professionals giving them care. The role prevents growth due to illness. The goal is to eradicate the barrier to growth and shorten the person's period of incapacitation.

Nursing homes are a paradox in the health care system. Persons who enter are not always acutely ill, but they often are molded into the roles of sick people in an institutional routine. The client's capabilities, potential, or possible discharge get little recognition. Not only is little beyond trivial

269

social amenities and provision for basic needs provided, but there is no attempt to encourage growth and continuation of socialization. Care is provided on the assumption that discharge will occur in case of death or transfer to a hospital and that only in the rarest instances will patients become independent again in the community.

OVERVIEW OF STATUS OF THE INSTITUTIONAL COMMUNITY

Nursing homes serve primarily the older citizens of the community. These institutions grew out of the almshouse concept of colonial America and have steadily increased in number since the early 1900s. They are represented in many modalities from boarding homes to mental hospitals.[1] Twenty percent are nonprofit, ten percent government sponsored, and the remainder are proprietary facilities.[2] There are approximately 25,000 nursing homes in the United States, sheltering two-thirds of the institutionalized elderly. Persons who enter such facilities often do so because they have no other recourse. On entering, they are usually over 75 years of age. They have lived alone, devoid of useful support networks, and half have had no close family ties, which is thought to be more closely related to admission than illness.[3]

Moss and Halamandaris' study of nursing homes concurs with these data. They add that, of admissions to an average nursing home, 66 percent come from their own homes, 31 percent from hospitals, and the remainder are transferred from other nursing care facilities. Their average stay is 2.4 years, after which time 80 percent die; only 20 percent ever return home. Many of the 20 percent return to nursing homes at a later date. Less than 50 percent of nursing home residents are ambulatory or mentally alert, and a third are incontinent.[4]

At any given time, slightly less than six percent of the population over 65 years of age lives in nursing homes. But, as Tobin points out, this statistic doesn't reveal the rapid increase in the probability of institutionalization as a person ages.[5] After a person reaches 65, there is about a one-in-four probability that institutionalization will eventually occur one or more times in the remainder of life. The rate more than doubles with 10-year increments of age; for example, from 65- to 74-years-old, 2 percent are cared for in nursing homes, mental hospitals, or personal care homes; from 74 to 84 years of age, the rate increases to 7 percent; and over 85 years of age, it is 16 percent. As a person advances in years after 65, independence becomes more expensive and difficult to maintain.[6]

Nursing home residence is not a popular choice with eligible candidates. Most people resist admission as long as possible, and usually every alternative is explored in preference to nursing home care. Contrary to myth, the nursing home population is not composed of those "deposited there by uncaring families;" there is little evidence to support this belief.[7] Institutionalization is not an indicator of family breakdown, as has been suggested, but for those 60 percent in nursing homes who receive no visitors at all, the appearance is difficult to rationalize.[8,9]

The entire concept of nursing home care is surrounded by negative attitudes. Many elderly state that admission is comparable to a "confession of final surrender, a halfway stop on the route to death."[10] Moss and Halamandaris found that:

> . . . [the] average senior citizen looks at a nursing home as a human junkyard, as a prison, a kind of purgatory, halfway between society and the cemetery, or as the first stop of an inevitable slide into oblivion. Nursing homes are not only synonymous with death, but with the notion of protracted suffering before death.[11]

Those with the most education about aging are the least willing to work in a nursing home, even with a pay differential. The turnover rate of personnel is about 70 percent a year. The programs at nursing homes are alleged not only to fall far short of meeting emotional needs of the clientele, but the environment is also depersonalized for the sake of efficiency in institutional tasks such as cleaning and ambulation. The high emphasis on routine in the environment creates a type of institutional neurosis that erodes individuality, minimizing any attempts at self-reliance by the client by unwittingly encouraging dependence on the staff.[12]

The effects of nursing homes on individuals have been thought to be psychologically deleterious. Empirical studies offer data that support this assumption. The process of institutionalization is thought to be destructive to its recipient population due to the social and cultural setting. Findings attributed to this include: (1) a greater degree of poor health (as might be expected); (2) more depression and negative self-images than in the general population; (3) poor adjustment, deprecatory personality patterns, and feelings of insignificance; (4) a decline in intelligence and abilities, and a low range of interests and activities; and (5) recipients more prone to death. These findings are not from long-term studies, however, but were only researched on patients already in nursing homes, which minimizes the value of the findings as compared against the general society.[13]

Lieberman argues against accepting these findings at face value, recognizing bias in selection of population samples and other artifacts of research methodology.[14] True, people in nursing homes are worse off, but there is no substantial proof of whether it is caused by living in nursing homes or is the major reason why independent living in the community was relinquished. At this point, stereotypes are perhaps overdrawn. Lieberman suggests that the degree of discrepancy between the adaptive response in the community and that of the nursing home (that is, radical environmental change) is a more important consideration. He states that ". . . the effect of an institution can be viewed less as a product of its quality or characteristics than of the degree to which it forces the person to make new adaptive responses or employ adaptive responses from the previous environment."[15]

A more open plan that allows more contact with the community and less closed congregate living might sustain effective use of prior adaptive responses and minimize deterioration in adaptive mechanisms of the clientele.

The level at which extremes in adaptive change might be required in moving from home to institution could be assessed more objectively by following factors devised by Bennett where, by examining the degree to which institutionalization occurred at home and in the nursing home, a person might more effectively assist the client in adapting.[16] A person would determine the degree to which:

- Present abode is considered to be a permanent residence.
- All activities are restricted to the residence grounds.
- All activities are scheduled sequentially for the residents as a group.
- Formal rules of conduct exist.
- There is continual observation and supervision.
- Rewards and punishment are standardized.
- Persons are not allowed to make decisions about personal property and use of time.
- Personal property is controlled by the individual.
- Residence is by choice.
- Congregate living is required.

Whether nursing homes are a major factor in deteriorating personalities in residents is a moot point, but nursing homes have a poor record of intent to create a home in which to live. Regimentation and minimal socialization, indifference, ignorance, and profiteering combine to reduce persons to a nonhuman status in order that they might "live" in the facility that dialectically negates living.[17]

Many indictments have been written of the negative conditions prevalent in nursing homes today. A major one is Mendelson's *Tender Loving Greed,* which concludes, from innumerable examples drawn from 200 nursing homes over a ten-year study, that nursing homes are, at the same time, big business and a tragedy.[18] They make unreasonable profits by capitalizing on federal bureaucratic failure to regulate, on powerlessness of the elderly, and on a facade of caring. Both profit and nonprofit institutions swindle the public under a paradoxical message of tender loving care based on inhuman practice and exorbitant prices. Mendelson gives no room for the exception, maintaining that ten years of observation failed to generate an exception, although nursing homes were "bad" in varying degrees.

Hendricks and Hendricks trace the paradox to federal legislation.[19] The goal of federal legislation has been to strengthen health care services through Medicare. The public overreacted to the new resources, and the result was an increased reliance on the nursing home process to solve minor problems of aging. Persons interested in business for profit opened numerous proprietary nursing homes, often with interests in direct conflict with the clientele they intended to "serve." As the programs became more prolific, complex, and obviously unsatisfactory, the government set more and more regulations, which evolved into a labyrinth, thickly entangled with opposition and limitation.

Many nursing homes have been closed, but many others halted services because they burned down first. Perhaps they don't alter client personalities, but the literature available paints a grim picture of findings. Abuses are widespread and unconscionable. Moss and Halamandaris point to good nursing homes and to people who are sincerely intent on creating a positive environment for the growth of elderly persons' potential.[20] However, the abuses disclosed in the Senate investigations under Senator Moss far outweigh the positive comments on various facilities to date. Abuses investigated and documented by the Senate investigations demonstrate the degree of profiteering, as well as ignorance and indifference, that seem to control the nursing home industry.

The abuses investigated and described before the Senate committee hearings were abuses against the human dignity of the elderly, and common among these were factors that also endangered the lives of the residents. There was negligence and deliberate physical injury, including improper use of restraints. Clients were slapped, punched, shoved, handcuffed, and strapped into beds, wheelchairs, and cubicles. Unsanitary conditions pervaded many homes, and there was often no protection for staff members or other clients from those who were suffering from contagious diseases, particularly tuberculosis. Housing was poorly maintained; heating and cooling were inadequate; and death by fire was well documented. In 1976, as many as 47 percent of the nursing homes did not comply with the minimum fire safety standards. Care was administered by untrained, unlicensed personnel about 80 percent of the time. The number of registered nurses fell far short of the number required. Other staff persons—aides and orderlies—were usually paid no more than minimum wage. It has been hypothesized that this condition attracts only a transient, uncaring, poor-quality worker. Others have argued that people cannot be persuaded to be sensitive and caring by pay alone.

Food was often of poor quality and meager quantity; horror stories substantiated the unbelievable accusations about the subsistence people endured. Cost and preparation of food were often cut to well below a dollar a day to cover all three meals and snacks per client; the implication was that lower food costs resulted in increased profit. Complaints brought reprisal to the elders who complained, rather than against the abusers. Profiteering has been a major charge leveled against nursing home operators who have misappropriated personal funds and solicited kickbacks from vendors and suppliers.[21]

The most common abuse and source of kickbacks was that of drug control. It was by far the most critical and widespread problem identified by the Senate committee. Records were poorly kept, and drugs erratically administered, often by untrained personnel. Twenty to 40 percent of the drug doses were given in error. There was a high incidence of adverse drug reactions and an indiscriminant use of tranquilizers. Prescriptions were outdated, falsified, and overpriced. Employees also had easy access to patients' drugs for personal consumption.[22]

All in all, Moss and Halamandaris concluded that 50 percent of the nursing homes were substandard, but few were closed. Moreover, the enforcement of federal regulations is inadequate, so that many homes have continued propagating horror stories and creating misery for the elderly clientele, who are needy and virtually powerless. This has brought a bad reputation to all nursing homes.

Poor working conditions, weak role models, and inadequate training make it difficult for staff members to carry out adequate care to the elderly in nursing homes, regardless of the level of care. Lack of policies and restrictions makes nursing care difficult to deliver. Poor administration, together with the isolation of nursing homes from other health care facilities in both policy and practice as well as resources, creates not only an unsavory place to work, but a setting for deviation from quality care.

Moss and Halamandaris do not categorically denounce nursing homes as does Mendelson. They maintain that for all the appalling findings of the

Senate committee "in almost any American city there is one nursing home offering excellent care."[23] All nursing homes have the potential for quality care, and the trigger for such change is in attitude.

> The lesson appears to be that it is an intangible—*esprit de corps*—a sense of motivation manifested in individualized treatment and maximized human dignity that marks the best nursing homes. Neither this *esprit de corps* nor Tender Loving Care can be imposed by government fiat. It must be the result of the desire and commitment on the part of the nursing home personnel.[24]

OPTIMAL FUNCTIONING IN INSTITUTIONAL SETTINGS

Residential changes are inevitable when dysfunctions occur either as a consequence of aging or disease processes. However, the new locale or habitation should not disrupt the continuance of meeting basic human needs. All elders should receive assistance appropriate to their remaining capabilities to achieve the highest possible level of health. Older people are characteristically individualistic since they have successfully survived to an advanced age by extending their personal coping and life styles.[25] Hence, the importance of individualized health promotion and maintenance care cannot be overemphasized, and these needs do not terminate with institutionalization.

Institutional care should aim for optimal level of functioning for each resident to counteract the prevailing attitude that institutionalization is a dying process rather than another way of living. For elderly people who have become more dependent on others to meet their activities of daily living, institutional care is necessary and vital to their welfare.[26,27] These individuals could have temporary disruptions of independent function, but often when improvement occurs, the possibility of returning to the previous noninstitutional life style is overlooked. Thus, the conclusion that institutionalization is the end of life's road is reinforced.

Currently, there is an urgent need to alter negative viewpoints to more positive ones focused upon the individual's well-being. If concerned care providers can subscribe to the philosophy of high-level wellness, some of the difficulties with negative outlooks about institutional life can be remedied. High-level wellness allows those who have restored abilities to return, with assistance from community support systems and relatives, to live in their homes or under other living arrangements within the community.

If institutional living becomes a permanent life style, the professional staff should take the leadership to make necessary changes for implementation of the high-level wellness concept. The care of the aged should begin with and be based on a comprehensive data base that views health holistically and incorporates the assets and liabilities of the individual.[28] The data base should contain a thorough health history and information from a physical examination, which should include major health deviations and their effects on the life style and coping abilities. Crucial to the process is the assessment of the psychological and sociological status since these factors are interrelated and influence the physical responses to bodily insults.

Psychosocial Aspects of Care

The three social-psychological needs of old people are identity, connectedness, and *effectance*.[29] Aged individuals tend to be looked upon negatively and measured by the apparent lack of productivity. There is a need to develop criteria for older groups that allow for a more positive identity. Connectedness indicates the desire for an individual to be a part of the social situation in which the person lives or dies. Whatever the social setting, individuals must possess feelings of belonging, have a relationship, and be connected to a group. Effectance is a social-psychological term that is now coming into use.[30] This requires having some influence on the environment and possessing the ability to make change. Institutional settings could begin to structure care modalities based on these social-psychological needs of older people. The new approach may begin with care givers putting themselves in the position of the aged by making a concerted effort to know them as individuals rather than as charges.[31] The objective is to identify the unique characteristics of each person so that special needs can be gleaned and used as a basis of care. It is also important that everyone working with the long-term care of elders examine their own feelings about aging. This process, combined with discussions of aging with their peers, allows care givers with strong negative feelings to develop a more tolerant understanding and thereby provide better service to meet older peoples' needs. Health workers involved with the care of the aged must be committed to the principle that human life is precious at any age, be sensitive to spoken and unspoken needs, show respect, and avoid stereotyping of people they are to serve.[32] These avenues for the care of the institutionalized elderly persons consider the attainment of realistic health goals, rather than imposing expensive therapy upon everyone.[33]

Another method for institutional staff members to become acquainted with the aged clients is suggested by Moos and his colleagues. They recommend using the Sheltered Care Environmental Scale (SCES) to assess the perceptions of the social environment of institutional settings by residents and staff.[34] This procedure can identify gross discrepancy between perceptions of the residents and staff members, thus pinpointing some indicators for potential tensions. The SCES is especially useful for new residents who are in need of more information about the facility to make a favorable adjustment. Allowing the residents to express their perceptions of the social environment is extremely useful to discover the optimal atmosphere sought and to devise appropriate interventions.

The health promotion and maintenance care of institutionalized elders is complex because of the social, emotional, and physical changes that limit input from the outside world.[35] An understanding of the mental health aspects of the aged is helpful for planning care to prevent isolation and loneliness. It is believed that the mental health problems affecting the aged are circular with a cause and effect pattern.[36] Apparently the human brain requires stimulation to effect responses, but if stimuli are not available, "cells may atrophy, memory and ability to manipulate the environment may fail, leading to profound sense of disorientation, anxiety, and fear."[37] These symptoms can lead to depression and apathy with further blocking of the stimuli receptors resulting in isolation behavior. This cycle continues, and the end result may be total cognitive failure if appropriate intervention with sensory stimulation does not take place.

Therefore, professionals responsible for health care of the institutionalized aged should not only focus care on the organic aspects, but also the environmental factors. Often the relationship between organic and functional components is interrelated and must be explored to determine cause of inadequate mental functions. This approach opens new avenues for the care and prevention of severe and nontherapeutic isolation behavior within institutional settings.

The environmental influences to health status are an important consideration. When elderly individuals move to an institutional setting from their own home environment, a major change is the decrease in the size of personal territory and an increase in the space shared with other people.

The concept of territoriality applies to the wellness status of not only humans, but also of other living species. Ardrey views territory as an area of space, water, earth, or air, which an animal or group of animals will defend as an exclusive preserve.[38] Moreover, territory is used to describe the inner compulsion by animate beings to possess and defend their space. Apparently possession of a territory enhances energy to the proprietor and, as accepted in the biological sciences, is believed to be a genetically determined form of behavior in humans and many species.[39] Territoriality is also a means for establishing and maintaining a sense of personal identity.[40]

According to Tate, the basic function of territoriality is to ensure that an individual has the necessary space to be free of physical discomfort and pain.[41] She asserts that aggressive and anxiety behavior are not uncommon when space is inadequate. Furthermore, territoriality is comprised of "the psychological identification with the place, symbolized by attitudes of possessiveness and arrangement of objects in the area."[42] These notions about territoriality significantly influence the behavior and well-being of older people. The loss of territory leads to some behavioral problems, such as social withdrawal following institutionalization, which suggests that this behavior may be a substitute for loss of privacy.[43]

It is necessary to possess territory as well as personal space to have privacy. Individual territory is much larger and a stationary entity, while personal space is carried wherever a person goes.[44] Because of its unique behavioral states, privacy is a part of the basic form of human territoriality and may be defined as an individual's right to decide which personal information will be shared and under what circumstances.[45] The function of privacy is to provide personal autonomy, emotional release that could have a safety valve effect, self-evaluation, and safekeeping of communication.

There are four basic degrees of privacy: solitude, intimacy, anonymity, and reserve.[46] Solitude is the most private state, where a person is isolated from others by choice. In long-term care settings, the lack of private rooms adds to the dilemma of meeting the solitude needs of older people.

Intimacy, thought to be a basic human need, allows a person to choose to become a part of a small group to attain close and relaxed relationships with others. Generally, the interactions are expedited when there are visual and other sensory controls to receive accurate information. The group must be isolated from others with appropriate environmental barriers in place. The physical structure of most institutions allows for intimacy, which should be encouraged among residents and family, friends, and other groups.

On the other hand, anonymity protects privacy by allowing a person to be in public view, but free from identification and scrutiny from others. Ease and relaxation in public areas is important for elderly people in supervised settings to allow for some independent activities not requiring staff involvement.

Reserve is one of the most complex states of privacy because of psychological barriers that are created to discourage unwarranted intrusions. This process allows a person to keep personal or shameful traits from others, particularly when the physical environment is not conducive to solitude or anonymity.

Degrees of privacy should be honored to meet not only the psychological needs of institutionalized people, but as a method to achieve high-level wellness. Tate contends that the internal geography of most long-term settings for elderly care has been decided by the needs of the staff rather than of the residents.[47] She suggests the following improvements of the physical environment for institutional settings:[48]

- Limit the size of nursing homes.

- Increase the number of private rooms.

- Build suites.

- Provide small dining areas to encourage more intimate dining groups.

- Provide smaller casual group areas, and place them near the rooms of the residents.

- Add private bathrooms with locks.

- Honor privacy.

- Arrange chairs and other furniture to maximize feelings of security and privacy.

In addition, allowing elderly individuals to take personal belongings, such as a favorite chair, dresser, and other small furniture, would be helpful in establishing territoriality in a new institutional environment. Familiar furniture may help make adjustment to relocation less painful by providing continuity from the previous life style to the new one.

As the discussion on territoriality and privacy indicates, each person has physical and nonphysical boundaries. It is more difficult to delineate the nonphysical boundaries, but often these aspects may be more or just as important as the physical boundaries. People need to maintain a zone around themselves no matter how crowded the area in which they temporarily live. The amount of personal space needed by each person will vary according to the emotional and physical status, cultural background, and position in the noninstitutional environment.[49] These factors should be considered in meeting the needs of older people in long-term care settings to assure that their self-esteem, identity, and independence are being supported. Appropriate interventions to fulfill territorial and spatial needs may allow: (1) the elderly person to select a comfortable distance from others; (2) judicious attempts to reverse isolation behavior by avoiding undue closeness; and (3) use of touch based on the type of relationship established so personal space is not violated.[50] The older person's preference for ample personal space should be incorporated in the health promotion needs.

The concept of personal space was introduced by Hall, an anthropologist who noted that cultural differences influenced the amount of interpersonal distance considered to be appropriate.[51] Study findings on attitudes toward others with whom a person shares special space indicate that there was a feeling of less crowdedness when physical closeness was with people who were liked and vice versa.[52] This finding has implications for residents in nursing homes, as older people are placed in the same environment or same room with total strangers, and elders in wheelchairs are placed next to each other without choice. Preliminary findings from another study on spatial-behavioral relationship showed that: (1) private rooms decreased aggression and increased cooperation among the elderly; and (2) semiprivate/semipublic space decreased aggression and increased cooperation, participation, social awareness, and public behavior.[53] These findings support Tate's suggestions that more private and semiprivate rooms should be made available in long-term institutional settings.

Modality of Care

The care in long-term facilities for more elderly persons should not necessarily be required to follow the procedures established for acute-care settings. The focus of care must be different because the objectives for the two types of health facilities are separate and distinct. The health care settings for the acute and the chronic sick roles assist to distinguish the appropriate modes of care.

The sick role concept was developed by Segrist and elaborated by Parsons to demonstrate the social role of acutely sick people. The sick role may be defined as: "the activity undertaken by those who consider themselves ill for the purpose of getting well. It includes receiving treatment from appropriate therapists, generally involves a whole range of dependent behaviors and leads to some degree of neglect of one's usual duties."[54] When a person is acutely sick, incapacitated, and unable to carry out normal functions, dependency on others who can assist them is expected until the person can assume self-care. This role is legitimized by society, and the sick person has a right to receive care. Society expects the person to accept this role however uncomfortable or undesirable, and the individual is obligated to get well as soon as possible.[55] Not everyone subscribes to these definitions and rationale, and adapts to the sick role. Factors that affect acceptance or rejection of the sick role are age, sex, race, marital status, religious and ethnic background, self-acceptance, methods of coping with anxiety, threshold for pain, and tolerance of disability.[56] Also, when the sick role as defined by Parsons is applied to chronically ill elderly persons, who can function independently some of the time, it is inappropriate to place them in a permanently dependent role contrary to health promotion and maintenance care. When a long-term facility uses the sick role concept as a guideline for care, it leads to dependency because chronic illness problems do not allow a complete recovery. Therefore, it is necessary that the chronic illness role, rather than the acute sick role, be the basis of care for the aged living in institutional settings.

Generally, the chronic illness role deals with a more complex health problem than the acute sick role, and the different dimensions that distinguish the former from the latter are as follows:

- Chronic illness is not, by definition, a temporary condition.

- The performance of dependency roles is more partial than total; the sick role may not be the dominant one throughout the illness.

- Because a prolonged sick role may pose a threat to other family members' roles, there is a difference in the degree of permissiveness in the care and other role obligation for the chronically ill person.

- The degree of alienation and dependency linked with chronic illness may vary from those resulting from the temporary role or acute illness.

- Chronic illness is more commonly a concern of advancing age.[57]

The major differences between the acutely and the chronically sick roles can be summarized as: First, the acutely sick role temporarily relinquishes normal roles and adopts a new role for the duration of the illness; the chronically sick role change is more partial, abandons the preillness role, adopts a new and less demanding role, and acquires the acutely sick role on a permanent basis in severe cases. Second, the acutely sick role is a sanctioned temporary dependency that allows the acceptance of help from a stronger and more adequate person; the chronically sick role allows a lesser degree of dependence to avoid threat to the role performance of family members. Third, medical treatment is urgent for the acutely sick role, and the lack of such service in this case is more threatening to life; in the chronically sick role, the lack of medical treatment is less of a threat, and delays of illness behavior and therapy may occur that have long-range implications for the patient's life and health when treatment is directed to control disease processes and rehabilitation. Fourth, the acutely sick role has clearly established societal norms for behavior; the chronically sick role has no established norms. Thus conflicts may occur between the demands of society and the person's own expectations. Fifth, the acutely sick role is primarily related to the younger groups; the chronically sick role is mostly associated with older people.[58]

Some may argue that the chronically sick role pertains mostly to the aged because the distinctions between illness and the typical expected aged role are difficult to distinguish.[59] Like the acutely sick role in the younger group, the elderly group cannot be held responsible for becoming chronically ill because persons are unable to stop the conditions from occurring as aging progresses.

It is beneficial for long-term institutional settings to base their care on the chronically sick role, rather than on the acutely sick role model, because the former considers the developmental needs of the aged population. Health promotion and maintenance care should include the following steps to achieve their goals to maximize optimal functions:

- Assist persons to function with remaining capabilities.

- Help persons to compensate for lost skills.

- Increase a person's abilities to achieve self-care.

- Improve a person's self-esteem and regain a sense of identity.

- Plan for discharge to home or other community settings.[60]

These functions emphasize the rehabilitation dimensions of care rather than complete recovery, which is the objective of the acute illness care approach. The thrust of rehabilitative care is high-level wellness while promoting a caring attitude at the same time.[61] Rehabilitation is a process that involves the concepts of prevention, maintenance, restoration, learning, and resettlement.[62] These concepts are central or pivotal to the optimal functioning of elderly individuals living temporarily or permanently in an institutional setting. Furthermore, care emphasizes support for independence and the maintenance of capabilities for as long as possible rather than fostering dependency behavior. Self-care to the extent of an individual's competence is encouraged and advocated.

Family and Community Participation

One means of keeping the older person in touch with the outside world is the continuation of family relationships, particularly after institutionalization. Family members' visits are vital to an elder's mental and physical health regardless of the frequent contacts with friends, neighbors, and others. This activity also reassures the elder that the new living arrangement does not mean abandonment. In most instances, contacts with family members by the older adults can be an intensive effort on their part to avoid institutional care. For the family members, visits to institutional settings provide opportunities to enhance previous relationships that may have deteriorated due to excessive demands placed upon them in an attempt to keep their elderly relative in the community. The fact that family members do everything in their power to maintain parents in their home is well documented; moreover, the development and maintenance of strong family ties and affection do not terminate with institutionalization. Institutional care does provide the technical health care needs, but does not replace the nontechnical aspects of care that only families can give.

Studies on family involvement with institutionalized elders have indicated that previously established visiting patterns continued.[63,64] Those offspring who had a sporadic visiting history maintained the same schedule. The studies also revealed that many family members did not enjoy visiting because of feelings of guilt and frustration regarding the admission of an elder relative to an institution. Long-term care agencies could develop programs to assist family members in coping with the negative feelings and to improve the quality of visits, which apparently deteriorates with the physical and mental status of the elderly relative.

Clearly, family members need more support and information about the health status of their institutionalized relative and what they could do during visits to make the experience more productive and satisfying. The information sharing may be formal or informal depending on the availability of the staff and needs of the families. Some useful topics to discuss may be the aging process, physical and mental changes, assistance that family members can provide during visits, family meetings for discussing common concerns, and general information about the institutional goals. Participation in these programs by the family members could eventually lead to a partnership between the families and the facility that articulates concerns and finds solutions for mutual problems. Other institutional programs that can assist family members in making meaningful visits are special holiday programs to which family members are invited; religious services open to families and friends; craft days to exhibit items made by the residents; and Sunday afternoon programs of musicals, plays, and other entertainment.[65] These special events offer a mechanism by which the institution and families not only can participate, but become better acquainted with each other. Generally the institution takes the initiative to create an atmosphere that is therapeutic to the residents and their families.

Long-term care facilities are an indispensable component of the aged's total health care needs in most communities. However, the general population is uninformed about the needs of institutionalized older people. This accounts for the limited community involvement and interest in offering volunteer programs that are so desperately needed to augment the services of the institution staff. A well-organized and dedicated volunteer effort, such as those provided in hospital settings by medical auxiliary, candy stripers, and so on, would be beneficial to both the aged residents and the volunteers. The latter would have the opportunity to interact with older people and not only learn about the unique needs of the elders, but also gain insights into their own aging process. A well-conceived program for orienting volunteers to the facility and providing information about the elderly group is essential to have a successful and gratifying experience.

Volunteers can assist with a number of activities to improve the quality of life for the residents. Helping older people in leisure activities, such as bingo, card games, dominoes, and other recreational pursuits, is particularly important to elders with physical disabilities. Letter writing, reading, and visiting are also valuable contributions by volunteers. Frequently, the elderly person may just enjoy conversing or taking a walk with a volunteer. The benefits derived by the older individuals from talking about their lives and sharing experiences are well known. The process is useful to allow self-expression and to receive feedback from others who are interested and willing to listen to them. Increased self-esteem and self-concept result from such interactions with the volunteers. Older people especially enjoy young volunteers who are in junior or senior high school because these students often remind them of their grandchildren. The boy and girl scouts, campfire girls, and other groups are also resources that can be used. Because each elderly resident must be considered as an individual with different characteristics and personality, all volunteers require an introduction and guidance to develop relationships with the older persons before undertaking their tasks and responsibilities.

Consumer groups who subscribe to the personal rights of institutionalized elders are another source of community contributors, and community-initiated advocacy functions directed toward ensuring the quality of care within the institutional setting are beginning to emerge. These types of support are welcome activities, as the issues of care problems are difficult tasks to pursue for most individuals or families. Relatives of resident elders are frequently hesitant to question care providers because of feelings of disloyalty to the institution that is freeing them from the day-to-day responsibilities for care. Some procedures should be made available to help families express their concerns without the threat of potential repercussions.

A well-organized advocacy movement that does not antagonize the facility's staff must be carefully planned. The objective is to mesh the efficient functioning of an institution without negating the idiosyncratic needs of each elderly individual. This means that the unique human needs of each person must be the basis of care. The advocate works within the system to resolve conflicts or difficulties through negotiation rather than by the use of threats. The ultimate objective is to ensure that elderly residents

receive care, which is imperative to their health promotion and maintenance needs.

NOTES

1. Ruth Bennett, "Isolation, Social Adjustment and Mental Disorder in Institutionalized and Community Based Aged," in Ruth Bennett, ed., *Aging, Isolation and Resocialization* (New York, N.Y.: Van Nostrand Reinhold Co., 1980), p. 56.
2. Sheldon Tobin, "Institutionalization of the Aged," in N. Datan and N. Lohman, eds., *Transitions of Aging* (New York, N.Y.: Academic Press, 1980), pp. 195–6.
3. Jon Hendricks and C. Davis Hendricks, *Aging in Mass Society* (Cambridge, Mass.: Winthrop Pub., 1977), p. 282.
4. Frank Moss and Val Halamandaris, *Too Old, Too Sick, Too Bad* (Germantown, Md.: Aspen Systems Corporation, 1977), pp. 5–8.
5. Tobin, pp. 195–6.
6. Hendricks and Hendricks, p. 66.
7. Ibid., pp. 282–7.
8. Kirsten Smith and Vern Bengston, "Positive Consequences of Institutionalization," *The Gerontologist* 19, no. 5 (October 1979): pp. 438–47.
9. Moss and Halamandaris, p. 8.
10. Hendricks and Hendricks, p. 282.
11. Moss and Halamandaris, p. 14.
12. Hendricks and Hendricks, pp. 283–5.
13. Bill Bell, ed., *Contemporary Social Gerontology* (Springfield, Ill.: Charles C. Thomas, 1976), pp. 357–61.
14. Morton Lieberman, "Institutionalization of the Aged: Effects on Behavior," in Bill Bell, ed., *Contemporary Social Gerontology* (Springfield, Ill.: Charles C. Thomas, 1976), pp. 369–79.
15. Ibid., p. 374.
16. Bennett, p. 56.
17. Dianna Shomaker, "Dialectics of Nursing Homes and Aging," *Journal of Gerontological Nursing* 5, no. 5 (Sept./Oct. 1979): 45–48.
18. Mary Adelaide Mendelson, *Tender Loving Greed* (New York, N.Y.: Vintage Books, 1974), pp. 233–45.
19. Hendricks and Hendricks, pp. 282–3.
20. Moss and Halamandaris, pp. 199–218.
21. Ibid., pp. 73–102.
22. Ibid., pp. 30–31, 57.
23. Ibid., p. 199.
24. Ibid., pp. 203–4.
25. Margo M. Griffin, "Holistic Approach to the Health Care of an Elderly Client," *Journal of Gerontological Nursing* 6, no. 4 (April 1980): 195.
26. Leticia Vincente, James A. Wiley, and R. Allen Carrington, "The Risk of Institutionalization Before Death," *The Gerontologist* 19, no. 4 (August 1979): 361–7.

27. Erdman Palmore, "Total Chances of Institutionalization Among the Aged," *The Gerontologist* 16, no. 5 (October 1976): 504–7.
28. Griffin, p. 195.
29. Vern L. Bengston, "The Aged and Their Social Needs," in Eugene Seymour, ed., *Psychosocial Needs of the Aged* (Los Angeles, Cal.: The University of Southern California Press, 1978), p. 36.
30. Ibid., p. 36.
31. Ibid., p. 38.
32. Priscilla W. Armstrong, "Comment: More Thoughts on Senility," *The Gerontologist* 18, no. 3 (June 1978): 316.
33. Ibid.
34. Rudolf H. Moos et al., "Assessing the Social Environments of Sheltered Care Settings," *The Gerontologist* 19, no. 1 (February 1979): 74–82.
35. Philip Ernst et al., "Isolation and Symptoms of Chronic Brain Syndrome," *The Gerontologist* 18, no. 5 (October 1978): 472.
36. Ibid.
37. Ibid.
38. Robert Ardrey, *The Territorial Imperative* (New York, N.Y.: Atheneum, 1966), p. 3.
39. Ibid., p. 5.
40. Juanita W. Tate, "The Need for Personal Space in Institutions for the Elderly," *Journal of Gerontological Nursing* 6, no. 8 (August 1980): 442.
41. Ibid.
42. Leon A. Pastalan, "Spatial Behavior: An Overview," in Leon A. Pastalan and D. H. Carson, eds., *Spatial Behavior of Older People* (Ann Arbor, Mich.: Univ. of Michigan, 1970), p. 212.
43. Martha N. Nelson and Robert J. Paluck, "Territorial Markings, Self-Concept and Mental Status of the Institutionalized Elderly," *The Gerontologist* 20, no. 1 (February 1980): 96–98.
44. Sharon L. Roberts, "Territoriality: Space and the Aged Patient in the Critical Care Unit," in Irene Mortenson Burnside, ed., *Psychosocial Nursing Care of the Aged* (New York, N.Y.: McGraw-Hill Book Co., 1980), p. 197.
45. Leon A. Pastalan, "Privacy as an Expression of Human Territoriality," in Leon A. Pastalan and D. H. Carson, eds., *Spatial Behavior of Older People* (Ann Arbor, Mich.: Univ. of Michigan, 1970), p. 89.
46. Tate, p. 439.
47. Ibid., p. 448.
48. Ibid., p. 442.
49. Roberts, p. 198.
50. Evelyn C. Gioiella, "Give the Older Person Space," *American Journal of Nursing* 80, no. 5 (May 1980): 898–9.
51. Paul M. Insel and Henry C. Lindgren, "Too Close for Comfort: Why One Person's Company is Another's Crowd," *Psychology Today* 11, no. 7 (December 1977): 100–6.
52. Ibid., p. 101.

53. A. J. DeLong, "The Spatial Structure of the Older Person: Some Implications of Planning the Social and Spatial Environment," in Leon A. Pastalan and D. H. Carson, eds., *Spatial Behavior of Older People* (Ann Arbor, Mich.: Univ. of Michigan, 1970), pp. 83–85.

54. David Mechanic, "The Concept of Illness Behavior," *Journal of Chronic Disease* 15, no. 2 (February 1962): 184–94.

55. Katherine M. Ness, "The Sick Role of the Elderly," in Irene Mortenson Burnside, ed., *Psychosocial Nursing Care of the Aged* (New York, N.Y.: McGraw-Hill Book Co., 1980), p. 231.

56. Stanisla Kasl and Sidney Cobb, "Health Behavior, Illness Behavior, and Sick Role Behavior," *Archives of Environmental Health* 12, no. 2 (February 1966): 246–66.

57. Gene C. Kasselbaum and Barbara Baumann, "Dimensions of the Sick Role in Chronic Illness," *Journal of Health and Human Behavior* 6, no. 1 (Spring 1965): 16–27.

58. Katherine M. Ness, "The Sick Role of the Elderly," pp. 236–7.

59. Ibid., p. 237.

60. Pauline L. Olsen, "A Nurse Administered Long-Term Care Unit," *Journal of Gerontological Nursing* 6, no. 10 (October 1980): 616–21.

61. Ann Rosenow and Janet M. Long, "Introduction," in Janet M. Long, ed., *Caring for and About Elderly People* (Rochester, N.Y.: Rochester Regional Medical Program and the University of Rochester School of Nursing, 1972), p. 5.

62. Ibid.

63. Kristen F. Smith and Vern L. Bengston, "Positive Consequences of Institutionalization: Solidarity Between Elderly Parents and Their Middle-Aged Children," *The Gerontologist* 19, no. 5 (October 1977): 438–47.

64. Jonathan Y. York and Robert J. Calsyn, "Family Involvement in Nursing Homes," *The Gerontologist* 17, no. 6 (December 1977): 500–5.

65. Rose Dobrof and Eugene Litwok, *Maintenance of Family Ties of Long-Term Care Patients: Theory and Guide to Practice* (Washington, D.C.: U.S. Government Printing Office, 1977), p. 44.

Chapter 16

Advocacy Role of the Professionals

Chiyoko Furukawa

There will always be individuals who are sensitive to the needs of the underprivileged and will devote their efforts to assist the less fortunate group. Within the last two decades, the aging population has been aided by the work of such participants in the White House Conference on Aging and the Administration on Aging, by selected United States senators and representatives, and by a variety of health and social service professionals. The major thrust of these persons has centered on improving services to the elderly group and instituting legislation to upgrade the aged's quality of life. The activities may be viewed as an ombudsman effort rather than one of advocacy because they did not seek the full participation of older people. The two terms "ombudsman" and "advocacy" are neither synonymous nor appropriate to use interchangeably.

The concept of ombudsman was invented in Sweden to manage the abuse of bureaucracy, to resolve grievances, and to keep the bureaucracy "honest."[1] The intent of the ombudsman process was to protect the people from bureaucratic administration and to prevent the public from being placed in a disadvantageous position. For example, the recipients of government benefits were allowed to employ a representative to purchase medical and rehabilitative services from health institutions by competitive bidding.[2]

Archer and Fleshman contend that an ombudsman is a mediator and does not intentionally take sides.[3] Conversely, the advocate speaks in favor of something and takes a definitive stand on issues.[4] As the aging population increases in the coming decade, the elderly people as a group should become more actively involved in the role of the advocate and be prepared to speak for their own needs. The elders and their families will be competing in the future with other societal groups for the same funds. Thus, as Streib suggests, older adults must become more militant so that they will receive attention and assistance for the problems they face.[5]

Most older individuals could be their own advocates if they were given the opportunity; however, several factors deter them from taking this role.[6] The complexities of the current service systems, particularly with government benefits, require comprehension of wordy directives and regulations just to complete the necessary application forms. These processes become severe obstacles to older people who have limited education, restricted mobility, and decreased stamina to fight the system. Most are reluctant to cause a commotion or actively seek to change the system because such demonstrations are considered to be contrary to their lifelong values. Furthermore, many professionals and laypersons often treat older individuals as nonpersons and tend to interact with them in a childlike manner. Thus, instead of their opinions and desires being listened to, elders often have forced upon them services that they may or may not want or need. Frequently this process leads to unnecessary dependency on the part of the older person, and inappropriate assistance is provided. These and other factors perpetuate the suppression of the elderly as a group and keep them from becoming their own advocates.

DEFINITIONS OF ADVOCACY

It is advantageous for health professionals to formulate or subscribe to a definition of advocacy to assist in the implementation of this concept. The classical definition of advocacy is: "the act of defending or pleading the case of another."[7] More recently, the meaning of advocacy has evolved beyond helping the disadvantaged, with goals to assist individuals or groups to become self-sufficient in seeking ways to overcome societal inequities. This approach is based on the existential philosophy, which stresses the principle of freedom for self-determination as the most fundamental and valuable human right.[8] This viewpoint acknowledges that the individual should be given the opportunity for making decisions that incorporate all of his or her values.

Berger's comprehensive, succinct, and contemporary definition of advocacy includes the influence of power, politics, and interest groups, and is stated as: "an activity through which people who are closely identified with the needs of some socially, politically, or economically deprived subgroup can promote changes in the nature of the power structure so as to improve the situation of their client group."[9] The theme underlying Berger's advocacy concept is that special interest group activities are designed to enable acquisition and the effective use of power to make desired changes in society.

The basis for the development of advocacy activities is the presence of unmet needs that society fails to recognize and the inability of disadvantaged groups to rectify inequities sufficiently through socially accepted channels. In the area of health promotion and maintenance, the role of professionals in supporting advocacy activities should be to guide and persuade older adults to become more assertive in achieving their needs for optimal levels of well-being.

HISTORICAL PERSPECTIVES

Advocacy for the aged is not a modern or recent happening. The family has played a major advocacy role since the beginning of time. From all indications, the elderly person's family will continue to help the aged receive their rightfully earned benefits. The family is usually the first line of defense and assistance for older people; however, the family will not be able to resolve the problems of aged relatives single-handedly as society becomes more complex.

As one of the first political action groups, the National Association of Retired Federal Employees sought to improve pension benefits for retired federal employees in 1920.[10] Later, Francis E. Townsend spearheaded a drive during the 1930s and 1940s primarily in California to obtain pension and other benefits for older people.[11] He proposed the Townsend Plan, which was designed to provide all Americans over the age of 60 with at least $150 per month financed by a national sales tax. However, the plan met its demise due to political bickering and charges of corruption, and was superseded by the Social Security Act in 1935.

The American Association of Retired Persons (AARP), an early advocacy group, was organized in 1946 by Ethel Percy Andrus to institute a low-cost health care plan for retired teachers.[12] This effort led to a 1955 agreement with the Continental Casualty Insurance Company to offer group health insurance for the National Retired Teachers Association (NRTA). Shortly thereafter, AARP and NRTA joined forces to share staffs and offices, but remained as separate entities. The support and growth of these organizations is indicated by reports that they have received as many as 2,000 membership applications in a single day.

Further concerns about the older population's health care gave impetus to the development of still another advocacy group, namely, the National Council of Senior Citizens (NCSC). This association was organized in 1961 following the White House Conferences on Aging and concentrated its efforts to enact the Medicare Act with the support of Walter Reuther, a renowned labor leader.[13] Advocacy activities by the NCSC lobby continued and were instrumental in obtaining increases in Social Security benefits in 1970.

The most recent advocacy group, known as the Gray Panthers, was started in 1972 under the leadership of Maggie Kuhn. The thrust of this group was older people working for their own cause to seek a better life style, freedom from worries, and more equitable distribution of goods and services.[14] These and other events have led to other benefits for the aged in many communities, such as reduced bus fares and property tax exemptions that are currently available in 48 states. Thus, elders have greatly benefited by the improved standards of livelihood, which would not have been possible without the advocacy assistance from several organizations.

The number of existing viable advocacy organizations indicates the progress that has been made to improve the status of elders. As major increases in the older population become a reality, the political strength of these groups may generate additional advocacy groups to achieve the goal of quality life for all individuals.

PROFESSIONAL ACTIVITIES

Older people are prone to feelings of powerlessness in their contacts with health care systems.[15] On the other hand, the right to self-determination is one of the fundamental human freedoms.[16] Therefore, professionals must acquire a sense of trust from older people before any attempts can be made to seek their involvement in advocacy movements. Clear communication between elders and advocates is also required to define the real needs and concerns, and unless an individual has actually experienced the same difficulties, understanding the needs from the perspective of the older person may be elusive. A confidante relationship should be developed so that elderly individuals can feel free to express their desires and share in the responsibility of resolving any wants or problems. It is essential that clients, even with severely lessened abilities to cope, choose to accept assistance, and their dignity and rights demand that professionals be patient and persistent in their interactions with each individual. Since the essence of advocacy is to help others to help themselves, the inclusion of the elders in the advocacy process dispels negative stereotypes and myths about aging by providing evidence of the positive attributes of older adults.[17]

Once the professional has become a confidante to an elderly person, the involvement of the family for assistance and support should follow. Family members require an accurate assessment about the potential resources available to support their elderly relative and to assure an effective working relationship with professionals. Shared interests, ideology, and justification for involvement give clues on whether or not family members are committed to advocacy activities. For instance, adult children may believe that their elderly parents' needs are adequately being met. They may be unwilling to participate in trying to get them more benefits. The children's rationale may be that the added services will only increase taxes, which are already high.

On occasions, some persuasion and bargaining by the professional may be necessary to gain full support from the family. A more detailed explanation of where the additional services can come from, what the cost will be, and who will be responsible for the added expense may be helpful. This information may help family members to decide to join an advocacy group so that improved services can be made available for their elderly relatives and other older people in the community.

Families with aged members are also in a position to give first-hand information about the plight of their elderly relatives to community leaders, legislators, and others. Often family members themselves are leaders in the community and occupy positions of stature that enable them to communicate the need for change. Special efforts should be made to reach other middle-aged persons who can assist in improving the elder's life status and consequently, their own lives in the future.[18] These direct interactions between the community, aging persons, and familes are essential to a successful advocacy process.

The role of an advocate involves representing the best interest of those who lack the expertise or are unable to seek solutions to their problems without some assistance. When this situation occurs, representation without assuming control may become extremely difficult.[19] This is especially evident when elderly persons are unable to express their desires and decisions any longer. The advocate must then be clear about the different personal values that form the basis for decision making. It may become necessary to recall past decisions made by the older individual under similar circumstances to obtain information or some idea about the client's life values. An advocate should make every attempt to view problems and decisions through the eyes of the elderly person.[20]

There will always be limitations to the advocacy role that professionals and family members can implement. A need for compromise exists when good intentions may not be accepted by the older person. For example, when an aged's physical and mental capabilities decrease, the potential for injury becomes greater, and a family's concern for the older relative's safety emerges. The aged individual may make the decision to continue independent living against the advice and wishes of the family. In this situation, the advocate should make certain that the elderly person understands the risk factors and is willing to take a chance rather than forego independent living. It is difficult to allow the person to make a choice, but surprisingly, many are able to manage and minimize hazards with supportive services and clear guidance.

A group of people who share the same concerns can be more effective than an individual. Elders as a unit are more likely to be heard on issues such as neighborhood safety. For example, they can negotiate with public officials to increase the neighborhood patrol. Senior power is beginning to wield influence in the public and political arena.[21] Professional activities to assist the causes of elderly groups may include getting accurate information, identifying individuals to approach for solutions to problems, planning strategies, and providing support.

IMPLEMENTING THE ADVOCACY ROLE

Advocacy is no task for the uncommitted and requires that professionals possess initiative, be innovative, and become action-oriented.[22] They should be prepared, if needed, to work overtime and engage in activities that may not have been a part of their educational background or training. Advocacy can be a complex process requiring skill, experience, sensitivity, persistence, tolerance for frustrations, and plain hard work.[23] It is no longer enough for professionals to provide only direct patient care. There is a priority on teaching and preparing clients to become independent decision makers and to be able to resolve future personal problems. Older people need to be informed, particularly regarding their rights, and given all the necessary information to make intelligent and advantageous decisions.

To assist older groups in their first advocacy activity, a small-scale problem with clearly defined goals that can be reached should be selected rather than a major issue that has greater possibilities for frustration, failure, and alienation by potential supporters.[24]

To date, advocacy activities for elders that are rooted in the local community appear to be the most effective.[25] Issues that can be taken directly to the sponsors in conjunction with other elderly group functions are believed to be worthwhile. Personal interaction with the aged and getting a first-hand account of problems and needs make an impact on the sponsors. The influence of grassroots politics has conjured responses from organizations in an effort to meet the demands of special interest groups.

An objective of advocacy activities is to reorganize or change conditions so that the power imbalance may be corrected.[26] This means that those not involved in decision making be given the opportunity to provide input. Advocacy movements evolve to remedy the dissatisfaction of groups who are concerned and who demonstrate the desire to change the situation. It is critical that when group efforts are used, the initial problem be a shared concern or need. There should also be an organization to plan and coordinate advocates' activities to expedite formation of a coherent relationship.

The elderly advocacy group must have an effective leader who is able to mobilize the individual participants and who possesses a comprehensive understanding of the power structure that is responsible for the denial of the aged peoples' rights.[27] This knowledge enables the leader to identify the system's political and economic basis for the decision-making process, which is important if the advocacy group is to be persuasive. This approach helps to select strategies that are useful to influence desired responses from the decision makers.

The professional and others, in developing a definitive strategy for the advocacy movement, must be cognizant of factors that may block progress, such as timing, the commitment of those involved, and the strength of the adversary.[28] The professional's roles are those of a facilitator, consultant, and teacher, particularly about the legislative process, political techniques, and other procedures related to the advocacy activity. The following steps should be considered in order to implement a methodical approach to an advocacy activity:

- Identify a problem, based on accurate facts, that has the group's collective support and commitment to seek change. The problem should be a longstanding, unmet need that affects the life style of the group.

- Determine objectives, with and for the advocacy group, that need to be achieved within a designated time frame.

- Formulate strategies to gain support and set up a cooperative working relationship with other community resources whose political powers could be beneficial to the group's cause.

- Study the adversary system, particularly the power structure and its workings and the people controlling the system; identify the necessary tasks to make the system respond to the group's need in a satisfactory fashion.[29]

- Prepare for confrontation by formulating a contingency plan in case an alternative must be used.

- Provide persistent leadership, organization, planning, and support to discouraged members as social and political changes often require more time than the group may realize. Recruit future leaders from the group for continuity and independent activity following the withdrawal of professional leadership.

Aside from informal citizen and professional groups, an agency may be established solely for purposes of advocacy functions. An agency that embarks on an advocacy mission has two distinguishing characteristics.[30] First, the agency must identify a clientele group, rather than the public-at-large, as the major focus for its activities. Second, the advocacy agency must accept as "one of its primary functions, the pro-active identification, pursuits, and marshalling of resources (in addition to those over which it has statutory authority) for the benefit of its clientele constituency."[31] An example of these activities is the influence exerted by an advocacy agency on legislation to benefit its clients directly.

The Administration on Aging (AOA), an organization created in 1965 through the enactment of the Older Americans Act (OAA), has been an important advocate of the aging. This advocacy establishment differs from a program agency in that its main function is to administer resources and programs mandated by legislation. Initially AOA served as a program and an advocacy agency because its latter role was not clearly defined; however, within the past decade, the involvement of the executive and legislative branches of the government contributed to changes in the agency's advocacy role. The 1971 White House Conference on Aging provided the impetus for clarifying AOA's advocacy role. One result was the codification of advocacy in the 1973 amendments, which gave a significant thrust to expand AOA's activities through legislative changes.[32] These changes mandated AOA to coordinate and assist with the planning and development of programs sponsored by both nonprofit and public agencies for the elders. The 1978 amendments to the OAA still did not totally clarify the advocacy role, but it did lead to the establishment of area agencies responsible to AOA for development of services. The involvement of national advocacy efforts with the local agencies led to a relationship through which the AOA can inform each area agency about new resources to tap, expedite articulation, and respond to the older people's needs at the grassroots level.

ADVOCACY FOR LEGAL ISSUES

As a person becomes older, it becomes virtually impossible to ignore the benefits of public and private institutions to maintain self-independence and for survival. Clearly, some older people must depend on government programs for the necessities of life and, in some instances, on private organizations for supplemental services. Depending on life circumstances, an elderly individual could potentially be involved with several health and social programs, for example, Medicare and Medicaid for health care needs, Social Security and private pension funds for income, Supplemental Security Income for additional financial assistance, and food stamps for nutritional requirements. There are many regulations that determine the eligibility for these benefits, and most older people cannot be expected to stay current with the frequent changes in the laws and guidelines. Moreover, the regulations are rarely written so that a single interpretation can be made, and when the benefits are terminated with or without cause, the legal issues pertaining to eligibility can be extremely complex.

Another position requiring legal interpretation, which the elderly individual may voluntarily or involuntarily become involved in, is the defense against guardianship, conservatorship, or commitment to institutions. Potentially, the aged can face an overwhelmingly complex legal issue with not only the bureaucracies, but also with relatives. It is difficult to understand, much less maneuver, the systems that are supposed to assist, rather than become adversaries to, elders. Unlike the younger population, many of today's elderly persons lack the experience of working effectively with bureaucratic organizations and have little or no involvement with the issues of individual legal rights.[33] Hence, a requirement for advocacy activities in the health promotion and maintenance care of older people is to ensure access to legal assistance. The advocacy role to prepare elders to resolve their legal disputes or questions independently may not be possible because legal functions require specialized educational training. However, an appropriate goal for the advocate is the timely recognition of the need for legal consultation and assistance, and providing informed advice on available resources to elderly clients.

The AOA, as one of the original advocacy groups, and the United States Congress have instituted services to provide legal support to the elderly group. Each state and local area planning for AOA is responsible for including legal services for the older population. To emphasize this activity, the Older Americans Act Amendment, legislated in 1975, created a legal service separate from other social programs and authorized funds to implement legal assistance to the aged.

Attorneys basically provide three types of advocacy services, namely, information and referral services, routine litigation, and law reform, in accordance with the Older Americans Act and other legislation designed to benefit the elderly group.[34] The information and referral services are unlike those offered by the social services and provide access to expert advice on the rights of clients. In particular, the purpose of these services is to study the eligibility requirements and benefits within the legal framework of the variety of assistance programs. A requirement for providing the services is a firm knowledge of the many laws pertinent to older people and concerning welfare, social security, consumer affairs, employment pensions, and owner/tenants. An advocacy activity, which can be conducted in conjunction with the services for interpreting the laws, is the preparation of educational materials to inform older people of their legal rights.

Routine litigation provides for specific defense of clients against evictions, in suits to enforce delinquent consumer contracts, or to repossess goods bought on credit.[35] One of the more important advocacy services for the still competent older person is in contesting involuntary commitment to institutions or the appointment of a guardian. A research finding suggests that the presence of an attorney acting in behalf of an individual prevents unwarranted guardianship or conservatorship.[36] Another advocacy activity is to offer routine legal assistance to elderly groups, such as in forming a nonprofit organization so that the full benefits of incorporation allow for tax exemption. This type of assistance is instrumental in providing elderly groups an opportunity to embark on major undertakings, or to build and finance housing projects or small businesses.

Law reform activities are the third basic legal advocacy function and are directed toward full and effective participation in legislative programs that are beneficial to the elderly clients. Legal advocates serve as monitors of programs to ensure that the intentions of each pertinent legislation are implemented. Two general law reform activities are representing a class of elderly people in test case litigations and seeking legislative or regulatory reform. More specifically, law reform efforts are involved in matters such as the inequities of Social Security benefits for divorced husbands, conditions in nursing homes that deprive the civil and constitutional rights of older clients, and challenges to the requirements for mandatory retirement.[37]

Advocacy activities on behalf of frail elders must be conducted within the existing statutes and laws of the community. Occasionally legislation is enacted without revisions to antiquated laws, which could usurp the rights of the aged. A case in point is the advocacy services of the Adult Protective Services (APS), which is an outgrowth of 1974 Title XX of the Social Security Act. The intent of the APS is to prevent abuse and exploitation of older people; however, because of the status of laws governing interventions in most states, some aged are unnecessarily losing their rights to decision making, control of their property, their privileges to execute legal documents, opportunities to express their political views or desires, and other functions.

Protective services are traditionally defined as "a system of preventive, supportive, and surrogate services for the elderly living in the community to enable them to maintain independent living and avoid abuse and exploitation."[38] According to Regan, two features characterize protective services: (1) the coordinated delivery of services to high-risk adults; and (2) the actual or potential authority to make substitute decisions for them.[39] The second feature involves the legal system because of the requirement for authority to intervene on behalf of the aged client. Problems related to the rights of the individual emerge from this feature because of the intervention laws. Often actions are decided in good faith to benefit the older person who is unable to participate in the decision making for a variety of reasons.

Guardianship and emergency civil commitment statutes are two interventions employable in most states. A serious shortcoming of guardianship is that the process requires the elderly person to be declared incompetent.

The court stresses two findings in declaring a person to be incompetent: (1) the individual has to be suffering from a condition that affects the mental capacity; and (2) functional disabilities, that is, inability for self-care or managing personal property, must result from the person's condition.[40] Unfortunately, there is more emphasis on the first condition because of reliance on the medical model approach, which views behavioral variances as being similar to physical diseases and giving the impression that the former can be quantified and labeled as pathological.[41]

As with any age group, elderly behavior has a wide range of normal behavior, but apparently this fact is not considered in the behavioral evaluation decisions. As a consequence, older people are at a disadvantage when competency is decided because "old age" is often equated to "senile" without ever considering the functional abilities still possessed by the elders. In addition, guardianship for the aged means the permanent loss of legal rights, and usually there are no provisions made to provide the appropriate amount of assistance in cases of gradual or partial loss of functions. The guardianship process is also costly and is known to have depleted the financial reserves of many older people. Several proposals, which have been suggested to remedy the state guardianship laws to preserve the rights of elderly individuals, include changes, such as the periodic review and renewal of guardianship by the court, that emphasize functional disability rather than mental illness in determining competency, promoting a stronger advocacy role for elders with representation by counsel, and restoring power to disabled persons in accordance with their functional abilities.[42]

SUMMARY

Advocacy is defined as "the act of defending or pleading the case of another" and also includes the more recently established goals of assisting individuals or groups to become self-sufficient in seeking ways to overcome societal inequities. The advocacy process, whenever possible, should strive to teach individuals and groups to speak against social injustices, and to become politically and economically astute to stage their own battles to make social changes and to provide input to the decision-making processes. Professional responsibilities require that assistance and support be given until the individual and group can function independently or interdependently to alleviate the situations that are impeding their rights to services and other needs.

Advocacy activities should have limitations so that the disabled or elderly individual's rights are guarded at all times. Advocates must make every effort to include their clients in decision making rather than taking the attitude of "we know what is best for you." Because of some state laws governing interventions, such as guardianship and declaration of incompetency, the Adult Protective Services may not adequately prevent abuses and exploitation of older people. Finally, several proposed changes to current guardianship laws are long overdue and are extremely necessary to preserve the rights of elderly individuals.

NOTES

1. Marvin B. Sussman, "Family, Bureaucracy and the Elderly Individual: An Organizational/Linkage Perspective," in Ethel Shanas and Marvin B. Sussman, eds., *Family, Bureaucracy and the Elderly* (Durham, N.C.: Duke University Press, 1977), p. 12.
2. Ibid.
3. Sarah E. Archer and Ruth P. Fleshman, *Community Health Nursing Patterns and Practices,* Second Edition (North Scituate, Mass.: Duxbury Press, 1979), p. 11.
4. Ibid.
5. Gordon F. Streib, "Old Age and the Family," in Ethel Shanas, ed., *Aging in Contemporary Society* (Beverly Hills, Cal.: Sage Publications, 1970), pp. 25–39.
6. Marcella B. Weiner, Albert J. Brok, and Alvin M. Snadowsky, *Working with the Aged: Practical Approach in the Institution and Community* (Englewood Cliffs, N.J.: Prentice-Hall, 1978), p. 203.
7. Mary F. Kohnke, "The Nurse as Advocate," *American Journal of Nursing* 80, no. 11 (November 1980): 2038.
8. Sally Gadow, "Advocacy Nursing and New Meaning of Aging," *Nursing Clinics of North America* 14, no. 1 (March 1979): 81–91.
9. Mark Berger, "An Orienting Perspective on Advocacy," in Paul A. Kerchner, ed., *Advocacy and Age* (Los Angeles, Cal.: The University of Southern California Press, 1976), p. 1.
10. Rochelle Jones, *The Older Generation: The New Power of Older People* (Englewood Cliffs, N.J.: Prentice-Hall, Inc., 1976), p. 218.
11. Steve Mehlman and Duncan Scott, "The Advocacy Role of NRTA-AARP," in Lorin A. Baumhoven and Joan D. Jones, eds., *Handbook of American Aging Program* (Westport, Conn.: Greenwood Press, 1977), pp. 161–77.
12. Rochelle Jones, *The Older Generation: The New Power of Older People,* p. 218.
13. Ibid.
14. Ibid., p. 234.
15. Joan C. Rogers, "Advocacy: The Key to Assessing the Older Client," *Journal of Gerontological Nursing* 6, no. 1 (January 1980): 33.
16. Sally Gadow, "Advocacy Nursing and New Meaning of Aging," p. 83.
17. Marcella B. Weiner, Albert J. Brok, and Alvin M. Snadowsky, *Working with the Aged: Practical Approach in the Institution and Community,* p. 204.
18. Ibid.
19. Ingeborg Mauksch, "Advocacy or Control: Which Do We Offer the Elderly?" *Geriatric Nursing* 1, no. 4 (November/December 1980): 278.
20. Ibid.

21. Neal E. Cutler, "Resources for Senior Advocacy: Political Behavior and Partisan Flexibility," in Paul A. Kerchner, ed., *Advocacy and Age* (Los Angeles, Cal.: The University of Southern California Press, 1976), p. 28.

22. Susanne S. Robb, Mark D. Peters, and Joseph W. Magy, "Advocacy for the Aged," *American Journal of Nursing* 79, no. 10 (October 1979): 1738.

23. Dorothy V. Moses, "The Nurse's Role as Advocate with the Elderly," in Adina M. Reinhardt and Mildred D. Quinn, eds., *Current Practice of Gerontological Nursing* (St. Louis, Mo.: The C. V. Mosby Co., 1979), p. 226.

24. Ibid.

25. Fred Cottrell, "Issues," in Mildred M. Seltzer, Sherry L. Corbett, and Robert C. Atchley, eds., *Social Problems of Aging* (Belmont, Cal.: Wadsworth Publishing Co., Inc., 1978), p. 321.

26. Mark Berger, "An Orienting Perspective on Advocacy," p. 7.

27. Ibid., p. 10.

28. Anita S. Harbert and Leon H. Ginsberg, *Human Services for Older Adults: Concepts and Skills* (Belmont, Cal.: Wadsworth Publishing Co., Inc., 1977), p. 234.

29. Mark Berger, "An Orienting Perspective on Advocacy," p. 12.

30. Dan Fritz, "The Administration on Aging as an Advocate: Progress, Problems, and Prospects," *The Gerontologist* 19, no. 9 (February 1979): 141.

31. Ibid.

32. Ibid., p. 143.

33. Paul Nathanson and John C. Lamb, "Advocacy and the Necessity of Legal Services," in Paul A. Kerchner, ed., *Advocacy and Age* (Los Angeles, Cal.: The University of Southern California Press, 1976), p. 126.

34. Ibid., pp. 128–133.

35. Ibid., p. 130.

36. Ibid., p. 131.

37. Ibid., pp. 132–3.

38. John J. Regan, "Intervention Through Adult Protective Services Programs," *The Gerontologist* 18, no. 3 (June 1978): 251.

39. Ibid.

40. Ibid.

41. Ibid.

42. Ibid., pp. 252–3.

Chapter 17

Self-Care and Health Teaching

Dianna Shomaker

INTRODUCTION

The health status of individuals and the extent of their personal commitment to continue preserving it are a multifaceted complex of factors; none can be isolated as dominant causal entities, and all must be considered as parts of the total unit of stimulating and suppressing actions of a momentary, unique process of living.

The consistent figure in this dynamic evolution is the individual. The behavior and decisions of that person are the major influence in the ultimate outcome of any action. Yet many people passively delegate authority for important actions to strangers and institutional policy. They are often influenced by the pressure of stereotypes, myths and lack of knowledge, and meeting externally imposed and often undesired goals of society. Many of these goals directly oppose a person's desires and capabilities. Once these goals are achieved, society moves on, and the unwilling recipient is left with greater unmet needs.

Rectification of such a plight lies in greater awareness of self and resources, deeper commitment to care, concern for personal maintenance and growth, and dynamic involvement in the direction and quality of life. Everyone is capable of this to some extent. For some it is not a conflict to flow with the dictates of society; for others it is counterproductive and diminishes self-esteem. Cause of such a position is long-term, evolving from habit, learning, and experiences that have accumulated throughout a lifetime. However, this position is not irreversible if alternatives are attainable, realistic, and satisfying.

The self-care concept is built on the premise that individuals have the capacity to increase the quality of life by decreasing dependence on others and strengthening interdependence if knowledge and resources are present. Health professionals can assist them by developing greater skill in encouraging creative interdependence between the care providers and the elderly. Professionals then become facilitators, teachers, mediators, and resource persons who support the client through a decision-making process of personal choice, not acquiescence. The means of achieving a deeper personal involvement, and commitment and awareness in identifying personal needs, goals, and priorities is through self-care. Clients develop their capabilities and discover the value of the self-care concept in improving personal use of drugs, diet, exercise and sexuality.

LEARNING

A common complaint of the elderly is memory problems.[1] A common assumption is that old people cannot learn. The question then arises, "To what extent does the older person have the capacity to learn and remember?" What value can be retrieved by the older person in health education, group discussions, and demonstrations of new material that would be useful for promoting self-care? Decrement of intellectual and cognitive functioning with age is not a new or obscure concept of aging, and studies of such functioning have often concluded that capacities are greater in earlier adult years of life. Recent studies are beginning to offer stimulating challenges to the validity of such a position.[2] No longer is it believed that IQ is fixed or that it declines with age.[3] The peak age range has gradually increased as various studies have been done, and it is yet to be proven that IQ declines with the biological processes of aging. Where differences in memory have been demonstrated, the authors state most frequently that there was no difference in primary memory by age, but loss was noted for older persons in the secondary or long-term memory process. Overall, however, there are too many problems with the scope and procedures to be secure in the findings. One of the more popular interpretations of recent data is that age has no effect on the rate of memory decay but does seem to influence retrieval of data from memory storage.[4] Caution is necessary in interpreting variables, unaccounted-for influences, and methodology in studies to date. Perhaps there are age-related changes in intellectual and cognitive functioning, but it is equally conceivable that they are minimal if a person adjusts for as-yet unknown interfering factors.[5] Observations offer some indications that: "Most elderly people continue to engage in learning throughout their lifetimes although learning style preferences and amount of learning actively pursued vary greatly from one individual to another.[6]"

Health care providers and educators need to capitalize on this learning style preference and the individual's unique potential.[7] Everyone is learning, but the difference between effectiveness of understanding and application often depends on wellness and illness, past experience, values, and other multiple factors important in each individual's life.[8]

Schaie noted that the elderly and the young performed differently, and postulated that abilities and skills in healthy people did not decline so much as they simply became obsolete.[9] The apparent declines were shown to be symptoms of inactivity and disuse, and the dormant skills retained the potential of being stimulated, and their use regained, through education. It is not irreversible deterioration. Schaie further showed that some individuals demonstrated improvement in levels of performance in their seventh and eighth decades, while others declined in their twenties and thirties. There is no indication the cause was different. Differences in performances were possibly due to health problems, environmental richness of experiences and resources, or willingness to experiment or take risks. Older people, when tested, were often more cautious and hence made errors of omission, whereas younger competitors made errors of commission because they were more willing to guess.

The literature, as a composite set of data, neither concurs with the age-decrement notion of learning ability nor proves learning ability is constant. For health educators, the rewards appear to be optimized by assuming that learning can take place, and then by integrating those known factors that have been employed when learning ability of the elderly was tested and shown to be capable of improvement. For instance, in 1963 and 1965 Canestrari and Eisdorfer produced results that indicated that reaction time was a factor that clouded performance results when the elderly were tested.[10,11] When elders were given more time for inspection and response, they benefited markedly in their scores.

In 1973, Botwinick proposed that learning ability is not comparable with performance.[12] One is not necessarily a measure of the other. Learning ability is an internal process, and performance is an external one. Behavior is not proof of cognizance, and factors other than degree of learning may limit a person's ability to perform.

Walsh, in summarizing three theories of age differences in learning and memory, pointed out that overarousal and the degree of task relevance among those tested influenced the older performer.[13] When elders used visual and verbal mediators, their performance increased and their recall improved on sorting-task trials. It has been postulated that elders do not process material as deeply if they do not consider it valuable or meaningful. Diminished recall could be the result of superficial processing.

Several guidelines can be drawn from these inconclusive studies, and, incomplete as they seem, the guidelines have merit when used in conjunction with other known factors relevant to the older population. The first is the increasing range of IQ peak, which has not been proven to have reached its maximum suggesting that potential growth has been increasing in proportion to increased richness of environmental experience and resources. The second is that people continue to learn throughout their lifetimes, but changes in learning preference must be taken into account. Those learning efforts are enhanced through visual and verbal mediators, and recall is greater when the time allowed to ingest the material and to respond is increased. Finally, learning seems to be greater when the importance of the material is ranked highly by the learner.

For the health care educator, presentation patterns to the older person must include the involvement of the client and the goals, priorities, and methods must be established in conjunction with the client. Information that is valuable will be more readily received by the client. These very factors, which have often been relegated to a position of diminished attention, are the basis of the self-care concept and are the means of encouraging the client to become more self-reliant and responsible for attaining goals of greater freedom in society.

SELF-CARE

Self-care is not a new concept. People have always practiced it in some form and to some degree; it has been necessary for survival. All manner of minor aches and pains, fevers, communicable diseases, and infections have been treated at home. Families have adapted to frailties and disabilities. Humans have learned to pasteurize milk, purify water, dispose of sewage, and refrigerate food in order to ensure health of a higher order.[14] Gradually, medical technology developed into a sophisticated system, with elaborate machines for detection, diagnosis, and prevention to monitor health status. Families slowly relinquished their autonomy in planning and deciding their fates to physicians, nurses, and social workers. Diseases were not as extraordinarily different, as were the improved means of diagnosis and care. Annual physicals and primary prevention were advocated. The basic patterns of illness were unchanged, but peoples' perceptions of their own competence in wellness and illness declined drastically in light of advanced technology and the public prestige accorded it.

Freedom and control by the public were subjugated to the health professions.[15] The populace gradually relinquished their home-oriented managerial roles of health maintenance and care of their sick to the hospital-based physicians; patients became passive, controlled receptacles in the health care system. Costs increased, control over personal goals of health waned, and people complained that the services were impersonal. Discouragement resulted and led to agitated rebellion against such outside intervention into personal responsibility.

Younger adults in particular wanted control over health care priorities and demanded a return of personalization to health care planning. As an alternative, many sought advice from the prolific do-it-yourself manuals that flooded the reader market. The 1960s witnessed the return of self-care in the form of communes. The social theme was warmth, caring, and sharing, and there was a strong trend against materialism, intellectualism, and formal institutions such as medicine, religion, and marriage. People banded together to help one another in home births, organic gardening, and vegetarian menus.[16] In the realm of medicine, besides wishing to have greater control over priorities and plans of health care, people became dissatisfied with the quality of medical care, the cost of it, and the seemingly futile increase in investment in health care that many claimed was not increasing the quality of health.[17,18]

This was the beginning of a new level of self-care. Individuals were demanding to have a share in responsibility for their care; to demystify the aura separating medical science and consumer ability, and to return autonomy to the public.[19] They wanted to join with the professionals controlling health care in defining rights, needs, priorities, options, and risk indices.[20] There was emphasis on the positive aspects of health and on attempts to prevent illness, in short, in helping clients develop the concept of a healthy state.[21]

Health is a dynamic, multidimensional concept that is most successful if the individual is involved in his or her own health maintenance and promotion.[22] Within the self-care concept, an individual would be an active participant, not passive or static as an object of health care directed by others.[23,24] Moreover, the systems in which the clients participate are those that they devise and control with the assistance of the health team in the community. Self-care is not merely letting people do for themselves in a system set up by the nurse.[25] Participation is the key to controlling personal preferred goals and needs, and ultimately to self-care. All persons have the right and the responsibility to care for themselves to the limits of their needs, abilities, and resources as they see justifiable within the limits of logic and practicality. That is the basic principle of self-care.

Orem defined self-care as: ". . . the practice of activities that individuals personally initiate and perform on their own behalf in maintaining life, health and well-being . . . [it] is an adult's personal, continuous contribution to his [or her] own health and well-being."[26] Zapka and Averill added that self-care is that "performance by consumers of activities traditionally carried out by health care providers."[27] Norris sees it as those processes that permit people and families to take initiative and responsibility, and to function effectively in developing their own potential for health.[28] Joseph points out that since self-care is controlled by the client, it will be strongly influenced by the individual's social and cognitive experiences, which are learned over time through interpersonal relationships.[29] Self-care has the ability to change self-esteem, self-image, and self-concept, and is governed by maturity, cultural practices, beliefs, experiences, skills, knowledge, values, illness, disability, energy needs, resources, social group involvement, and family and other support systems. It is truly positive and holistic action, incorporating the medical system into an individual's personal world, which is integrated with practical and continuous patterns of daily living.[30] However, self-care is broader than the illness orientation that has dominated the greater part of health education in the past. Its broader scope encompasses the total environment, delegating many functions now held by the professionals to the clients.[31] It can be therapeutic or adaptational for universal needs or to alleviate a crisis, but all degrees of self-care require a degree of thought, choice, and decision.

There are several levels of self-care, one of which is therapeutic. Therapeutic self-care is seen by Orem as those activities that support life and promote normal function, growth, and development, as well as maturation, and that prevent, control, or cure disease and injury processes.[32] Universal self-care actions that incorporate therapeutic planning span several areas of basic human need where individuals are aware of the significance of these self-care actions for life and health, and of the implications of their own behavior on other human beings. In Table 17-1, Orem identifies areas

Table 17-1 Areas of Self-Care and Potential Action

Area	Potential Self-Care Action
1. Air, water, and food needs for health and normal body functioning	1. Adjust ways of meeting daily requirements.
2. Excretion needs as well as social importance of proper disposal	2. Implement new techniques for self-care.
3. Activity and rest for optimum stimulation and involvement	3. Revise daily routine; modify self-image.
4. Solitude and social interaction conducive for reflection; stability of mental health; development of positive, realistic self-care concept; and validation of values and goals	4. Revise daily routine; modify self-image.
5. Hazards to life and well-being that can be reduced by decisions regarding interpersonal relationships; self-protection; rejection of harmful foods and drugs; modification of environmental factors	5. Change life style.
6. Health deviation that interrupts integrative functions of daily living	6. Cope with health deviation.

Source: Compiled from ideas found in Dorothea Orem, *Nursing: Concepts of Practice* (New York, N.Y.: McGraw-Hill, 1971), pp. 27–30.

where some action may be required for change, and he also identifies the action that may be taken in a self-care modality.

Norris categorizes the activities of self-care carried out by the client as:

- monitoring, assessing, and diagnosing health status in such behaviors as attention to diet, breast examination, self-education, and home treatment;

- supporting life processes through good personal hygiene; regular, balanced meals; concern for growth; and adequate relationships with others;

- instituting therapeutic and corrective care even in terminal illness, maximizing positive aspects of existence, seeking information on intervention, and making decisions for growth and improvement within personal capabilities;

- preventing disease and maladjustive states, and coping with stress and debilitation through increased knowledge and capabilities, for example, CPR classes;

- specifying perceived personal health needs individually defined, but seeking further knowledge where necessary to better understand personal perceptions;

- auditing and controlling treatment programs toward a goal of stability outside the institutions of health care, for example, nursing homes and hospitals;

- joining self-initiated health care where individuals share treatment and emotional support of one another, for example, Alcoholics Anonymous, Weight Watchers, and smokers' clinics.[33]

Orem maintains that decisions for self-care are deliberate, voluntary acts that are self-initiated and self-directed.[34] Self-care today does not presume to return to a situation where all scientific medical knowledge and bearers of it are rejected, but it does presume to improve the use of both facets of health care by integrating them into a program where professionals assist, facilitate, and coordinate resources and programs that reflect preestablished patient priorities, goals, resources, and abilities. Joseph's placement of nursing applies to all other health care providers in the self-care team:

. . . nursing is to help individuals engage in and accomplish self-care, thereby promoting health, facilitating recovery from disease, or permitting a peaceful death. The role of the nurse is to facilitate and increase the self-care abilities of the patient.[35]

For those clients whose impairments limit performance, professionals will assist, educate, teach procedures, and facilitate modification to each unique individual.[36] In all situations action initiated must be pursued until the person attains the desired results. This requires knowledge, motivation, commitment, ability, and energy whereby the client draws upon the community resources to augment personal needs and resources.[37]

Application of the self-care concept is practical in the clinic setting as well as on an individual basis. The two are easily combined. Zapka and Averill initiated the "Self-Care Colds Clinic" at the University of Massachusetts. It is a prepaid ambulatory care program, established to reduce inappropriate use of the medical staff and simultaneously increase individual self-reliance by increasing involvement, responsibility, and initiative. This process encourages the individual to assess symptoms and make decisions regarding care preferred. This was fostered by increasing patient knowledge of symptoms, care, medications, and preventive measures related to colds. Symptoms were assessed against a checklist. (See Chapter 18.) When necessary, clients requested increased information and direction from the clinic medical staff.

This program, in its fourth year of existence, has created a process that allows clients to save both the facility and themselves time and money while caring for personal needs that, in the past, required the attentions of a physician. The services are low-cost; over the first two years the program has saved the clinic an estimated $46,120.[38] The program is readily accessible, flexible, and educational. Moreover, self-care requires fewer staff members and the clients less medical care.

Kosidlak reports another approach to self-care for senior citizens. This approach evolved from an awareness that there often exists a poor understanding between chronic disease and its relationship to symptoms experienced by the client. This group established a 30-hour course for a moderate-size group of elderly. The objectives were: (1) to encourage acceptance of individual responsibility for self-care; (2) to teach skills and symptoms of illnesses predominant in their age group; (3) to increase their understanding and awareness of health problems; and (4) to teach them to use resources more appropriately and effectively toward the goal of better self-care in common illnesses and injuries. For these persons health became a satisfying, participant process.[39]

Drug Education

Elderly men and women use more drugs than any other age cohort.[40,41] Twenty-five percent of all drugs manufactured are consumed by the elderly.[42] They use them preventively as well as therapeutically. Users, however, tend not to be healthy. Each year they consume a staggering number of doses of prescription medicines, and nonprescription or "over-the-counter" (OTC) drugs. A user rate for prescriptions has been estimated at three times as great as for younger persons or even healthy peers.[43] The mean number of OTC drugs in the home is between 17.2 and 24.4 drugs per household.

OTC drugs are often used before seeking medical advice. Cause for this has been speculated to be due to lower income and decreased mobility. The drugstore is closer; drugs are more accessible; cost is initially less; and waiting is minimal. This does not negate the use of prescription drugs, but rather increases the number of OTC and prescription drugs used in conjunction for exponentially more chronic and long-term drug needs. Perhaps they are not used for the same symptom, but they may be used for the same illness.[44] Everyone uses OTC drugs to some extent, but, like prescription medication, when they are used without adequate knowledge they not only can create serious hazards to a person's health, they can alter and possibly jeopardize the desired effects of prescription drugs. This is the source of drug problems of as yet unrealized dimensions. A drug history of patients does not always include use and frequency of use of nonprescription drugs. For many clients they are not considered to be medicine, and so they do not think to tell the physician, nurse, pharmacist, or others about such medications. Many do not recognize the dangers. For example, aspirin is the drug of choice for arthritis and simple pain. It is low cost and ubiquitous, and these very qualities render it safe in the minds of many. Due to advertising, an inappropriate OTC drug may become a substitute in popularity. Tylenol is a good example. When used in place of aspirin for arthritis, it is ineffective because it lacks the anti-inflammatory characteristics of aspirin. On the other hand, aspirin has side-effects too, such as lowering of blood-sugar, cholesterol and platelet aggregation, increase of gastric distress and bleeding, and aggravation of insulin hypoglycemia.[45,46]

There are dangers for those on restricted sodium diets. Over-the-counter medications of bulk laxatives often contain as much as 250 mg. of sodium per package. In addition, antacids create problems with sodium retention. They increase the pH of the stomach, but also delay or decrease the absorption of iron, nutrients, and other medications, such as digoxin and tetracycline. Hence, clients may find themselves needing two drugs, OTC or prescription, that are deleterious to one another.

Alcohol is scarcely given attention as a drug. Of course, it is a drug and it offers complications of its own besides inebriation. It can cause central nervous system (CNS) depression when combined with hypnosedatives, antihistamines, antidepressants, antipsychotics, antimanic drugs, and barbiturates. In addition, paralytic ileus is a risk when alcohol is used with antidepressant drugs.[47]

The potential for dangerous combinations of OTC and prescription drugs is much greater and has been unpredictable because millions of elderly Americans with multiple chronic conditions, who live outside the institutional system, are responsible for self-medication, many with minimal awareness of drug actions.[48]

Aging is a major influence of undefined proportions in the dynamics of drugs. Involutional changes affect the therapeutic effectiveness in several ways. The absorption, distribution, excretion, and metabolism of drugs among the elderly is recognized to be different than the actions of the same drug in a younger person, but to date such processes have not been well researched. Unfortunately, some drug reactions in the older age group can occur even when using the recommended dosage. Other reactions and toxicities are due to slower excretion rates, and of course, some are from overt abuse of all types of drugs.[49] The only guideline is knowing that it might create untoward reactions in older clients because of metabolism and receptor-tissue sensitivity changes that accompany aging. (See Chapter 18.)

Whether drug problems stem from involutional changes relating to prescription medicines, home remedies, or OTC drugs, the problem remains the same: there has been an overall increase in client responsibility, while supervision by health care providers has not grown proportionately.[50] Health care providers have scarcely begun to provide stimulating, personalized counseling to the elderly in any important degree of comprehensive community drug-use programs. Professionals are often more concerned with prescription drugs to the exclusion of OTC drug potential hazards. It has been asked, "How much responsibility can be delegated to the client, and how much supervision must accompany it?" This is an important consideration because of the possibility that pill-taking for the elderly with multiple chronic illnesses can become a fulltime occupation. A person can conceivably swallow 30 or more pills a day: that amounts to 210 pills a week.[51] Comfort suggests that care providers have their clients put a day's supply of pills in a plastic bag. The results are often astounding.[52]

It is not difficult to imagine that patients become confused about what to take and when, or about pills reacting against the purposes of each other. Health care providers can assist clients in constructing a tailormade drug education and monitoring program that would reduce medication errors by incorporating precautions known to be most effective in reducing medication errors.

Research has shown four major causes of error. First, the most consistently common cause of medication error is omission of drugs:

- The patient simply forgot.

- The medication was never purchased because of expense or inconvenience.

- The patient was somehow prevented from taking the medicine.

To illustrate the final point, envision the perplexity of a moderately crippled arthritic attempting to remove the cap from a bottle or pill container. Difficulties and frustrations could easily lead to omission.

The second most common abuse of drugs is inappropriate self-medication.[53,54] The reasons seen here are also common; they evolve from practicality and expedience:

- use of someone else's medicine

- exchange of drugs with friends

- use of personal or spouse's old prescription leftovers

- arbitrary self-selection from whatever is available

- use of outdated medications

- compensation for an earlier omission by taking two doses

- experimentation at random

- misunderstanding of directions

The third category of drug abuse leading to medication errors is incorrect dosage or timing.[55] This is not uncommon among people with physical limitations. The crippled arthritic who cannot remove the cap, when finally successful, may pour all the medicines in a saucer for future convenience. Others, who cannot stabilize hand tremors long enough to swallow from a teaspoon, drink from the medicine bottle, that is, one gulp equals a teaspoonful. Those with poor vision or the adventuresome who bypass turning on the light at night have the misfortune of occasionally medicating from the wrong bottle. Other examples include forgetting when the last medication was taken, making an erroneous interpretation of "with meals" (some eat six times a day, some fast for 12 hours), and obtaining the same prescription by another name from a second physician, thus guaranteeing a double dose. Being without restrictive physical limitations or lack of cognizance, however, is little assurance that the errors will be avoided or costs kept to a minimum, but there is some evidence to indicate that education and devices for remembering do decrease human errors and result in more cognizance in use. Researchers will have to discover how to eliminate internal reaction problems.

The final category is that of inaccurate knowledge. There are two prongs to this dilemma. One is incomplete or inaccurate knowledge on the part of the physician, who may then give the patient automatic refills or telephone prescriptions without medical evaluation.[56] The other prong is inaccurate knowledge on the part of the client. Confusing directions may lead the client to misuse or omit drugs from his or her regimen. Accuracy and clarity are crucial in both health teaching and client implementation.

Individualized drug education can assume an infinite variety of dimensions and styles of presentation; it transcends largely printed labels and words of caution. It must consist of finding the elderly, and assessing their needs, capabilities, and resources; tailoring the medications to their individual situations, consistently and repeatedly; and approaching patient teaching in a more imaginative, thoughtful style, perhaps slowing down, asking for feedback, using visual aids, and most importantly, involving the client. One client lamented, "Plan with us, not for us, and we'll not make so many mistakes."[57] Brock envisions the care provider's role as one of educator, supervisor, and monitor in collaboration with the client, family, physician, pharmacist, and other persons who provide service to the client.[58] Optimal preparation will expedite maximum safety in drug therapy, allowing safeguards against toxicity, overdose, and idiopathic reactions. Such a role should also involve a dual advocacy to both the client and the prescribing physician. Planning should flow from full assessment of the client's motivation and understanding of the drugs, as well as physical capabilities and limitations. Several devices for better health education have begun to take this into account, and there is now more sensitivity in comprehensive strategy.

People with poor eyesight cannot see labels and diagrams unless there are good lighting, big letters, and accurate prescription lenses. For example, a diabetic with poor vision has an immediate potential of drug misuse. Why not suggest to that person the use of a mounted magnifying glass, which can be purchased at any dime store; a 150 watt light bulb; preset syringes; and a body chart for maintaining a rotating injection site record. The body chart is simple. The elder can choose seven sites for injection, then he or she can make a list according to days of the week. It no longer is a matter of where it was given last, but of what day of the week it is. Monday is always the right arm, Tuesday the left arm, Wednesday the right leg, and so on.

Devices to assist in remembering the pill schedule have also become sensitive to the needs of individual elderly. Creativity has blossomed in devising pill boxes, calendars, clocks, charts, and so on.[59] Graphic instructions, such as a clock on the prescription label or a sticker on the container if all medicines must be taken before discontinuing the regimen, have increased compliance and decreased medication error. Many studies report greater compliance when there is also some form of written information accompanying the prescription. Consumers indicate increased knowledge of side effects, special directions, and precautions. Morris and Halperin report that about 95 percent of the population read the written material dispensed with the prescription, and at least two-thirds of them remember what they have read.[60] It has been argued that drug inserts are a good source of information and should be given out with each prescription, but those who oppose such a scheme maintain that it leads to inappropriate self-medication, suggestion-induced side effects, alarm among clients, or pill sharing and exchanging. Eighty percent of clients polled felt the inserts were a positive aid and should be continued.

Modifications of inserts have been affected by giving out brochures, summary sheets, programmed instruction booklets, and one-page handouts. Some pharmacists, doctors, and manufacturers have devised short slide-tape presentations. Results indicate that medication errors decrease as teaching increases due to greater consumer awareness and knowledge, but often compliance is questionable. Increased knowledge has not always been enough to alter pill-taking behavior, but clients have demonstrated better understanding of the medication and quicker recognition of side effects, and there have been fewer hospitalizations. Written information as a sole means of improving medication consumption is much less effective than when educational intervention is multifaceted and designed to improve drug compliance behavior.

The greatest degree of reduction in medication errors was when verbal and written instructions were employed simultaneously, and the instructions were simple. This success can be intensified with follow-up contacts for clarification and encouragement within three to five days after the initial issue of the medications.[61]

The implication of a community-based health maintenance plan would be the creation or improvement of the team concept among the professionals, the family, and the resources available to the client, encompassing the desires and needs of the client as primary to action and success. Three major issues not fully addressed to date would be improvement of self-care, reduction of medication errors, and promotion of a higher degree of holistic care and client responsibility. An ideal multidisciplinary approach would be advantageous, but would require a highly organized, mobile group with groomed channels of communication where professionals within the community collaborated to encourage reciprocal responsibility, knowledge, and satisfaction by the client.[62] In contrast, the physician has limited time, and the pharmacist has sporadic contact with the client.

In view of time and budget realities, someone must coordinate the communication. The most likely candidates who could serve such a function are persons who visit the client in the home, such as the community health nurse, the outreach worker, or the social worker. Everyone would have to have a firm understanding of the gerontological process. They would then have to initiate case conferences to share information. Often, even though there has been health teaching from the physician, the nurse, and the pharmacist, the knowledge received from each remains separate and isolated, as if it were for three different patients. Intercommunication is vital.

Assessment is the third area where all involved persons should collaborate to share their findings and establish an accurate client drug profile. Schwartz advocates taking a 24-hour medication history similar to a dietary history.[63] The inquiries should glean an accurate list of all OTC and prescription medications. The drug profile, in conjunction with the coordinated case conferences, will decrease duplication and conflict in medicine and detect change, toxicity signals, and new symptoms that result from drug combinations.

What models might be used for tomorrow? Research in pharmacy is needed to determine how the dosage list differs with age. The issues of possible altered mechanisms of drug metabolism, drug action, distribution, and toxicity need to be addressed.[64] Also needed are greater drug assessment sensitivity, recognition of the value of over-the-counter drugs in interaction with daily prescribed medicines and diet, and development of more creative and realistic routines that will increase responsible independence in the home.

Dietary Behaviors

Proper nutrition is the best preventative of poor health regardless of age, but becomes increasingly important as a person ages.[65] Even so, dietary practices that reflect lifelong habits are more often influenced by economics, attitude, and environment than by logic and sound nutrition.[66,67,68] Good nutrition is a major determinant of both good health and recovery from surgery and illness.[69,70]

Ideally, everyone should have sound nutritional habits. Habits are formed and improved during early childhood. In relationship to aging, retirement extracts similar demands for dietary preparation as it does for economies. A person needs to maintain an appropriate diet throughout life to prepare for retirement.[71] However, the lifelong diet demonstrates long-term food patterns, which are capable of jeopardizing health in later life and are compounded by the complexities of aging. Just as optimum health can prevent illness, ill health can create malnutrition. It can result from chronic illness, long-term nutritional deficiencies, endocrine imbalances, and physical handicaps.[72] Malnutrition and poor dietary habits, which cause a person to be underweight, can occur for many of the same reasons that lead to obesity. Health risks are less likely to be related to overburdening the body, than to depriving it of needed nutrients and fluid. Many who do not eat enough food have reported causes such as inability to get to the store, indifference, loneliness, limited budget, and misconceptions about the components of an adequate diet. In addition, they may also be experiencing chronic difficulty with chewing because of poor dentures. Poor habits of eating, fluid intake, activity, drug use, and urinary and bowel elimination create illness, dehydration, and altered blood chemistry.

"The symptoms of malnutrition are often varied, insidious, and hard to pick up,"[73] but observation of nutritional status is important and easily implemented. It is only a gross gauge, of course, but it serves as the initial impression of overall health status. The ratio of height and weight immediately indicates the degree of tissue deficiency or excess; refinement of observation can later be measured. Texture, complexion, tone, and turgor are other indicators. The hair and nails are a third measure, in which a person examines quality of texture, color, pliability, and lustre.[74] The condition of the tongue and fissures at the corner of the mouth will reveal anemia or vitamin deficiency. A second set of indicators of health and diet is assessed through client description of personal attitude, activity level, energy, interest, and body functioning.

Malnutrition among the elderly is greater than has been assumed. Deficiencies of calcium, iron, and B_{12}, as well as protein are common.[75] Undernutrition can be further assessed by several laboratory tests, the most common being hematocrit, hemoglobin, and serum albumin tests.[76]

Leahy, Cobb, and Jones challenge the community health nurse to encourage the client to develop an interest in all aspects of the meal.[77] This includes learning to recognize good eating habits; important factors in the environment that enhance or distract the consumer at meals; patterns of meals; and regularity of eating, picking, snacking, and skipping meals. The nurse should teach the client the fundamentals of the Four Basic Food Groups, interpreting the physician's prescription so that it is realistic and meaningful and pointing out that vitamins do not correct an imbalanced diet. The nurse should also assist the client in finding substitutes for items that must be omitted, such as sugar and salt. Finally, the nurse should encourage perusing daily advertisements for food sales nearby, purchasing in small amounts for freshness and, similarly, cooking in small amounts for greater benefit of vitamins and minerals.

Body nutritional requirements are known to alter as people age. Exact changes and needs are still being researched, but it has been determined that older people need fewer calories, but more vitamins, minerals, and proteins.[78] Young and Scrimshaw report on studies at the Massachusetts Institute of Technology (MIT) addressing the protein needs of the elderly. They published data to assist in dispelling the myth that the elderly need less food because their metabolism is slower, and their activity is reduced.[79] Protein requirements are no less than for younger adults. Moreover, the elderly probably need a greater margin of safety because there is probably less protein absorbed and greater protein loss from the body due to past and present disease conditions. The body requires more protein intake to assure minimum body cell maintenance than when younger. Also, in contrast to previous assumptions, Slesinger et al. found that older people, as with all age groups, eat as much meat as the minimum requirement recommended for the daily standard.[80] The area of deficiency in this study was in the consumption of milk, which was far below any other age group. Seventy-five percent drank less milk less often, and 45 percent claimed to drink no milk at all.

Calcium is the most commonly deficient mineral element in older adults. The low use of milk results in a low calcium diet and predisposition to osteoporosis in women 59 years of age and older. It has been posited that a lifelong pattern of little or no calcium intake after childhood does not allow for calcium stores in early adulthood, against which a person can draw as aging takes place.[81] The aging process includes changes in hormone levels and the consequent effect upon the blood's calcium level; if the level is not kept constant through calcium intake, then calcium is drawn out of the bone stores. Therefore, bone loss in old age, which is evidenced in increased incidence of bone fragility, is possibly related to skeletal mass at maturity and the drawing down of calcium stores.

Diet is one of the universal units of self-care. A person may assume that it is relatively stable, but actually diet changes over time as a person's body needs change and the choice among alternatives for meeting such needs is not always therapeutic. The primary examples of unsatisfactory choices are obesity and deficiency malnutrition. The therapeutic style of self-care includes an awareness of significance of diet to life and health. Consumption should meet, but not exceed, required body needs in an attempt to preserve the anatomical and physiological integrity of body function, that is, a healthy state.[82] Either extreme of consumption is unhealthy and threatens the integrity of the human organism.

"It is typical (though not desirable) for humans to increase their weight with age."[83] Extreme weight gain brings about far greater social castigation than does extreme weight deficiency. In addition, extreme weight gain is considered a chronic disease that involves and jeopardizes all systems of the body. Obesity responds poorly to medical treatments.[84] Price and Pritts list the following eight systemic complications linked to obesity:

1. atherosclerosis, hypertension, hyperlipidemia, ischemic heart disease
2. greater susceptibility to colds and other respiratory problems
3. increased incidences of gallbladder problems
4. greater abnormalities of menstrual cycles
5. cardiovascular disease
6. diabetes
7. osteoarthritis of weight-bearing joints
8. increased morbidity and mortality[85]

Since obesity also jeopardizes a person's self-esteem, self-image, and social success, it is reasonable to assume that there will be a strong psychological component in treating it. It is beneficial to encourage self-care by the client in the form of behavior modification, which can result from professional group therapy or from community-based organizations such as Weight Watchers and TOPS (Take Off Pounds Sensibly), which are based on group-level reinforcement.[86]

Professional personnel working with obese elderly could serve as facilitators, educators, and support systems for the clients, offering a data base for the client's decisions. The responsibility for changing the behavior and diminishing the problem must come from the client.[87] As parts of a therapeutic goal, the obese person should attempt to develop: (1) a realistic concept of self and values; (2) stable mental health; (3) autonomy; (4) comfortable group membership; and (5) a personality that would avoid impairment of self because of food dependencies.[88]

Obesity is more effectively eradicated by individuals who assume responsibility for self-care than by those who prefer to rely on other means. To illustrate, exercise is superior to appetite suppressants for weight loss. Anxiety increases caloric intake, and the use of tranquilizers to relieve it is far more dependency-oriented and ineffective for weight loss and self-control than an adequate exercise program that stresses self-reliance; diet adjustment and exercise are preferable to laxatives, the same functions in relation to constipation. Studies that tested the use of bran and dietary fiber as a secondary means of alleviating constipation do not report positive findings either, primarily because of other complications created in the body. Reports suggest that dietary fiber increases the amount of fecal fatty acid and decreases protein digestion and absorption, plasma protein, zinc, magnesium, and phosphorus.[89] In general, any attempts to control the body are superior if they advocate self-reliance rather than drugs, food, or alcohol.[90]

Emphasis has been upon the overweight, not to the exclusion of problems that face those who are underweight, but because the majority of elderly are more prone to obesity. Berger stated that a 1973 survey "revealed that 71 percent of the women and 84 percent of the men over 50 were obese."[91] In oversimplicity, both overweight and deficiency can be corrected by the amount of proper food put into the mouth. The reason that is simplistic has to do with consideration of behavior patterns of longstanding that are difficult to change. Much of the problem is in implementing the change.

Exercise

Until recently, it was assumed the amount a person could exercise diminished with age and that the deterioration was not reversible. Recently, these assumptions have been challenged. Physiologists are not claiming a reversal of the aging process, but there has been sufficient evidence to indicate that physical activity favorably influences mortality, a person's state of emotional health, and the level of physiological functioning.[92] Muscle strength does decline with age, but the decline is not as significant as might be thought. At 60 years, there is usually not more than a 10 to 20 percent loss. The fatigue rate is greater and more significant.

With regard to muscle retraining, muscles can be improved through exercise. Weg reports one study in which, within six to eight weeks of supervised continuing exercise, men in the 60 to 90 age group regained some degree of muscle strength and tone, and better cardiovascular efficiency and aerobic ventilation.[93] The improvement was similar to that of younger counterparts, but of course was measured from lower achievement levels. In other studies, women did not improve as much, but there was some improvement. Moreover, with neither older men nor women was there a correlation between improvement and athletic commitment as youth.[94]

Exercise in an older adult can improve the cardiovascular and respiratory systems. It will also help decrease blood pressure, body fat and weight, and risk factors—such as coronary heart disease—and reduce cholesterol, tension, back pain, joint pain, stiffness, and loss of calcium from bones.[95,96,97] Exercise is not a panacea, but it does eliminate some negative aspects of old age associated with sedentary behavior. People report feeling better, sleeping better, feeling less anxious or depressed, and enjoying an improvement in their self-image.[98]

Exercise programs should not be undertaken indiscriminately. A physical examination is absolutely necessary before beginning any concerted exertion. For older people it is better to have the regimen prescribed by an exercise physiologist or a physician. There are also other guidelines to be heeded. Kosidlak started a self-care program for older adults, 90 percent of whom had chronic medical problems.[99] It was an all-encompassing program to increase self-reliance and awareness, of which one segment of attention was on exercise and the possible positive results. Participants were cautioned to exercise in pairs, to learn to listen to body messages, and to be able to describe them. Not only would they be able to handle common minor illnesses and injuries, but they would be able to alleviate several problems to some extent by being more active in exercise.

Many people do not exercise, and elderly people encouraged by stereotype and caution to assume a sedentary life style are very much a part of that sedentary segment of society. Exercise programs should be designed for the capabilities, limitations, priorities, and goals of each person.

Price and Luther recommend exercising three nonconsecutive days a week in a plan that allows 10 to 15 minutes to warm up, stretch, and condition; 15 to 60 minutes of exercise, the amount inversely related to the intensity of the exercise; and a 5- to 10-minute period to cool down.[100] For many, walking briskly will be the exercise activity of choice. Aerobic exercise is vital.

Walking, running, and swimming are excellent aerobic exercises using large muscle masses. DeVries, in his studies of physiology of aging, advises that "exercise programs for older people should maximize the rhythmic activity of large muscle masses and minimize (1) high activation levels of small muscle masses; and (2) static (or isometric) contractions."[101] DeVries maintains these restrictions are necessary due to occlusion of bloodflow in small muscles during isometric exercises and the increase in systemic blood pressure, whereas rhythmic movement of large muscle masses allows periodic relaxation and blood flow. "Active leg muscle contraction—as occurs in walking—yields 30 percent or more of the power required to sustain the movement of the blood, thus reducing the work of the heart by a corresponding amount."[102] DeVries advises that people be taught to take their own pulse, and that individual plans for exercise be based on allowable maximum heart rates calculated by age.[103]

For persons resuming walking after an illness, exercise should be gradually increased with focus on increased mobility and should include exercising two times a day. Indoor exercises with a similar degree of range of motion as gained in outdoor exercises are valuable replacements during poor weather or as complements to other programs.[104]

Exercise increases both oxygen and nutrients transported to the tissue, and elimination of wastes due to increased bloodflow.[105] It can be a benefit to many elderly people, but some feel DeVries' program is too vigorous for those who are less fit.[106] However, DeVries advises everyone to plan carefully with their physician before beginning an exercise program. That is a caution that cannot be dismissed lightly, even by those who consider themselves to be in good health, who prefer independence, or who have always exercised.

Exercise is another universal of self-care that provides for basic daily needs. To plan beneficial exercise is a deliberate action based on informed judgment. It is ideally self-initiated, self-directed, and self-controlled. A visit to the physician and discussion of the assets and hazards of exercise builds a basis for valid judgments of needs, priorities, and capabilities.[107]

Sexuality

Sexuality, more than drugs, diet, and exercise is clouded with myths and subjectivity, and is controlled by cultural norms. Further, it has been assumed that physical changes in the body, for example, wrinkles and gray hair, plus the absence of the need to procreate also mean the lack of sexual need and ability. However, studies show the contrary to be true. Elderly people do have the need, the right, and the potential for a pleasant and active sex life.[108]

Aging is a normal process of development, stimulated by acquisition of knowledge and experience. This is a continual growing process. Unfortunately, the body is changing as a person ages, and this is seen as decline and decay by many, often to the extreme that they falsely equate it with a disease process. The result is to withdraw all privileges of past enjoyments and to deal with "the disease," which will eventually kill the individual. There are many physical and physiological changes, but on close scrutiny none of the normal physical changes are so drastic as to become barriers to sexual activity. They are such changes as decrease in height, muscle mass, strength, elasticity of skin, and thinning of skin due to decrease in number of cells; and hormonal changes and increase in adipose tissue. These in turn result in sagging breasts, wrinkles, thicker lower trunk, and a decrease in the length, width, and expansive ability of the vaginal barrel.[109,110]

Physiologically, the plasma level of sex hormones changes, and the Bartholin glands are less active. The fallopian tubes are smaller and lose some motility factors. The involutional process is evident, but that is not a corollary to impotence or inability to function successfully, sexually. Neither are the flaccid testicles, thickened seminiforous tubules, or the decline in viable sperm that is seen in males. The clitoris is still sensitive for women; their sex drive and ability are still as intense as in earlier years. Men do not have erections as frequently as in their youth, but they now have control over ejaculation, which makes sex far better at 50 than it was at 20. "This means that older men can remain erect and make love longer before coming to orgasm. There is also the advantage of lovemaking experience gained throughout a lifetime."[111]

Physiologically there are few valid reasons to eliminate sexual activity, but many report that they no longer engage in it. The outstanding reasons cited are impotence and disinterest by men, and lack of a partner or a partner who is uninterested by women. This diminishing interest and potency seem to stem far more frequently from psychological factors than from biologically-based causes. Only ten percent of impotence cases need be considered permanent.[112] Those caused by hormone deficiency can be alleviated by hormone therapy; the other factors generally require psychological counseling. However, whether the problem is organic or psychological, reversal of the condition is often difficult.

Masters and Johnson outline three phases of intercourse, termed the excitement, plateau, and orgasmic phases.[113] The first phase takes longer, requiring a greater degree of caressing and play. The erection and testicular elevation is not as great, but, as mentioned earlier, this is compensated for by a prolonged plateau phase where pleasures are increased with age. The orgasmic phase and subsequent resolution are of shorter duration.[114,115,116] In summary:

> There are indeed physiologic changes with aging, but they are not coterminous with cessation of intercourse unless an individual wishes it so. Those who have ceased sexual activity for some time are not prohibited from resumption if the desire and occasion arise.[117]

Many of the restrictions of sexual activity occur because of heavily enforced social codes. In this regard, social norms identify who shall be allowed the privilege of sex. These norms are taught to children from birth, socializing them according to a specific set of values and mores. Items and factors taught are accepted, altered, or rejected throughout a lifetime, but as a person ages, the socialization is nearly complete, stabilized into a relatively consistent pattern of behavior and beliefs. Today's older generation was socialized at a time when sex was only thought to be permitted between married younger persons who needed to procreate children; sexual relations were not assumed to be a part of retirement recreation. Sexual desires do not die after a particular age in life. The perplexity is that couples do not grow old together and die simultaneously. One almost always precedes the other. Most commonly, women are left as widows in a social ratio of males and females that does not have the capacity to absorb single older women. But the need for love, touch, warmth, and sharing socially and sexually remains, often clouded in embarrassment, shame, and frustration, and controlled by diversion, repression, or sublimation. "The need for love, and by extension, sex, in our society is considered to be a basic human need which does not begin or end with the ability to procreate. The need lasts throughout one's life and there is a physiological foundation for such behavior."[118]

The role of the professional in providing guidance and information to the older client is more complicated than to younger clients, because of the increased incidences of ill health, disease, and widowhood compounded by beliefs in the myths and stereotypes of young and old, and the very personal, sensitive nature of the subject. But, as with all other topics in this chapter, sexuality in a person's life is, perhaps more than other factors, determined by that person's decisions based on a very personal perception of the data. For those older couples with only slight problems and no major physical limitations, counseling is fairly simple, discussing goals, facts, and emotions. However, when an imbalance of relationships is introduced, the incapacity of one imposes doubly complex issues interwoven with past known values and future unknown conditions and fears. Inequality intercedes; what was known is now unfamiliar, unresponsive, and frightening, and many of the predictabilities of an ongoing relationship are destroyed. A stroke immobilizes muscles and emotions, blinding and barricading channels of love, communication, and movement. The flaccid hand, awkward speech, or altered personality are overwhelming to the values of both the victim and the spouse. Often the concern and counseling are focused only on the victim, not the victim's spouse.

The self-care concept is just as valuable in these emotional instances as it is in diet, drug use, and exercise. Both individuals need to set goals in light of resources, limitations, and needs. The guilt and frustrations of partners in unbalanced situations are every bit as serious as those of the widow who no longer has a sexual partner, perhaps even more so since the victim is changed markedly from past patterns of love and sharing. The values an individual holds strongest can be those that prevent change and necessary adaptations in relationships. There is no area of sexual counseling where values and culture do not merge with physiological concepts, but the approach need not be complicated. For many, the opportunity to discuss in forums is readily accepted; for others, smaller groups or individual discussion is necessary. But for all, the major therapeutic pattern seems to be one of talking out the issues, ventilating emotions, and reevaluating norms, needs, and knowledge. Questions never considered become important, and resolution is urgently desired.

Communication skills and active listening techniques are necessary as in all areas of interviewing and counseling. Again, the professional's role is that of facilitator and resource person, not a decision maker. For those couples where disease and time have created a disparate relationship, a facilitator can guide them toward establishing mutually acceptable goals and provide a positive atmosphere where feelings can be shared and clarified without threat to one another.[119]

Group discussions in a warm, open, matter-of-fact forum have been successful for many elderly couples, and there is a gradual increase in requests for more information by the elderly.[120] Sviland and Wood offer pragmatic guidelines for such forums of self-care planning.[121,122] Discussions and counseling begin at the client's level of understanding and readiness to avoid afront and withdrawal. All discussions should be based on fact, use assessment skills, clarify assumptions, and allow the clients to come to their own conclusions. This is the client's series of decisions. This is a personal subject, and conclusions will come to rest with the person who must live with them. Professionals are there to present data, interpret its ramifications, and keep communication channels open for the client.

Each person is unique, and so to each one are the problem and resolution. Self-care involves identifying and attending to health and social deviations that impose on norms of sexual relationships created by aging, illnesses, and death. The greater the demands, the greater will be the necessary effort if the person is to achieve new stability.

NOTES

1. Terence M. Hines and James L. Fozard, "Memory and Aging: Relevance of Recent Developments for Research and Application," in C. Eisdorfer, ed., *Annual Review of Gerontology and Geriatrics,* Volume 1 (New York, N.Y.: Springer Publishing Company, 1980), p. 110.

2. David A. Walsh, "Age Differences in Learning and Memory," in D. Woodruff and J. Birren, eds., *Aging* (New York, N.Y.: D. Van Nostrand, 1975), pp. 116–7.

3. Carl Eisdorfer, "Intellectual and Cognitive Changes in the Aged," in S. Han and M. Gehe, eds., *Readings in Gerontology* (Ann Arbor, Mich.: Institute of Gerontology, 1976), pp. 614–5.

4. Hines, pp. 97–110.

5. Eisdorfer, p. 618.

6. P. Pierce, "Intelligence and Learning in the Aged," *Journal of Gerontological Nursing* 6, no. 5 (May 1980): 270.

7. Ibid.

8. M. Haro et al., *Explorations in Personal Health* (Boston, Mass.: Houghton Mifflin Co., 1977), p. 14.

9. K. W. Schaie, "Age Changes in Adult Intelligence," in D. Woodruff and J. Birren, eds., *Aging* (New York, N.Y.: D. Van Nostrand Co., 1975), pp. 111–24.

10. R. E. Canestrari, Jr., "Paced and Self-Paced Learning in Young and Elderly Adults," *Journal of Gerontology,* 18, no. 2 (1963): 165–8.

11. Eisdorfer, pp. 612–8.

12. Jack Botwinick, lecture, in Geriatric Program for Mental Health Outreach, "Memory and Aging," 1980, Albuquerque, New Mexico.

13. Walsh, pp. 116–7.

14. Dorothea Orem, *Nursing: Concepts of Practice* (New York, N.Y.: McGraw-Hill, 1971), p. 15.

15. Catherine Norris, "Self-Care," *American Journal of Nursing* 79, no. 3 (March 1979): 486–9.

16. Ibid.

17. Ibid., p. 487.

18. Jody Bennett, "Symposium on the Self-Care Concept in Nursing," *Nursing Clinics of North America* 15, no. 1 (March 1980): 129–30.

19. Haro et al., p. 13.

20. Norris, p. 486.

21. M. Lucille Kinlein, "The Self-Care Concept," *American Journal of Nursing* 77, no. 4 (April 1977): 601.

22. Janet Kosidlak, "Self-Help for Senior Citizens," *Journal of Gerontological Nursing* 6, no. 11 (November 1980): 668.

23. Haro et al., p. 14.

24. Bennett, p. 129.

25. Kinlein, p. 598.

26. Orem, pp. 13–39.

27. Jane Zapka and Barry Averill, "Self-Care for Colds: A Cost Effective Alternative to Upper Respiratory Infection Management," *American Journal of Public Health* 69, no. 8 (August 1979): 814.

28. Norris, p. 487.

29. Lynda Sacco Joseph, "Self-Care and the Nursing Process," *Nursing Clinics of North America* 15, no. 1 (March 1980): 131–43.

30. Orem, pp. 14–19.

31. Norris, p. 487.

32. Orem, p. 20.

33. Norris, pp. 487–9.

34. Orem, p. 31.

35. Joseph, p. 132.

36. Ibid.

37. Orem, pp. 34–36.

38. Zapka and Averill, pp. 814–6.

39. Kosidlak, pp. 663–8.
40. Anna Brock, "Self-Administration of Drugs in the Elderly: Nursing Responsibilities," *Journal of Gerontological Nursing* 6, no. 7 (July 1980): 398.
41. P. Bush and D. Robin, "Who's Using Non-prescription Medicines?" *Medical Care* 14, no. 12 (December 1976): 1014–23.
42. D. Lenhart, "The Use of Medications in the Elderly Population," *Nursing Clinics of North America,* no. 1 (March 1976): 135–44.
43. Ibid.
44. Bush and Robin, pp. 1014–23.
45. L. S. Goodman and A. Gilman, *The Pharmacological Basis of Therapeutics,* Fifth Edition (New York, N.Y.: Macmillan, 1975), pp. 331–3.
46. Irene Burnside, *Nursing and the Aged* (New York, N.Y.: McGraw-Hill, 1976), p. 373.
47. G. S. Avery, "Drug Interactions That Really Matter: A Guide to Major Important Drug Interactions," *Drugs* 14 (1977): 132–46.
48. Kosidlak, p. 667.
49. Dianna Shomaker, "Use and Abuse of OTC Medications," *Journal of Gerontological Nursing* 6, no. 1 (January 1980): 21–23.
50. D. Schwartz, "Safe Self-Medication for Elderly Outpatients," *American Journal of Nursing* 75, no. 10 (October 1975): 1809.
51. Ibid.
52. Alex Comfort, *Family Practice News,* December 1, 1977.
53. Schwartz, p. 1809.
54. M. M. Basen, "The Elderly and Drugs—Problem Overview and Problem Strategy," *Public Health Reports* 92, no. 1 (Jan/Feb 1977): 43–48.
55. Schwartz, pp. 1809–10.
56. Basen, p. 44.
57. Schwartz, p. 1809.
58. Brock, pp. 398–404.
59. Ibid., p. 404.
60. Louis A. Morris and Jerome Halperin, "Effects of Written Drug Information on Patient Knowledge and Compliance: A Literature Review," *American Journal of Public Health* 69, no. 1 (January 1979): 4752.
61. Ibid.
62. Judith A. Sullivan and F. Armiguacco, "Effectiveness of a Comprehensive Health Program for the Well-Elderly," *Nursing Research* 28, no. 2 (Mar./Apr. 1979): 71–74.
63. Schwartz, pp. 1809–110.
64. Basen, pp. 44–47.
65. Kosidlak, p. 667.
66. Kathleen Leahy, Marguerite Cobb, and Mary Jones, *Community Health Nursing,* Second Edition (New York, N.Y.: McGraw-Hill, 1972), p. 206.
67. Jane Hentzler and Alice Henneman, "Where Can You Go for Nutritional Assistance?" *Journal of Gerontological Nursing* 6, no. 9 (Sept. 1980): 551.
68. Doris Slesinger, Maxine McDivitt, and Florence O'Donnell, "Food Patterns in an

Urban Population: Age and Sociodemographic Correlates," *Journal of Gerontology* 35, no. 3 (May 1980): 432–3.

69. Vernon R. Young and Nevin S. Scrimshaw, "Protein Needs of the Elderly," *Urban Health* 4, no. 4 (August 1975): 37.

70. Hentzler and Henneman, p. 551.

71. Leahy, Cobb, and Jones, p. 205.

72. Hentzler and Henneman, p. 551.

73. Karen L. Combs, "Preventive Care in the Elderly," *American Journal of Nursing* 78, no. 8 (August 1978): 1340.

74. Virginia Byers, *Nursing Observations,* Second Edition (Dubuque, Iowa.: William C. Brown, 1968), p. 14.

75. Ruth Murray, Marilyn Huelskoetter, and Dorothy Driscoll, *The Nursing Process in Later Maturity* (Englewood Cliffs, N.J.: Prentice-Hall, 1980), pp. 512–3.

76. Ruth Weg, "Changing Physiology of Aging: Normal and Pathological," in D. Woodruff and J. Birren, eds., *Aging* (New York, N.Y.: D. Van Nostrand, 1975), pp. 239–40, 251.

77. Leahy, Cobb, and Jones, pp. 205–7.

78. Weg, p. 251.

79. Young and Scrimshaw, pp. 37–39.

80. Slesinger et al., pp. 439–40.

81. Ibid., p. 439.

82. Orem, p. 21.

83. Herbert A. DeVries, "Physiology of Exercise and Aging," in D. Woodruff and J. Birren, eds., *Aging* (New York, N.Y.: D. Van Nostrand, 1975), p. 261.

84. James Price and Cathy Pritts, "Overweight and Obesity in the Elderly," *Journal of Gerontological Nursing* 6, no. 6 (June 1980): 342–4.

85. Ibid., p. 343.

86. Ibid., p. 345.

87. Ibid., pp. 345–6.

88. Orem, p. 25.

89. Ethel Battle and Carolyn Hanna, "Evaluation of a Dietary Regimen for Chronic Constipation," *Journal of Gerontological Nursing* 6, no. 9 (Sept. 1980); 527–32.

90. Kosidlak, p. 667.

91. Ruth Berger, "Nutritional Needs of the Elderly," in Irene Burnside, ed., *Nursing and the Aged* (New York, N.Y.: McGraw-Hill, 1976), p. 116.

92. Bernita M. Steffl, "Prevention Measures and Safety Factors for the Aged," in Irene Burnside, ed., *Nursing and the Aged* (New York, N.Y.: McGraw-Hill, 1976), p. 476.

93. Ruth Weg, "Changing Physiology of Aging: Normal and Pathological," in D. Woodruff and J. Birren, eds., *Aging* (New York, N.Y.: D. Van Nostrand, 1975), p. 251.

94. Herbert DeVries, "Physiology of Exercise and Aging," in D. Woodruff and J. Birren, eds., *Aging* (New York, N.Y.: D. Van Nostrand, 1975), pp. 257–72.

95. Ibid., p. 267.

96. Kosidlak, p. 666.

97. J. Price and S. Luther, "Physical Fitness: Its Role in Health for the Elderly," *Journal of Gerontological Nursing* 6, no. 9 (Sept. 1980): 517–9.

98. Ibid., pp. 518–20.

99. Kosidlak, pp. 663–8.

100. Price and Luther, pp. 521–2.

101. DeVries, pp. 271–2.

102. P. S. Timiras, *Developmental Physiology and Aging* (New York, N.Y.: Macmillan, 1972), p. 418.

103. DeVries, pp. 268–72.

104. Murray, Huelskoetter, and O'Driscoll, pp. 469–516.

105. Timiras, p. 419.

106. Morton Puner, *To the Good Long Life* (New York, N.Y.: Universe Books, 1974), p. 82.

107. Orem, pp. 13–15.

108. W. Masters and V. Johnson, *Human Sexual Response* (Boston, Mass.: Little, Brown and Co., 1966), pp. 223–70.

109. Dianna Shomaker, "Integration of Physiological and Socio-Cultural Factors as a Basis for Sex Education to the Elderly," *Journal of Gerontological Nursing* 6, no. 6 (June 1980): 314–5.

110. N. Wood, *Human Sexuality in Health and Illness,* Second Edition (St. Louis, Mo.: C. V. Mosby, 1979), pp. 48–74, 95–106, 287–322.

111. R. Butler and M. Lewis, *Aging and Mental Health* (St. Louis, Mo.: C. V. Mosby, 1977), pp. 112–8.

112. M. Sviland, "A Program of Sexual Liberation and Growth in the Elderly," in R. Solnick, ed., *Sexuality and Aging* (Los Angeles, Cal.: USC Press, 1978), pp. 96–114.

113. Masters and Johnson, pp. 223–70.

114. Wood, pp. 48–74, 95–106.

115. Butler and Lewis, pp. 112–8.

116. Shomaker, "Integration of Physiological," pp. 315–6.

117. Ibid.

118. Ibid., p. 313.

119. Ibid., p. 317.

120. Sviland, pp. 96–114.

121. Ibid.

122. Wood, pp. 107–92, 323–63.

Part IV

Tools, Guidelines, and Resources

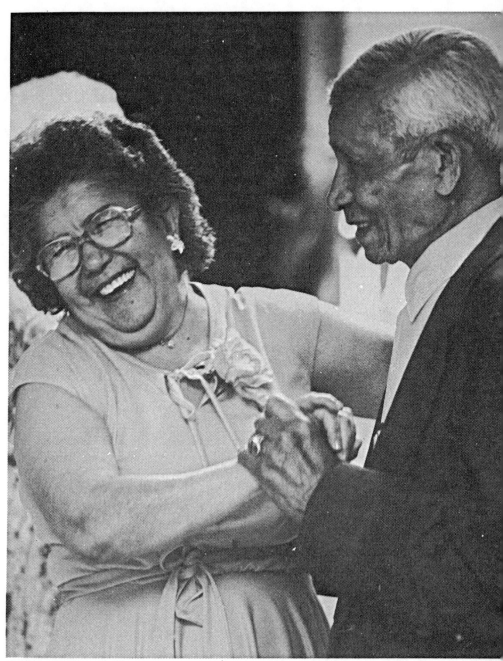

Courtesy Albuquerque News

Chapter 18

Tools, Guidelines, and Resources

Chiyoko Furukawa and Dianna Shomaker

The information presented in this section comes from many sources; therefore, it has not been used in one setting as a composite approach to care. The items are intended to be employed as they appear or to serve as a model for the development of tools, protocols, and guidelines to benefit the health promotion and maintenance care of the aged. The materials were also selected to represent many of the various components and philosophies of care outlined in this book.

The compilation of the information is by no means complete or comprehensive. The user is encouraged to seek additional resources to clarify specific information and to broaden the scope of the suggested tools and guidelines.

These information materials are arbitrarily categorized into two sections: health promotion and maintenance information, and assessment guides.

HEALTH PROMOTION AND MAINTENANCE INFORMATION

Table 18-1 Anatomic Changes to Consider in Care of Aged

	Functional Change	Outcome
Heart	Decreased stroke volume; slower heart rate	Drop in cardiac output
	Estimated left ventricular work declines at rest	
	Blood flow through the coronary arteries decreases	
	Myocardial ability to use oxygen decreases[1]	Heart less well equipped to handle stress; with coexisting heart disease, cardiac failure and death may result

333

Table 18-1 continued

	Functional Change	Outcome
Blood Vessels	Smooth muscle replaced by fibrous and hyaline tissue causing decreased vascular elasticity	Increased pulse pressure and systolic blood pressure
Kidney	Renal blood flow drops at a steady rate, starting at age 40[2]	Proportional reduction in glomerular filtration rate (usually measured as creatinine clearance)
	Decreased fluid intake leads to decreased ability to concentrate urine	Normal GFR at age 40 of 120 ml./min. falls to 60 or 70 ml./min. at age 85[3]
	Ability to dilute urine decreases	BUN rises from a normal value of 9.5 mg./100 ml. at age 20 to 15–20 mg./100 ml. at age 70–80[3]
Lungs	Reduction in vital capacity and increase of residual volume; reduction of pulmonary diffusion; loss of lung recoil; and maldistribution of pulmonary ventilation/perfusion ratios—all due to change in type or quantity of fibrous proteins, collagen, and elastin in lung matrix[4]	Decrease in arterial oxygen tension, less respiratory reserve in major illnesses, surgery, or trauma
	Progressive weakening of respiratory muscles	Reduced negative and positive intrathoracic pressure on forced inspiration and expiration; this plus reduced expiratory flow rates account for decrease in maximum breathing capacity
GI Tract	Decreased motility of stomach and intestines	Constipation
	Reduction in intestinal blood flow[5]	Possible delay or slight reduction in drug absorption
	Increase in gastric pH	Affects solubility of some drugs
	Number of absorbing cells may be decreased and active transport systems may be modified	No data to support major change in drug absorption[6]

Table 18-1 continued

	Functional Change	Outcome
Musculoskeletal System	Decrease in number and bulk of muscle fibers; muscle fibers are replaced by nonmuscular fibrous tissue	Decrease in muscular strength, endurance, and agility
	Density of bone decreases; in women after middle age may be related estrogen deficiency, insufficient dietary intake, and perhaps abnormalities in calcium, protein, and amino acid metabolism[7,8]	Osteoporosis, osteoarthritis
Hematological System	Iron deficiency anemia, probably caused by malnutrition and malabsorption[9]	Iron and folate deficiency and a change in oxygen-carrying capacity
	Anemia due to chronic diseases such as infection, arthritis, malignant disease	Mild, normocytic and normochromic anemia
Endocrine System	Insulin response or peripheral sensitivity to insulin release may be reduced	Return to fasting level in glucose tolerance test is slower[3]

[1] Harris, R. Special features of heart disease in the elderly patients. In *Working With Older People—A Guide to Practice, Vol. 4, Clinical Aspects of Aging,* ed. by A. B. Chinn. (Public Health Service Publ. No. 1459) Washington, D.C., U.S. Government Printing Office, 1971, pp. 81–102.

[2] Papper, Solomon. The effects of age in reducing renal function. *Geriatrics* 28:83–87, May 1973.

[3] Cole, W. H. Medical differences between the young and the aged. *J. Am. Geriatr. Soc.* 18:589–614, Aug. 1970.

[4] Williams, M. H. Special problems in respiratory diseases. *Geriatrics* 29:67–71, June 1974.

[5] Bender, A. D. Effect of age on intestinal absorption: implications for drug absorption in the elderly. *J. Am. Geriatr. Soc.* 16:1331–1339, Dec. 1968.

[6] Crooks, J., and others. Pharmacokinetics in the elderly. *Clin. Pharmacokinet.* 1(4):280–296, 1976.

[7] Trotter, M., and others. Densities of bones of white and Negro skeletons. *J. Bone Joint Surg.* (Am.) 42-A:50–58, Jan. 1960.

[8] Yoshikaw, M., and others. Osteoporosis in Japan, a clinical and experimental study. In *Proceedings of the Eighth International Congress on Gerontology.* Washington, D.C., Federation of American Societies for Experimental Biology, Vol. 1, 1969, p. 225.

[9] Evans, D. M. Hematological aspects of iron-deficiency in the elderly. *Gerontol. Clin* (Basel) 13:12–30, 1971.

Source: Copyright © 1978, American Journal of Nursing Company. Reproduced with permission from the *American Journal of Nursing* 78, no. 8 (August 1978): p. 1349.

Table 18-2 Basic Food Groups

Food Group	Recommended Servings Per Day for People Over 50	Contribution to Diet
fruit and vegetable	4	vitamins A, C; fiber
bread and cereal	4	B-vitamins, fiber
meat and legumes	2–3	protein, iron, vitamin B_{12}, folacin
milk and milk products	2	calcium, protein
fats, sugars	as needed	calories, essential fatty acids

A diet that consistently includes these servings, with extras to provide sufficient calories, should be adequate nutrition for well older adults.

Source: Reproduced with permission from Geriatric Nursing, American Journal of Care for the Aging, May/June, 1, no. 1 (May/June 1980): p. 71. © 1980, American Journal of Nursing Company.

GUIDELINES FOR MEDICATION AND FOOD COMBINATIONS

These guidelines are general suggestions and may not apply in all situations. Your physician may give you different instructions. See your physician, pharmacist, nurse, or dietitian/nutrition advisor for further information.

I. Some Drugs Prevent Proper Use of Nutrients

Laxatives: such as mineral oil, dulcolax, phenolphthalein
Antacids: gelusil, Maalox, milk of magnesia
Cholesterol lowering agents: Atromid-s, questran
Stool softeners: colace, surfak
Alcohol:
Anti-infective agents when used long-term
Diuretics:
(If you must take these medicines, you should ask your doctor.)

II. Some Drugs Should Be Taken on an Empty Stomach

Oral penicillins: Penicillin g, ampicillin, nafcillin, oxacillin, dicloxacillin, Cloxacillin
Tetracycline
Lincocin
Cleocin

III. Some Drugs Should Not Be Taken with Milk or Milk Products

(The calcium in milk can reduce the effectiveness of the drug.)
Bisacodyl (dulcolax)
Potassium Chloride solutions
Potassium Iodide
Tetracyclines (except vibramycin and minocin)
(Generally speaking, all antibiotics should be taken at least one hour before or two hours after a meal.)

IV. Some Drugs Should Be Taken with Meals

Indocin	Macrodantin	Motrin
Phenylbutazone	Iron salts	Furadantin
Oral Corticosteroids	Potassium supplements	
Metronidazole	Reserpine	
Aspirin (large doses)		
Any nonsteroidal anti-inflammatory		

(Again, when the doctor prescribes medicine, ask about taking it with or without food!)

PRECAUTIONS FOR USE OF OVER-THE-COUNTER AND PRESCRIBED DRUGS

Over-the-Counter Drugs

Aspirin

analgesic, inexpensive, and easily accessible

- The patient should know its advantages. Many scoff because it is so readily available; therefore it must not be any good.

- Patient needs to know the toxic signs and, if using it in large doses daily (for example, arthritis), occasional blood tests should be run to determine leukocytosis.

- Patients need to be aware of other drugs contained in pills, along with aspirin, which might be contraindicated by another condition, for example, caffeine, phenacetin, antacids that are implicated with kidney problems when used chronically.

Tylenol

This analgesic lacks the anti-inflammatory properties that make aspirin effective in arthritis.

Alka Seltzer

contraindicated in low sodium diets

• Watch for edema and congestive heart failure.

Baking Soda and Antacids

sodium retention factor, commonly used to treat gastrointestinal complaints

• They cause an increased pH in the stomach; therefore, the absorption of acidic drugs, iron, some nutrients, and some antibiotic medicines is delayed.

Mineral Oil

retards gastric emptying and impedes absorption of minerals and fat soluble vitamins

• There is a danger of aspiration pneumonia in debilitated patients.

• By causing loss of vitamin K, it is a potentiating factor for anticoagulants.

• A dependency on laxatives is a common situation created by routine use of such things as mineral oil. It would be wiser to have a good diet, adequate fluid intake, and plenty of exercise.

Vitamins

• C—Some say over 1 gram a day prevents colds, but causes diarrhea and precipitates uric acid crystals and potential kidney stones.

• D—Some advocate large doses to increase resistance to colds, but it also causes hypercalemia, weakness, fatigue, headaches, nausea, diarrhea, and vomiting.

Alcohol

• Large dose reduces cerebral oxygen uptake and potentiates the action of tranquilizers, hypnotics, and antihistamines.

Prescribed Medicines

Cardiac Drugs

- Side effects: vomiting, diarrhea, diuretic deplete potassium, which causes the myocardium to be more sensitive to digitalis, creating arrhythmias, and digitalis toxicity

Diuretics

- Reserpine and Ismelin cause hypotension, orthostatic hypotension, and bradycardia.
- Potassium loss requires Potassium supplements.
- Aldactone spares Potassium but causes headaches, drowsiness, or diarrhea.

Aspirin and other Arthritic Drugs

- Butazolidin not used with elderly for arthritis, because it causes gastric ulcers, edema, hepatitis, and nephritis in documented cases.
- Indocin causes gastrointestinal distress and in some cases psychic disturbances. It also aggravates Parkinsonism and asthma.
- Zyloprim is used for gout but can cause skin reactions and cataracts.
- Motrin is effective in much the same way as aspirin. It is a nonsteroid that relieves pain, stiffness, and swelling.

Urinary Tract Infections

- Furadantin has the side effects of headache, vertigo, hemolysis of red blood cells.

Peripheral Vascular Dilators

- Papavarine, Nicotinic Acid for treatment of circulatory problems occasionally causing flushing and headaches; contra-indicated in glaucoma.

Ointments and Lotions

- Those that contain steroids create a hazard when significant amounts are absorbed into the system through the skin.

Antibiotics and Antihistamines

- If used for cough and sore throat in some elderly because of the increased chance of secondary pneumonia from relatively minor ailments.

Antihistamines: hypersensitive reaction, drowsiness, blurred vision, central nervous system depression

- All of these are even more noticeable when one drinks alcohol.

Psychotropic Drugs

- **Valium/Librium:** affects coordination and ambulatory function. Especially dangerous for those who are predisposed to falls.
- **Ritalin:** confusion, paranoia, lowered convulsive threshold
- It also causes psychosis, and addiction.
- **Tricyclic Anti-depressants:**
- (Tofranil, Norpramin, Pertofrane and Aventyl) are atropine-like in action, for example, dry mouth; contra-indicated in glaucoma.
- **MAO Inhibitors:**
- Parnate and Marplan are antidepressants. They can cause confusion, restlessness, liver toxicity, and prolong and intensify actions of anesthetic, barbiturates, and insulin.
- If a patient is on these drugs he/she should avoid (a) agents that elevate blood pressure; (b) cheese; (c) pickled herring; (d) cold preparations; and (e) alcoholic beverages.
- All these drugs enhanced by use of alcohol.

Figure 18-1 Flow Diagram Leading to Unpredictability of Drug Effects in the Aged

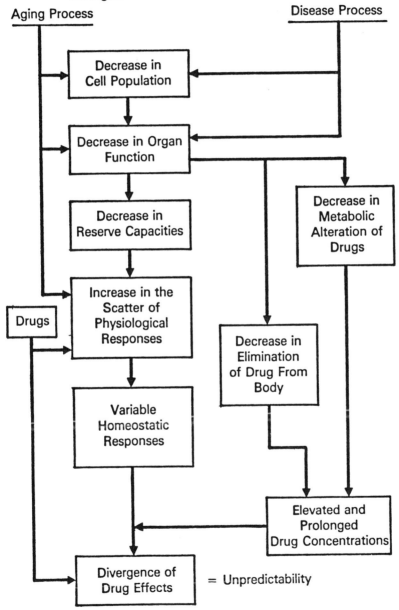

Source: Reprinted by permission from Gene A. Riley, "How Aging Influences Drug Therapy," *U.S. Pharmacist* (November/December 1977), p. 36

The following five figures are schematics of significant adverse drug interactions. This information should be used with other current drug literature and personal drug profiles of clients.

The interaction classification numbers below correspond to the superscript numbers in the right hand boxes of the figures.

Clinical Significance of Adverse Drug Interactions

Interaction Classification	Clinical Significance
1	These interacting drugs ordinarily should NOT be administered concurrently
2	Concurrent administration of these drugs often leads to therapeutic difficulties
3	These potentially interacting drugs can be\administered concurrently. if appropriate adjustments in dose or method of administration are made
4	Clinical evidence is inconclusive or controversial

* *Source:* Reprinted with permission from Lawrence H. Block, "Drug Interactions and the Elderly," *U.S. Pharmacist* (November/December 1977): 46, 47, 48, 50, 52, 53.

Figure 18-2 Selected Interactions of Drugs Affecting the Central Nervous System

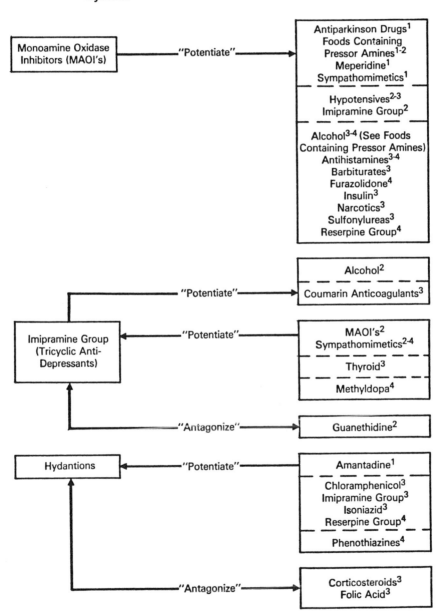

Figure 18-2 continued

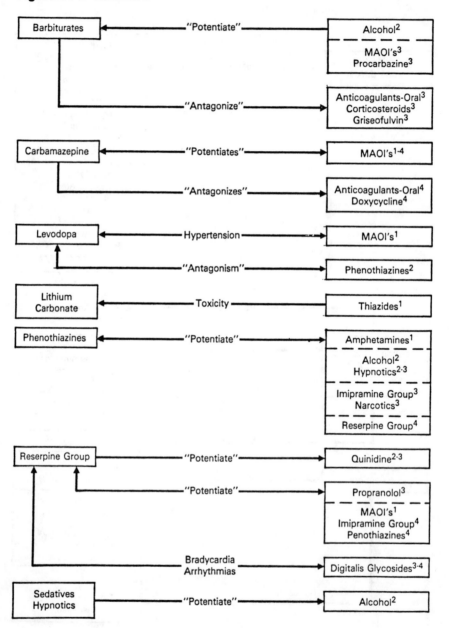

Figure 18-3 Selected Interactions of Cardiovascular Drugs

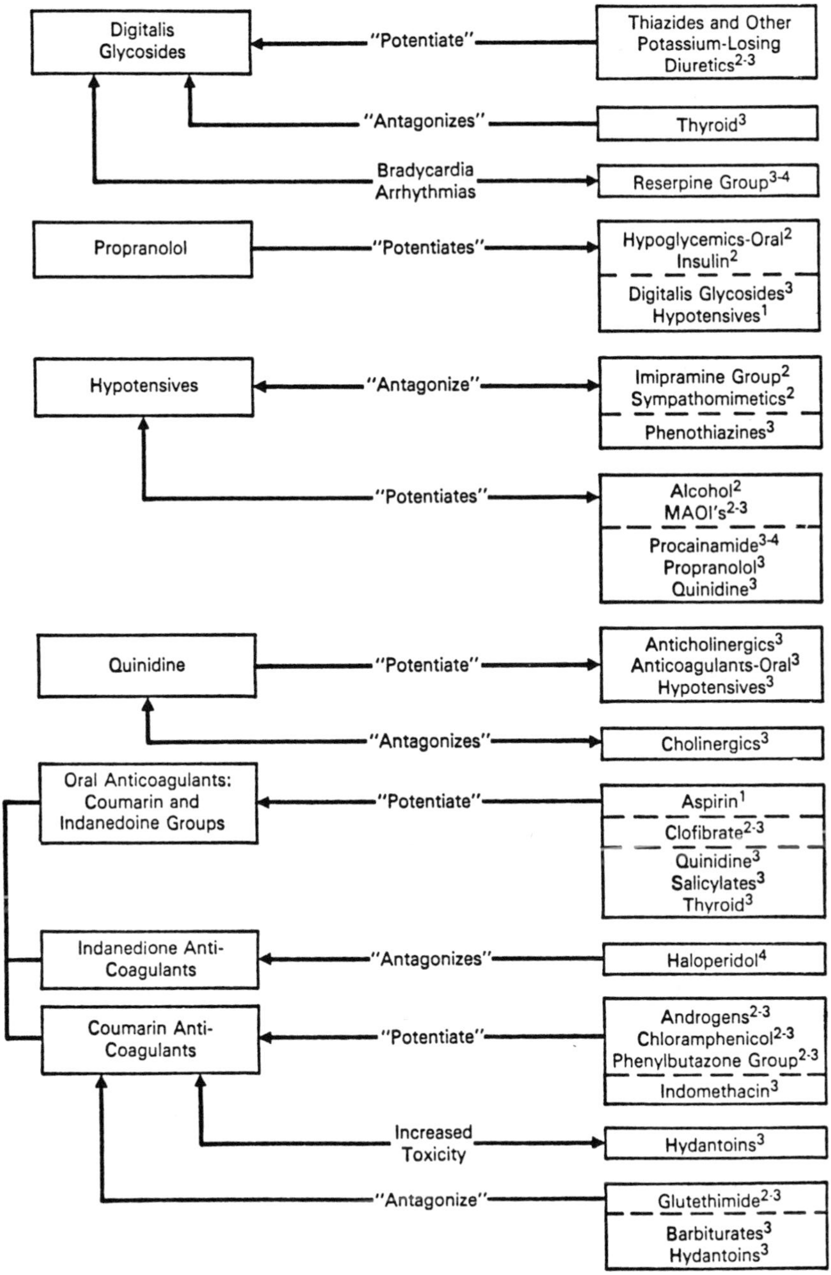

Digitalis Glycosides	◄— "Potentiate"—	Thiazides and Other Potassium-Losing Diuretics[2-3]
	"Antagonizes" —	Thyroid[3]
	Bradycardia Arrhythmias	Reserpine Group[3-4]
Propranolol	"Potentiates" —	Hypoglycemics-Oral[2] Insulin[2]
		Digitalis Glycosides[3] Hypotensives[1]
Hypotensives	◄— "Antagonize"—	Imipramine Group[2] Sympathomimetics[2]
		Phenothiazines[3]
	"Potentiates"—	Alcohol[2] MAOI's[2-3]
		Procainamide[3-4] Propranolol[3] Quinidine[3]
Quinidine	"Potentiate"—	Anticholinergics[3] Anticoagulants-Oral[3] Hypotensives[3]
	"Antagonizes"—	Cholinergics[3]
Oral Anticoagulants: Coumarin and Indanedoine Groups	◄— "Potentiate"—	Aspirin[1]
		Clofibrate[2-3]
		Quinidine[3] Salicylates[3] Thyroid[3]
Indanedione Anti-Coagulants	◄— "Antagonizes"—	Haloperidol[4]
Coumarin Anti-Coagulants	◄— "Potentiate"—	Androgens[2-3] Chloramphenicol[2-3] Phenylbutazone Group[2-3]
		Indomethacin[3]
	Increased Toxicity	Hydantoins[3]
	"Antagonize"—	Glutethimide[2-3]
		Barbiturates[3] Hydantoins[3]

Figure 18-4 Selected Antibiotic—Anti-Infective Interactions

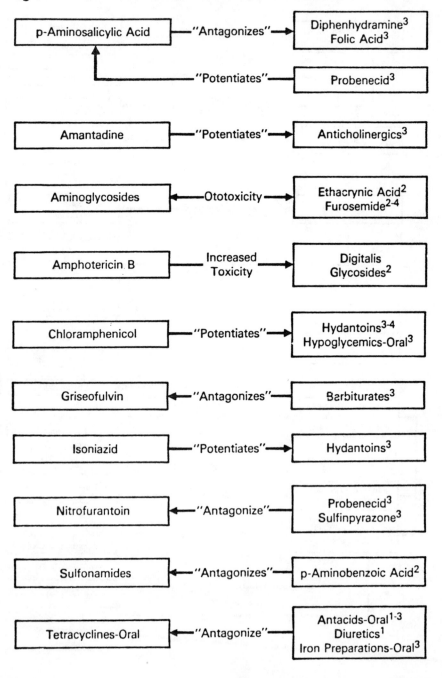

Figure 18-5 Miscellaneous Drug Interactions

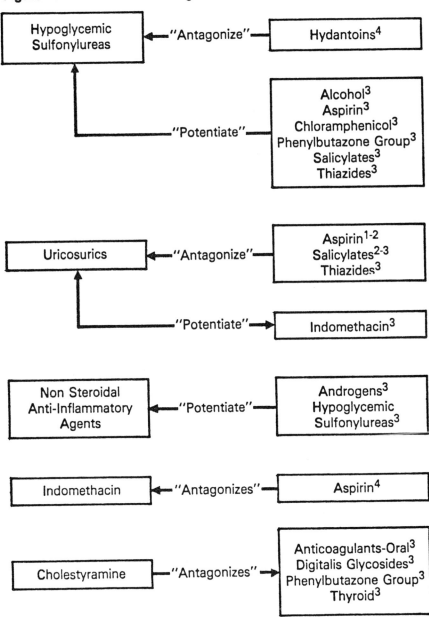

ASSESSMENT GUIDES

Suggested Guidelines for Components of Health Assessment of the Aged

1. Physiological dimension
   a. Past medical and health history and review of body systems—illnesses, hospitalizations, surgeries, traumas, fractures, diagnostic tests, frequency of medical care, date and purpose(s) of last visit, vision and hearing examinations, immunizations, allergies.
   b. Medication patterns—prescriptions, over-the-counter, herbs, ointments, suppositories, laxatives, dosages, length of time on medication, time of day medication is taken, mode of medication intake
   c. Nutrition and fluid intake—number of meals per day, food preferences and dislikes, amount and type of beverage intake per day, description of appetite, food allergies, weight gain or loss, usual weight, preferred weight, height, body type
   d. Sleep and rest patterns—number of hours per night, number of naps per day, interrupted sleep, difficulty getting to sleep
   e. Elimination pattern—urinary pattern (day/night), bowel habits (regular/irregular), diarrhea, constipation
   f. Reproductive—number of children, pregnancy complications, sexual activities, and satisfaction and dissatisfaction
   g. Family health history—medical problems (cancer, hypertension, diabetes, stroke, heart problems), other familial conditions (sickle-cell anemia, hemophilia, and so on
   h. Activity level—amount of exercise, ambulation problems, recreational participation and preference (golf, swimming, tennis, cards, and so on)
2. Psychological dimension
   a. Adaptation/coping—aging process, retirement, decreased income, loss of friends/family member, response to change and stress, self-control, anxiety, anger, depression, loneliness
   b. Family relationship—marital, offspring, relatives, residence of family members
   c. Support person(s)—relative, friend, health professional, neighbor, and so on (primary and secondary support persons)
   d. Mental status—orientation, attention span, memory, and recall
   e. Sexuality—opportunity for expression, preference, and so on
   f. Life and health goals—short- and long-term

3. Sociocultural dimension
   a. Ethnicity—primary language, cultural values and beliefs
   b. Educational background—future goals, and so on
   c. Place of birth
   d. Marital history
   e. Past work experience and income source(s)—income adequate/inadequate
   f. Religious preference—ability to attend church services
   g. Living arrangement—type of home (apartment, home, boarding house, and so on), own, rent, others living in household
   h. Hobbies and interest(s)—new or lifelong and established
   i. Activities and outings from home—daily, weekly, monthly, and so on
4. Environmental dimension
   a. Rural or urban—type of neighborhood, relationship with neighbors
   b. Accessibility—to medical care, recreational facilities, grocery store, relatives, friends, other life essentials
   c. Pollution problems—water, air, garbage and trash, noise, chemicals
   d. Transportation—private, public, other
   e. Home safety—stairs, bathroom facilities, type of cooking facilities, ventilation, heating and cooling, home and yard maintenance
   f. Screening results—blood (hemoglobin, blood glucose), urine (sugar, albumin, nitrite)
5. Subjective Data
   a. Chief complaints or concerns expressed
6. Objective Data
   a. Vital signs—blood pressure, pulse, respiration
   b. Physical examination findings

Table 18-3 Functional Assessment of Elderly People

Physical Classification

I. a. Capable of unlimited and unsupervised activity
   b. Fully ambulatory; able to go about the city independently in safety
   c. Has no physical condition requiring medical supervision or closeness to emergency medical care
   d. No evidence of heart disease in any form
   e. No evidence of prior cancer except cured skin cancer
   f. No complaints except those that cannot be related to any known disease entity

Table 18-3 continued

Physical Classification

II. a. Capable of moderate activity; ambulatory without supervision for activities in own home or immediate vicinity
   b. Can manage without help for care, and otherwise requires minimal supervision
   c. Physical condition may require medical supervision, but frequent or special treatment or closeness to medical or nursing care not required
   d. May have had a previous illness that has left no residuals, e.g., healed myocardial infarction without angina or ECG abnormalities other than healed infarctions, cancer with no evidence of recurrence, or mild diabetes (diet-controlled)
III. a. Limited capabilities
   b. Dependent on others for bedmaking and baths and general supervision of activities
   c. May or may not need a walking aid (cane) but can carry on routine activities without additional personal service
   d. Generally requires escort on the outside
   e. May require regular periodic medical care; availability of emergency medical or nursing care desirable
   f. These people have moderate incapacities such as angina, arthritis, which does not limit them to a wheel-chair, chronic respiratory disease, or diabetes requiring medication
IV. a. Limited capabilities requiring assistance for personal care and daily living activities
   b. Must be in a protected environment because of need for general nursing supervision
   c. Closeness to emergency medical care desirable
   d. Requires periodic medical care at close intervals
   e. Practically housebound
   f. Angina or intermittent heart disease limits physical capacities, arthritis prevents ambulation, and there are severe hearing or visual impairments, but these patients still have the capacity to be independent for daily activities after orientation
V. a. Chronically ill and confined to the vicinity of their own rooms
   b. Require a large amount of personal service and constant supervision
   c. Should be near their own dining and toilet areas, and have a nurse on call at all times
   d. Physical condition requires 24-hour nursing care or intensive medical treatment
VI. Persons requiring hospital-type care:
   a. Bed patients requiring intensive medical and nursing care
   b. Patients with infectious or contagious disease

Source: Reprinted by permission from M. P. Lawton, "Functional Assessment of Elderly People," *Journal of American Geriatrics Society* 29, no. 6 (June 1977): 469

Table 18-4 Scale for Instrumental Activities of Daily Living

Males Score		Females Score
	A. Ability to use telephone	
1	1. Operates telephone on own initiative; looks up and dials numbers, and so on	1
1	2. Dials a few well-known numbers	1
1	3. Answers telephone but does not dial	1
0	4. Does not use telephone at all	0

Table 18-4 continued

Males Score		Females Score
	B. Shopping	
1	1. Takes care of all shopping needs independently	1
0	2. Shops independently for small purchases	0
0	3. Needs to be accompanied on any shopping trip	0
0	4. Completely unable to shop	0
	C. Food preparation	
	1. Plans, prepares, and serves adequate meals independently	1
	2. Prepares adequate meals if supplied with ingredients	0
	3. Heats and serves prepared meals, or prepares meals but does not maintain adequate diet.	0
	4. Needs to have meals prepared and served	0
	D. Housekeeping	
	1. Maintains house alone or with occasional assistance (e.g., heavy work domestic help)	1
	2. Performs light daily tasks such as dishwashing and bedmaking	1
	3. Performs light daily tasks but cannot maintain acceptable level of cleanliness	1
	4. Needs help with all home maintenance tasks	1
	5. Does not participate in any housekeeping tasks	0
	E. Laundry	
	1. Does personal laundry completely	1
	2. Launders small items; rinses socks, stockings, and so on	1
	3. All laundry must be done by others	0
	F. Mode of transportation	
1	1. Travels independently on public transportation or drives own car	1
1	2. Arranges own travel via taxi, but does not otherwise use public transportation	1
0	3. Travels on public transportation when assisted or accompanied by another	1
0	4. Travel limited to taxi or automobile, with assistance of another	0
0	5. Does not travel at all	0
	G. Responsibility for own medication	
1	1. Is responsible for taking medication in correct dosages at correct time	1
0	2. Takes responsibility if medication is prepared in advance in separate dosages	0
0	3. Is not capable of dispensing own medication	0
	H. Ability to handle finances	
1	1. Manages financial matters independently (budgets, writes checks, pays rent and bills, goes to bank); collects and keeps track of income	1
1	2. Manages day-to-day purchases, but needs help with banking, major purchases, and so on	1
0	3. Incapable of handling money	0

Source: Reprinted by permission from M. P. Lawton, "Functional Assessment of Elderly People," *Journal of American Geriatrics Society* 29, no. 6 (June 1977): 472

Table 18-5 Physical Self-Maintenance Scale

		Score
A.	Toilet	
	1. Cares for self at toilet, completely; no incontinence	1
	2. Needs to be reminded or needs help in cleaning self or has rare (weekly at most) accidents	0
	3. Soiling or wetting while asleep, more than once a week	0
	4. Soiling or wetting while awake, more than once a week	0
	5. No control of bowels or bladder	0
B.	Feeding	
	1. Eats without assistance	1
	2. Eats with minor assistance at meal times, with help in preparing food, or with help in cleaning up after meals	0
	3. Feeds self with moderate assistance and is untidy	0
	4. Requires extensive assistance for all meals	0
	5. Does not feed self at all and resists efforts of others to feed him or her	0
C.	Dressing	
	1. Dresses, undresses, and selects clothes from own wardrobe	1
	2. Dresses and undresses self, with minor assistance	0
	3. Needs moderate assistance in dressing or selection of clothes	0
	4. Needs major assistance in dressing, but cooperates with efforts of others to help	0
	5. Completely unable to dress self and resists efforts of others to help	0
D.	Grooming (neatness, hair, nails, hands, face, clothing)	
	1. Always neatly dressed and well-groomed, without assistance	1
	2. Grooms self adequately, with occasional minor assistance, e.g., in shaving	0
	3. Needs moderate and regular assistance or supervision in grooming	0
	4. Needs total grooming care, but can remain well groomed after help from others	0
	5. Actively negates all efforts of others to maintain grooming	0
E.	Physical ambulation	
	1. Goes about grounds or city	1
	2. Ambulates within residence or about one block distant	0
	3. Ambulates with assistance of (check one): *a* ( ) another person; *b* ( ) railing; *c* ( ) cane; *d* ( ) walker; or *e* ( ) wheelchair:	0
	1___gets in and out without help	
	2___needs help in getting in and out	
	4. Sits unsupported in chair or wheelchair, but cannot propel self without help	0
	5. Bedridden more than half the time	0
F.	Bathing	
	1. Bathes self (tub, shower, sponge bath) without help	1
	2. Bathes self, with help in getting in and out of tub	0
	3. Washes face and hands only, but cannot bathe rest of body	0
	4. Does not wash self but is cooperative with those who bathe him	0
	5. Does not try to wash self, and resists efforts to keep him clean	0

Source: Reprinted by permission from M. P. Lawton, "Functional Assessment of Elderly People," *Journal of American Geriatrics Society* 29, no. 6 (June 1977): 471

Exhibit 18-1 Initial Screening Physical Examination Form

Physical Exam

Client's Initials:_____   Date:_____
       Age:_____

Vital Signs on Progress Note

General survey	Skin Hair Nails

Eyes   Acuity
  EOM (Extra Ocular Movements)
  Fundi
  Pupils
  Visual fields
	Head
	Ears
	Nose
	Hearing
	Sinuses

Mouth
Throat
Tongue
Teeth
Gums
	Neck
	  Thyroid
	  ROM (Range of Motion)
	  Trachea

Lymph Nodes Occipital Pre- and postcuricular Supraclavicular Axillary Inguinal	Breasts Nipples Axilla
Lungs (include rate)	Heart (include rate) PMI (Point of Maximum Intensity) S_1 S_2 Carotid, Femoral, Dorsal, Pedis, Radial

Abdomen
  Liver
  Masses
  Spleen	

Exhibit 18-1 continued

Physical Exam

Neurological
  Cranial nerves
  Motor (drift, toe stand)
  Coord (F→N, Romberg)
  Reflexes
  Sensation (touch, vibration, prop)

Pyschological	Musculo-skeletal
Affect	
Orientation: time, place, person	ROM (Range of Motion)
Mood	
Thought content	Strength
Memory	
Serial sevens	Gait

See Problem List and Progress Notes for summary of problems.

Signature

Source: Reprinted with permission from Corina Casias, R.N., M.S., C.F.N.P., College of Nursing, University of New Mexico, Albuquerque, New Mexico, 1981.

The following four exhibits were devised by a team of nurse practitioners, pharmacists, physicians, and others in Albuquerque, New Mexico, for use in an outpatient care setting for the elderly. The Personal Health Record is a booklet approximately three by five inches that the client retains and carries to the clinics and to other health care settings.

Exhibit 18-2 Personal Health Record

Personal Health Record
of

_____

Name

_____

Social Security Number

_____

Medicare Number

_____

Address

_____

Telephone Number

Past History

Problem List

Physical:

Psychological:

Social Cultural:

Environmental:

Exhibit 18-2 continued

Birth Date:	Marital Status:
Date	Notes

Medications
Dates:

Tests/Procedure

Date	Test	Result

Source: Reprinted with permission from Corina Casias, R.N., M.S., C.F., N.P., College of Nursing, University of New Mexico, Albuquerque, New Mexico.

Exhibit 18-3 24-Hour Dietary Inventory Interview Form

Date:

Client's Name:

   Major questions to client: Beginning with yesterday morning, tell me the first thing you ate and the environmental circumstances. After the first food, tell me other foods sequentially until this a.m. (Total 24 hours)

Time when you got up _____ a.m. or p.m.

First food	Amount of food eaten	Preparation					Persons present				Atmosphere				
		Self	Cold	Restaurant	Meal Site	Other	Alone	Family	Friend/Ngb.	Other	Silence	TV	Radio	General Noise	Other

---

How do you decide type of food and quantity to be eaten?

How many meals do you eat in a day? 1 2 3 4 5 6

How many snacks do you eat in a day? 1 2 3 4 5 6

Do you ever skip meals?   Yes ___ No ___

Which do you skip most often?   N/A ___ Bkf ___ Lunch ___ Dinner ___

Reasons for skipping meals:

    ___ not hungry (physiological)   ___ unable to cook

    ___ no food   ___ didn't feel like eating (psychological)

    ___ sick   ___ habit

    ___ busy   ___ other

Is this a typical 24 hour pattern?   Yes ___ No ___
   How does it deviate?

Are you on a special, prescribed diet? Yes ___ No ___
   If so: what kind?

   Prescribed by whom?

Recommended weight _____   Actual weight _____

Recommended caloric intake _____   Actual caloric intake _____

                                        Difference _____

Exhibit 18-4 Assessment Guide of Foot Care

Date:
Client's name:

1. What have you been told about how to take care of your feet?

2. What are the reasons for taking special care of your feet?

3. Do you usually wear:

	Yes	No
Shoes	____	____
Slippers	____	____
Tight fit	____	____
Fit well	____	____
Good repair	____	____
Other comments:		
Socks or Stockings	____	____
Fit well	____	____
Clean	____	____
Without holes	____	____
Hose supports	____	____
Tight fit	____	____
Other comments:		

4. Do you bathe your feet daily? Yes ___ No ___
   If no, please state how often you do bathe your feet.
   What water temperature do you use to bathe your feet? Hot ___
   Warm ___
   What kind of soap do you use to wash your feet?
   Do you dry your feet and toes thoroughly? Yes ___ No ___
   Do you inspect your feet and toes for cracks, blisters, cuts, sores, swelling, color change?
   What do you do when you find problems with your toes or feet?

5. Do you cut your own toe nails? Yes ___ No ___
   Do you cut your toenails straight across even with your toes? Yes ___
   No ___

6. Do you have corns and callouses? Yes ___ No ___
   If yes, who takes care of them?

7. If your feet get cold how do you get them warm? Please explain.

Exhibit 18-5 Check List for Symptoms for Colds

yes no

___ ___ Do you think you have a fever? (Shaking chills, periodic especially at night, headache)

___ ___ Have you been exposed to strep throat?

___ ___ Has your sore throat been present longer than three days?

___ ___ Is your sore throat causing severe discomfort?

___ ___ Have you noticed that your tonsils are enlarged, or have white spots on them?

___ ___ Do you have a history of recurrent strep throats or rheumatic fever?

___ ___ Have you noticed any enlarged lymph nodes or bumps on the side or back of your neck?

___ ___ Have you had a cough for over one week which is becoming worse?

___ ___ Do you cough up greenish or bloody sputum?

___ ___ Do you have a history of tuberculosis or a recent change to a positive TB test?

___ ___ Are you short of breath with mild exercise such as climbing stairs?

___ ___ Do you have chest pains or a wheezing cough?

___ ___ Do you have ear pain or facial pain?

___ ___ Has the fatigue or runny nose lasted over 10 days?

___ ___ Have you vomited or had diarrhea during the past two days?

___ ___ Have you had rheumatic fever or rheumatic heart disease?

If you answered "yes" to any question, symptoms may indicate a condition requiring professional care.

Source: Reprinted with permission from Jane Zapka & Barry Averill, Amherst University 1981

Index

Note: Italicized page numbers indicate references to tables and figures.

About the Authors

CHIYOKO FURUKAWA, R.N., B.S.N., M.S., is currently Assistant Professor of Nursing (Community Health) at the University of New Mexico College of Nursing in Albuquerque. While serving as community health nurse at the Boulder, Colorado, County Health Department in 1972, she initiated health promotion and maintenance services to the aging population. Later, she taught community health nursing at Wright State University School of Nursing in Dayton, Ohio. Presently, Ms. Furukawa also serves as a consultant to the Albuquerque Visiting Nurse Service and to the Bernalillo County Health Department, and as a member of several advisory committees for agencies and groups serving the elderly population.

DIANNA MCDONALD SHOMAKER, R.N., B.N.S., M.N., M.A., is Assistant Professor of Nursing at the University of New Mexico College of Nursing in Albuquerque. She also has been a public health nurse in Taos County, New Mexico, and a research assistant for Washington State Health Department, where she studied the health problems of migrant laborers. Ms. Shomaker, who authored *Tool to Develop Teacher Effectiveness in Diploma Schools of Nursing* when she was a research coordinator for Hotel Dieu School of Nursing in El Paso, currently serves on the Board of Directors of "Share Your Care" day care center for the frail elderly in Albuquerque. She is presently studying for a Ph.D. in anthropology at the University of New Mexico.